INTERNATIONAL PERSPECTIVES IN HEALTH INFORMATICS

Studies in Health Technology and Informatics

This book series was started in 1990 to promote research conducted under the auspices of the EC programmes' Advanced Informatics in Medicine (AIM) and Biomedical and Health Research (BHR) bioengineering branch. A driving aspect of international health informatics is that telecommunication technology, rehabilitative technology, intelligent home technology and many other components are moving together and form one integrated world of information and communication media. The complete series has been accepted in Medline. Volumes from 2005 onwards are available online.

Volume 164

Recently published in this series

ISSN 0926-9630 (print)
ISSN 1879-8365 (online)

International Perspectives in Health Informatics

Edited by

Elizabeth M. Borycki

School of Health Information Science, University of Victoria, Victoria, British Columbia, Canada

John A. Bartle-Clar

Shotbolt Consulting, Victoria, British Columbia, Canada

Mowafa S. Househ

College of Public Health and Health Informatics, King Saud Bin Abdulaziz University for Health Science (KSAU-HS), Riyadh, Kingdom of Saudi Arabia

Craig E. Kuziemsky

Telfer School of Management, University of Ottawa, Ottawa, Ontario, Canada

and

Ellen G. Schraa

School of Health Policy & Management, Faculty of Health and School of Administrative Studies, Faculty of Liberal Arts & Professional Studies, York University, Toronto, Ontario, Canada

IOS
Press

Amsterdam • Berlin • Tokyo • Washington, DC

ISBN 978-1-60750-708-6 (print)
ISBN 978-1-60750-709-3 (online)
Library of Congress Control Number: 2011921028

Publisher
IOS Press BV
Nieuwe Hemweg 6B
1013 BG Amsterdam
Netherlands
fax: +31 20 687 0019
e-mail: order@iospress.nl

Distributor in the USA and Canada
IOS Press, Inc.
4502 Rachael Manor Drive
Fairfax, VA 22032
USA
fax: +1 703 323 3668
e-mail: iosbooks@iospress.com

International Perspectives in Health Informatics
E.M. Borycki et al. (Eds.)
IOS Press, 2011

Preface

Around the world developed and developing countries are using health information systems to improve the health of populations, the quality of healthcare, reduce medical error rates and improve access to health information and health services. Health information systems are becoming key to country delivery of healthcare and health services, and health informatics is now recognized as a separate and unique area of disciplinary study and professional practice in many countries throughout the world. Countries and governments are supporting the education of health informatics professionals and engaging researchers to promote the advancement and integration of health information systems into healthcare.

World wide governments and healthcare organizations are choosing to implement health information systems such as the following:

- Electronic Health Records
- Clinical Decision Support Systems
- Clinical Information Systems
- E-learning Systems
- Personal Health Records
- Systems that support Online communities
- Public Health Information Systems
- Telehealth and Tele Intensive Care Unit Systems
- Mobile Health Information Systems

Governments, regional health authorities and other healthcare organizations from around the world are also evaluating the clinical and cost effectiveness of these health information systems. The goals of this work have included improving the quality of healthcare while at the same time ensuring the effective use of scarce healthcare resources (i.e. human, monetary and technological) to ensure the long-term sustainability of healthcare systems. Researchers are designing and developing health information systems, conducting research, developing new methods for evaluating health information systems and moving the science of health informatics forward.

Globally, the situations of countries and regional health authorities are not unique. Many countries are addressing key issues at the intersection of technology and healthcare such as privacy, ethics, patient safety, efficiency and effectiveness. Researchers are studying these issues and developing solutions in conjunction with country, regional and local healthcare organizations. There are many lessons that have been learned and many more that will be learned in the coming years. Many health informatics issues are not unique to one country or one organization. Many of these issues are present throughout the world – in each country, involving differing healthcare delivery systems and differing types of health information systems. There is a need for researchers to exchange ideas within this global context and, learn from each other so that knowledge can be transferred and international solutions and best practices form the basis of health informatics work. The improvement of our healthcare systems using health information systems and technologies is dependent upon these international exchanges and solutions to address many of the real-world problems we encounter today and into in the future.

The Information Technology and Communications in Health (ITCH) conference was first held in 1987 to promote the global exchange of ideas in health informatics. The conference is hosted by the School of Health Information Science at the University of Victoria. The theme of the 2011 conference is Health Informatics: International Perspectives. The conference provided a unique opportunity to share lessons learned by both developed and developing countries. In addition this ITCH conference was special as it honoured Professor Denis Protti's leadership and contributions to the field of health informatics. Professor Denis Protti was the founding Director of the School of Health Information Science at the University of Victoria and has contributed his knowledge and expertise to guiding health informatics education, projects and initiatives in Canada and internationally.

It is hoped that the exchange of knowledge among the participants at ITCH 2011 will lead to increased dialogue and greater improvements to health information systems and technologies leading to more sustainable healthcare systems worldwide today and into the future.

Elizabeth Borycki
School of Health Information Science
University of Victoria
Victoria, British Columbia
Canada

ITCH 2011 Steering Committee

Chair – Abdul V. Roudsari

Program Chairs – Andre Kushniruk and Abdul V. Roudsari

Student Poster & Practitioner Poster Co-ordinator – Pasquale Fiore

Workshop Co-ordinator – Alex Kuo

Promotion and Business Co-ordinator – Leslie Wood

Sponsor and Exhibitor Co-ordinators – Al Schyf and Nancy Gault

Proceedings Editors – Elizabeth Borycki and John Bartle-Clar

Technical Co-ordinator – John Bartle-Clar

Members at Large – Jim McDaniel and Colin Partridge

ITCH 2011 Scientific Program Committee

James Anderson
Purdue University, USA

Riccardo Bellazzi
University Pavia, Italy

Maged Boulos
University of Plymouth, UK

Joe Cafazzo
University Health Network, Canada

Robert Calnan
Vancouver Island Health Authority, Canada

Susan Clamp
Leeds University, UK

Enrico Coiera
Australia

Dominic Covvey
University of Waterloo, Canada

Eric Eisenstein
Duke University Medical Center, USA

Paul Fisher
Universidade Federal do Rio, Grande do Sul, Brazil

Marilynne Hebert
University of Calgary, Canada

Don Juzwishin
Alberta Health Services, Canada

David Kaufman
Columbia University, USA

Jonathan Kay
Oxford John Radcliffe Hospital, UK

Craig Kuziemsky
University of Ottawa, Canada

Kevin Leonard
University of Toronto, Canada

Selma Limam Mansar
Carnegie Mellon University, Qatar

Jim McDaniel
University of Victoria, Canada

Christian Nøhr
Aalborg University, Denmark

Anthony Norris
New Zealand

Grace Paterson
Dalhousie University, Canada

Francesco Pinciroli
Politecnico di Milano, Milan, Italy

Denis Protti
University of Victoria, Canada

Jan Talmon
Maastricht University, Netherlands

Robyn Tamblyn
McGill University, Canada

Joseph Tan
McMaster University, Canada

Minhong (Maggie) Wang
University of Hong Kong, Hong Kong

Jens Weber
University of Victoria, Canada

Jeremy Wyatt
Digital Healthcare, UK

Contents

Evaluation

Health Records

Health Informatics Initiatives in Developing Countries

Healthcare Modeling and Simulation

Human Computer Interaction

Initiatives in International Health Informatics

Clinical Decision Support

International Perspectives in Health Informatics
E.M. Borycki et al. (Eds.)
IOS Press, 2011
doi:10.3233/978-1-60750-709-3-3

Decision Support and Automation Bias: Methodology and Preliminary Results of a Systematic Review

Kate GODDARD [a,1], Abdul ROUDSARI [b], Jeremy WYATT [c]

[a] *Centre for Health Informatics, City University, London, UK*
[b] *School of Health Information Science, University of Victoria, Victoria, British Columbia, Canada*
[c] *Institute for Digital Healthcare, University of Warwick, UK*

Abstract. Automation bias – or a tendency to over-rely on automation – is a subject which has been studied in a variety of academic fields. Clinical Decision Support Systems (CDSS) aim to benefit the clinical decision making process. Although most research shows overall improved performance with use, there is often a failure to recognize the new errors that CDSS can introduce, and as such the healthcare field has a gap in this research. This paper summarizes the methodology and preliminary results of a systematic review over a broad range of fields into the effects of over-reliance on automation. Results indicate that though automation bias is a significant phenomenon, it is not well defined, and there is a gap in the research which must be addressed to optimize the use of decision support

Keywords. automation, human judgment, cognition, reliance, systematic review

Introduction

Clinical Decision Support Systems (CDSS) aim to provide clinicians and healthcare professionals with intelligently filtered information centered on the patient. This occurs with the provision of Alerts and Reminders, Image Recognition, Diagnostic Assistance, and Therapy Planning and Critiquing.

Globally, the role of IT is increasingly important in healthcare, including increasing interest in Clinical Decision Support. As an emerging market, it is imperative that effective and efficient CDSS is generated as a product robustness, scalability, and extensive testing before deployment.

Although most CDSS are 80-90% accurate, it is known that occasional incorrect advice given may tempt users to reverse a correct decision, and thus introduce new errors. These errors can be termed *automation bias (AB)*, where users tend to accept computer output without sufficient thought. For example, Friedman et al [1], noticed that in some cases, clinicians would override their own correct decisions in favor of the erroneous advice from the CDSS – in 12% of cases the CDSS caused the physician to

---

[1] Corresponding author: Centre for Health Informatics, City University, Northampton Square, London, EC1V 0HB, UK, Email: kate.goddard.1@city.ac.uk

put the correct diagnosis on their list, but in 6% of cases their own correct decisions were dropped in favor of the erroneous computer-generated advice – a net gain of 6%.

Research is required to identify factors involved to mitigate risk and refine the appropriate usage of CDSS to maximize benefits gained from CDSS implementation. A systematic review is being carried out at City University, London, to survey the literature available.

1. Aims

The overall review aim is to systematically review the literature surrounding DSSs and automation bias, particularly in the field of healthcare. The specific review objectives are to answer the following questions:

- What is the rate of AB and what is the problem
- Does it vary in different studies and settings? Focus on causes, risk factors, barriers and facilitators, and types of users.
- Is there a way to avoid AB? What is the impact?

2. Methodology

Systematic literature reviews aim to clearly identify and document the comprehensive strategies used to locate relevant literature, critically appraise methodological issues and synthesize the resulting evidence. Given that initial searches indicated there is a relative paucity of healthcare specific evidence it was decided that a number of databases and research domains would be included and wide parameters for inclusion/exclusion to ensure all relevant articles are identified were maintained. The caveat was included that similar underlying cognitive processes were at work in automation bias within different research fields.

2.1. Sources of Papers

The search took place between September 2009 and January 2010. The following sources were searched to identify articles relevant to this review: MEDLINE/PubMed, CINAHL, PsycInfo, IEEE Explore and Web of Science.

2.2. Search Strategy

Combinations of subject-specific free text and index terms were used to search electronic databases. No timeframe limit was set for any database, the language filter was set to English language studies only. The study types included within the PubMed/Medline filter were Randomized Controlled Trials, and Comparative studies. All funding types were included in the search. Non-PubMed/Medline searches used these criteria if available, otherwise studies were chosen by hand

Search terms surrounded the three themes of automation and clinical decision support, human factors (such as human engineering, psychological phenomena and processes), and performance and error factors (such as diagnostic error, sensitivity and specificity).

2.3. Eligibility criteria

It is clear from preliminary searching that the research should not be limited by a specific field. Investigations into decision support and automation from non-healthcare disciplines have valuable input to highlight factors in human-computer systems, the formation of cognitive biases and recommendations on how to debias individuals. Included were:

- Papers that examined human interaction with automated decision support were included from various fields (such as aviation, motoring and cognitive psychology). In particular, the field of healthcare was the focus of interest.
- Papers that studied empirical automation use were included, including those which had a subjective participant questionnaire or interview element.
- Papers which looked at the appropriateness and accuracy of the participant use of DSS were included

    Purely technical papers were excluded e.g. detailing DSS development, as they omitted much of the human element. Non-English language papers were excluded.

3. Selection process

The selection process is outlined in Figure 1.

3.1. Data extraction

To help clarify the research question, a PICO (Population, Intervention, Comparison, and Outcome) taxonomy is used. For the results, the results will be organized and tabulated according to an extended PICO framework to capture extra information. The primary variables are outlined below:

- Population: all participants, any demography or background e.g. from naïve to field experts
- Intervention/exposure: Automated decision support, real or simulated; Interruptive versus non-interruptive versus adaptive, and Presentation mode: visual, textual, both
- Comparison/ Design: Groups not using automated decision support, or different forms of decision support (non-automated or automated but a different design), or before and after design. Randomization and controls.
- Outcome: Extent of advice use, participant performance (participant decision accuracy, timings), errors in automation use, user awareness of automation reliability or failure, cross verification behaviors

    To assess the papers for quality, a generic set of criteria was adapted from relevant items from the CONSORT (for Randomized Trials [2]) checklist.

3.2. Reliability

The final papers were tested for reliability of extraction using Cohen's kappa statistic. The crude rate of agreement between 2 raters on sample of 100 papers with a pseudo randomized number of "hit" papers was 87%. Cohen's kappa was 0.8436; according to

Landis and Koch [1], who formulated a table for assessing Kappa significance, this result implies "almost perfect agreement".

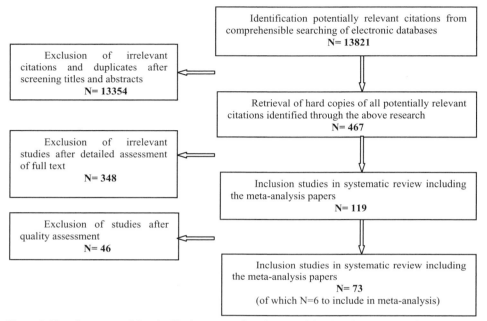

Figure 1. Flowchart summarizing the filtering process for relevant articles (based on PRISMA flowchart [2]

4. Preliminary Results and Discussion

Though some studies do exist which demonstrate the AB effect, there appears to be very few definitive and deliberate studies into looking at how inaccurate DSS advice affects the user's decision. Where studies do exist, a lack of homogeneity in terms of study domain, DSS type and experimental design affects ability to directly compare rates of overreliance and effects of potential causal factors. The AB finding is also generally incidental to other primary aims, though may be available in raw data, it is a rarely analyzed and reported finding. Some of the emerging results are outlined below.

Even though the nature of automation bias is not clear, enough studies, discussion papers and anecdotal evidence exists to imply that it is a consistent effect. It is postulated frequently but lacks a strong empirical evidence base. AB appears to differ by field and DSS type; apparent rate differs by interruptive or non-interruptive nature of DSS and nature of fault. Omission errors may be more prevalent in interruptive systems, with higher error rates generally.

AB has been most explicitly explored in aviation field. Within the clinical field Computer Aided Detection followed by Electrocardiogram support have seen the most investigation. Fewer studies were found with "traditional" CDSS (such as QMR, Iliad). AB is both reported a pronounced problem [4] which may render DSS not useful overall, and conversely a small issue where it is still worthwhile given the benefits [5].

Relative task inexperience may cause AB [6]. Other factors include clinician under confidence[7], or over trust in automation [8]. Individual differences in reliance have been found e.g. potential for complacency [9]. More complex tasks are also posited to increase reliance [10]. Training appears to aid AB prevention[11]. Too much on-screen detail makes people less conservative (target cuing task) [12], thus increasing biases. Increasing accountability [13] also decreased rates of AB.

5. Conclusion

The factors involved in the phenomenon of automation bias are complex, however despite the high risk associated with medication error there is little direct research into overreliance on technology within the healthcare and CDSS field. This systematic review (including a meta-analysis of 6 papers with adequately homogenous designs and outcome measures) will help elucidate the nature of AB according to the aims, its scope, and ultimately how to better design decision support systems to reduce it.

References

[1] C.P. Friedman, A.S. Elstein, F.M. Wolf, G.C. Murphy, T.M. Franz, P.S. Heckerling, P.L.Fine, T.M. Miller, V. Abraham, Enhancement of clinicians' diagnostic reasoning by computer-based consultation: a multisite study of 2 systems, *JAMA* **282** (1999), 1851-1856.

[2] D. Moher, A. Liberati, J. Tetzlaff, D.G. Altman, The PRISMA Group. Preferred Reporting Items for Systematic Reviews and Meta-Analyses: The PRISMA Statement, *PLoS Med* **6** (2009).

[3] J.R. Landis, G.G. Koch, The measurement of observer agreement for categorical data, *Biometrics* **33** (1977), 159-174

[4] S.D. Hillson, D.P. Connelly, Y. Liu, The Effects of Computer-Assisted Electrocardiographic Interpretation on Physicians' Diagnostic Decisions, *Medical Decision Making* **15** (1995), 107-112.

[5] S.T. Quek, C.H. Thng, J.B.K. Khoo, W.L. Koh, Radiologists' detection of mammographic abnormalities with and without a computer-aided detection system, *Australasian Radiology* **47** (2003), 257 – 260.

[6] K. Marten, T. Seyfarth, F. Auer, E. Wiener, A Grillhösl, S. Obenauer, E.J. Rummeny, C. Engelke, Computer-assisted detection of pulmonary nodules: performance evaluation of an expert knowledge-based detection system in consensus reading with experienced and inexperienced chest radiologists, *European Radiology* **14** (2004), 1930-1938.

[7] S. Dreiseitl, M. Binder, Do physicians value decision support? A look at the effect of decision support systems on physician opinion, *Artificial Intelligence in Medicine* **33** (2005), 25-30.

[8] D.P. Biros, M. Daly, G. Gunsch, The Influence of Task Load and Automation Trust on Deception Detection, *Group Decision and Negotiation* **13** (2004), 173-189.

[9] L.J. Prinzel, H. De Vries, F.G. Freeman, P. Mikulka, *Examination of Automation-Induced Complacency and Individual Difference Variates*, Technical Memorandum No. TM-2001-211413, NASA Langley Research Center, Hampton, VA., 2001.

[10] N.R. Bailey, M.W. Scerbo, *The effects of operator trust, complacency potential, and task complexity on monitoring a highly reliable automated system*, Dissertation Abstracts International: Section B: The Sciences and Engineering, US, ProQuest Information & Learning, 2005.

[11] A.J. Masalonis, *Effects of training operators on situation-specific automation reliability, Systems, Man and Cybernetics,* IEEE International Conference, 2003.

[12] M. Yeh, Display Signaling in Augmented Reality: Effects of Cue Reliability and Image Realism on Attention Allocation and Trust Calibration, *Human Factors: The Journal of the Human Factors and Ergonomics Society* **43** (2001), 355-365.

[13] M.D. Burdick, L.J. Skitka, K.L. Mosier, S. Heers, The ameliorating effects of accountability on automation bias, *Proceedings of the 3rd Symposium on Human Interaction with Complex Systems* (1996), 142.

8

International Perspectives in Health Informatics
E.M. Borycki et al. (Eds.)
IOS Press, 2011
doi:10.3233/978-1-60750-709-3-8

Automated Recognition and Post-Coordination of Complex Clinical Terms

Philip GOOCH[a], Abdul ROUDSARI[b]

[a] Centre for Health Informatics, School of Informatics, City University, London, UK
[b] School of Health Information Science, University of Victoria, Victoria, British Columbia, Canada

Abstract. One of the key tasks in integrating guideline-based decision support systems with the electronic patient record is the mapping of clinical terms contained in both guidelines and patient notes to a common, controlled terminology. However, a vocabulary of pre-coordinated terms cannot cover every possible variation - clinical terms are often highly compositional and complex. We present a rule-based approach for automated recognition and post-coordination of clinical terms using minimal, morpheme-based thesauri, neoclassical combining forms and part-of-speech analysis. The process integrates MetaMap with the open-source GATE framework.

Keywords. natural language processing, interoperability, clinical decision support

Introduction

Application of natural language processing (NLP) techniques for recognition of biomedical and clinical terms has recently been driven by increased demand for information retrieval and extraction tools for standardising and exchanging data between electronic medical record (EMR) systems[1].

While there are a number of approaches to this task, including rule, dictionary, and statistical based approaches[2], there are essentially three steps involved:

1. *recognize* the text string as a possible term (*candidate term* identification)
2. *classify* the candidate term (e.g. chemical compound, part of body, disease)
3. *map* the term to a single concept (*pre-coordination*) or to qualified, multiple concepts (*post-coordination*) within a standardised vocabulary or ontology.

The last step is essential for semantic interoperability of data between EMR systems. For guideline-based clinical decision support (CDS) to provide point of care recommendations within an EMR, patient data must be mapped to the terminology and data model (a *virtual medical record*) employed by the guideline knowledge base[3].

The UMLS Metathesaurus from the National Library of Medicine (NLM)[4] is a large, multi-lingual vocabulary of biomedical concepts classified according to one or more types from a semantic network. The Metathesaurus comprises over 100 reference terminologies, such as HL7 v3, SNOMED CT and LOINC, which have been adopted as international standards for patient data encoding, and form the basis of the information model adopted by at least one formalised guideline model[3]. MetaMap is a tool for discovering UMLS Metathesaurus concepts in free text[5], and is considered to be the 'gold standard' for this task[6]. It allows complex clinical terms to be mapped to individual concepts within UMLS source vocabularies.

Composition of Clinical Terms

The naming of chemical and biological terms frequently involves the use of Latin and Greek *morphemes*. Such terms are known as *neoclassical compounds*. Computational analysis of neoclassical compounds can help identify unknown terms and provide classification for human review[7]. In this paper, we present a purely rule-based application utilising neoclassical combining forms (NCF), part-of-speech (POS) analysis and lexical rules for recognition of complex clinical terms. A post-coordination module annotates the clinical terms with metadata from MetaMap and provides output in HL7 v3 CDA XML.

1. Method

We constructed an NLP pipeline within the GATE framework[8]. The pipeline consists of generic modules for tokenization, POS tagging and noun-phrase identification. Modules were also developed for identification of neoclassical compounds; anatomical terms; chemical nomenclature; proteins, drugs and enzymes; temporal expressions and quantities; and clinical term post-coordination. A MetaMap plugin for GATE was developed in Java using the MetaMap Java API[9]. The transducer modules were written in the GATE JAPE grammar.

1.1. Identification of Potential Clinical Terms

Following approaches suggested by [7],[10], we created lists of neoclassical morphemes and classified them as prefixes, roots and suffixes relating to bodily concepts (e.g. *gastr-*, *haem-*, *derm-*), clinical signs (*cirrh-*, *glauc-*, *-itis*, *-asis*, *-lytic*) and descriptive and positional terms (*ankyl-*, *pachy-*, *inter-*, *intra-*). Suffixes considered to be strongly indicative of a clinical term without an accompanying neoclassical prefix or root were grouped separately (e.g. *-itis*, *-ostomy*). Regular expressions were written to combine the morphemes into patterns that represent a complete neoclassical compound.

1.2. Recognition of Anatomical Terms

Anatomical terms tend to be highly compositional. We created gazetteers from which to construct regular expressions for identification of complete anatomical structures, using functional prefixes (*adductor, extensor*), positional prefixes (*anterior, posterior, distal, dorsal*); anatomical parts and surfaces (*bursa, cortex, fossa, fascia*), organs and organ parts. Complete anatomical terms can then be recognised, for example:

Endothoracic$_{\text{neoclassical}}$ **fascia**$_{\text{part}}$ **of anterior**$_{\text{position}}$ **thoracic**$_{\text{neoclassical}}$ **wall**$_{\text{part}}$

Right$_{\text{position}}$ **posterior**$_{\text{position}}$ **cusp**$_{\text{part}}$ **of aortic**$_{\text{neoclassical}}$ **valve**$_{\text{part}}$

1.3. Recognition of Chemical Compounds

Using lists of chemical element names, ions and alkane prefixes we created combinatorial rules that implement the IUPAC nomenclature[11, 12] for organic and inorganic compounds. Systematic combination of chemical morphemes allows a variety of compounds to be identified, for example:

di$_{multiplier}$**sodium**$_{element}$**hypo**$_{oxidation\_prefix}$**chlor**$_{ion\_root}$**ite**$_{oxidation\_suffix}$

tri$_{multiplier}$**chlor**$_{ion\_root}$**ometh**$_{alkane\_root}$**ane**$_{alkane\_suffix}$

2,3-di$_{multiplier}$**eth**$_{alkane\_root}$**yl**$_{alkane\_suffix}$**pent**$_{alkane\_root}$**ane**$_{alkane\_suffix}$

Additional production rules were created by combining chemical morphemes with neoclassical terminals such as -*ase* (enzymes: e.g. acetylcholinesterase), -*ein*, -*in*, -*ine*, -*an* (biological molecules: e.g. ferritin).

1.4. Candidate Term Post-coordination

Prepositional terms comprise two or more noun phrases joined by the prepositions 'or' or 'to'[13], e.g. 'carcinoma of the lung'.

Such compound phrases require an initial normalisation process so that they can be properly post-coordinated with qualifier concepts from the Metathesaurus.

After experimenting with different noun-phrase combinations to see which combinations gave the best results in MetaMap, we devised the following heuristic:
1. Remove non-negating determiners (*a*, *the*, *this*) from each noun phrase
2. Store the first noun phrase
3. Reverse the order of the remaining noun phrases
4. Add the last token of the first noun phrase to the end
5. Add the remaining tokens of the first noun phrase to the beginning

Example: 'an ipsilateral fracture of the left femoral neck'
    Step 1: {ipsilateral fracture}{left femoral neck}
    Step 2: {ipsilateral fracture}{left femoral neck}
    Step 3: {left femoral neck}
    Step 4: {left femoral neck}{fracture}
    Step 5: {ipsilateral}{left femoral neck}{fracture}
Although this form is not exactly equivalent semantically to simply reversing the order of the noun phrases[13], this method produces the desired qualified concepts from MetaMap:

```
Meta Mapping (875):
   637 Ipsilateral {SNOMEDCT} [Spatial Concept]
   637 Left {SNOMEDCT} [Spatial Concept]
   884 Femoral Neck Fracture (Femoral neck fracture {SNOMEDCT}) [Injury or
Poisoning]
```

From this HL7v3 CDA XML can be generated by mapping UMLS semantic types to their corresponding qualifiers in SNOMED.

2. Results

The NCF transducer was evaluated against a corpus of 500 MedLine abstracts that had previously been annotated solely with MetaMap (Table 1).

Candidate terms identified by the neoclassical rules were submitted to MetaMap for concept mapping; comparing only the candidate terms against those validated by MetaMap yielded the results shown in Table 2.

The performance of the entire pipeline has not yet been formally evaluated: we are currently refining the rules against an NLP research data set from i2b2[14].

Table 1. Recall and precision of neoclassical combining forms(B) vs MetaMap(A): whole abstract

Annotation	Match	Only A	Only B	Overlap	Recall	Precision	F1.0lenient
Medical_Term	7682	14953	1358	4466	0.45	0.90	0.60

Table 2. Recall and precision of neoclassical combining forms(B) vs MetaMap(A): candidate terms only

Annotation	Match	Only A	Only B	Overlap	Recall	Precision	F1.0lenient
Medical_Term	9597	861	1358	2551	0.93	0.90	0.92

3. Discussion

The high precision but moderate recall of the NCF rules shows that they are useful but insufficient for identifying clinical terms in unstructured text. Additional rules are required for matching anatomical terms, biochemical compounds and complex phrases.

3.1. Related Work

[15] presented a module for recognising medical terms using neoclassical forms, although they validated candidate terms against a general lexicon (EuroWordNet), rather than a specialist biomedical thesaurus. [10] suggested a methodology for medical term recognition using NCFs, but an implementation was not described.

[13] proposed a similar approach to normalising prepositional terms, although they used simple noun-phrase order inversion. However, our approach seemed to produce more useful results from MetaMap, although this requires more formal evaluation.

[16] developed the open-source Health Information Text Extraction (HITEx) tool using GATE. As with our approach, this combined standard GATE modules for POS tagging and noun-phrase chunking, and a regular expression based term identifier. They used the UMLS Metathesaurus directly, although their tool provided similar concept mapping functionality to MetaMap. Additionally, they used a machine-learning component, currently missing from our approach. It is not clear whether they used neoclassical combining forms to assist in term identification. Also, their rules are written in a compact, undocumented syntax, whereas our rules are written in JAPE, which is well documented, easy to modify and extend.

4. Conclusion

We have developed a rules-based approach for clinical term identification, concept mapping and post-coordination within the GATE framework that integrates with

MetaMap. Our approach provides high precision with moderate recall when evaluated against general biomedical texts. However, with rule refinement for specific domains (such as clinical notes and clinical guidelines), recall should improve.

We aim to release the code as an open-source project so that the rules can be shared and enhanced by other researchers working in the field.

Acknowledgements

We thank Angus Roberts, Natural Language Processing Group, Department of Computer Science, University of Sheffield, for assistance with GATE and in developing the MetaMap plugin. Deidentified clinical records used in this research were provided by the i2b2 National Center for Biomedical Computing funded by U54LM008748 and were originally prepared for the Shared Tasks for Challenges in NLP for Clinical Data organized by Dr. Ozlem Uzuner, i2b2 and SUNY.

References

[1]   W.W. Chapman, K.B. Cohen, Current issues in biomedical text mining and natural language processing, *J Biomed Inf* **42**(5) (2009), 757-759.
[2]   M. Krauthammer, G. Nenadić, Term identification in the biomedical literature, *J Biomed Inf* **37** (2004), 512-526.
[3]   S.W. Tu, J.R. Campbell, J. Glasgow, M.A. Nyman, et al., The SAGE Guideline Model: Achievements and Overview, *J Am Me Inform Assoc* **14**(5) (2007), 589-598.
[4]   National Library of Medicine, *UMLS® Reference Manual*, Bethesda, MD, National Library of Medicine, 2009.
[5]   A.R. Aronson, F.M. Lang, An overview of MetaMap: historical perspective and recent advances, *JAMIA* **17** (2010), 229-236.
[6]   N.H. Shah, N. Bhatia, C. Jonquet, D. Rubin, et al., Comparison of concept recognizers for building the Open Biomedical Annotator, *BMC Bioinformatics* **10(Suppl 9)** (2009), S14.
[7]   A.T. McCray, A.C. Browne, and D.L. Moore, *The Semantic Structure of Neo-Classical Compounds*. 1988, National Library of Medicine.
[8]   H. Cunningham, D. Maynard, K. Bontcheva, V. Tablan, *GATE: A Framework and Graphical Development Environment for Robust NLP Tools and Applications*, Proceedings of the 40th Anniversary Meeting of the Association for Computational Linguistics (ACL'02), Philadelphia, 2002.
[9]   National Library of Medicine, *Overview (MetaMap API)*, [Accessed 01 July 2010], Available from: http://mmtx.nlm.nih.gov/javaapi/javadoc/, 2009.
[10] S. Ananiadou, *A methodology for automatic term recognition.*, Proceedings of the 15th conference on Computational linguistics, Kyoto, Japan, Association for Computational Linguistics, 1994.
[11] IUPAC, *Nomenclature of Organic Chemistry, Sections A, B, C, D, E, F, and H*, Oxford, Pergamon Press, 1979.
[12] IUPAC, *A Guide to IUPAC Nomenclature of Organic Compounds (Recommendations 1993)*, Oxford, Blackwell Scientific publications, 1993.
[13] G. Nenadić, S. Ananiadou, J. McNaught, *Enhancing automatic term recognition through recognition of variation*, Proceedings of the 20th international conference on Computational Linguistics, Geneva, Switzerland, Association for Computational Linguistics Morristown, NJ, USA, 2004.
[14] Ö. Uzuner, Y. Juo, P. Szolovits, Evaluating the state-of-the-art in automatic de-identification, *JAMIA* **14**(5) (2007), 550-63.
[15] R. Estopà, J. Vivaldi, M.T. Cabré, *Use of Greek and Latin forms for term detection*, Second International Conference on Language Resources and Evaluation, Athens, Greece, 2000.
[16] Q.T. Zeng, S. Goryachev, S. Weiss, M. Sordo, et al., Extracting principal diagnosis, co-morbidity and smoking status for asthma research: evaluation of a natural language processing system, *BMC Med Inf Dec Mak* **6** (2006), 30.

International Perspectives in Health Informatics
E.M. Borycki et al. (Eds.)
IOS Press, 2011

13

doi:10.3233/978-1-60750-709-3-13

Study of the Effects of Clinical Decision Support System's Incorrect Advice and Clinical Case Difficulty on Users' Decision Making Accuracy

Kamran GOLCHIN[a], Abdul ROUDSARI[a,b,1]

[a] *Centre for Health Informatics, School of Informatics, City University, London, UK*
[b] *School of Health Information Science, University of Victoria, Victoria, British Columbia, Canada*

Abstract. Different Clinical Decision Support Systems (CDSS) are reported to have different effects on clinicians' performance and various factors have been shown to be responsible for that (e.g. system's advice correctness, case difficulty, users' expertise...). The aim of this study is to determine how "advice correctness" and "case difficulty" affect users accepting/rejecting the comments of the system and consequently making a right or wrong decision. It was shown that in difficult cases, users level of making mistakes in clinical decision making was significantly higher when the comments were wrong. But there was no statistically significant difference between easy and difficult cases in how users accepted/rejected correct advice.

Keywords. clinical decision support system, advice correctness, case difficulty, user performance

Introduction

Clinical Decision Support Systems are "active knowledge systems which use two or more items of patient data to generate case-specific advice"[1] and support decision making in clinical processes from diagnosis to treatment, so by definition they play an important role in reducing medical errors. On the other hand, as physicians are quite susceptible to following the decision support systems' comments [2], correct advice is theoretically helpful to them while the systems' wrong suggestions are potentially a risk factor for worsening physicians' performance. Thus DSS's effect on physicians' performance is not always the same and different factors such as system's advice correctness, case difficulty and users' expertise have been shown to affect the final outcome [3- 8]. This article addresses whether case difficulty and advice correctness can affect physicians response to DSS, focusing on the following objectives:

---

[1] Abdul Roudsari, School of Health Information Science, University of Victoria, BC, Canada; Email: abdul@uvic.ca

1. How far are general practitioners (GPs) capable of identifying system's incorrect advice (in difficult cases)?
2. How GP's performances differ between easy and difficult cases (when the system advice is correct)?

1. Methodology

A clinical decision support system simulator was developed as a web application[2], in which the system's comments or advice could be manipulated as desired, and in accordance with the difficulty level of the patient scenarios. Hence, researchers can set the accuracy of the system by defining the percentage of the comments which will be wrong (which is not possible in studying real decision support systems). A relational database was designed and used to store clinical cases in the form of questions, and each question was related to one correct and some incorrect answers in the form of advice or system comments. The cases were also divided into three categories according to their difficulty for general practitioners; easy, intermediate, and difficult.

The DSS simulator published online, and 29 general practitioners participated in the study. When each GP logged into the application, fifteen randomly selected questions, five from each category, were presented to him in the form of a quiz with each question being randomly accompanied by either correct or incorrect advice. Accuracy of the system was set to 100% for easy case, 80% and 60% for intermediate and difficult cases respectively. Finally, users were asked whether they agreed with the advice or not and their answers were recorded by the application.

GPs' decisions were divided into "Right Decision" (agreeing with correct advice or rejecting incorrect advice), and "Wrong Decision" (agreeing with incorrect advice and rejecting correct advice), and this study tried to measure whether the making of right or wrong decisions is related to the correctness of system comments and/or the difficulty level of the cases.

2. Results

The first step in the analysis of the found data is data validation and filtering the outlier data. Pearson Chi square test was used to compare the correctness of the responses between the participants. The resulting P value was 0.278 with df=28, which is not statistically significant, and shows that no outlier response is present in this dataset.

To compare the effect of incorrect advice on GPs' decisions to difficult questions, the frequency of right/wrong responses (Table 1) were compared using Kendall Tau b test (both variables were ordinal). This test resulted in P=0.031 which is statistically significant, and shows that for difficult questions, wrong advice caused more mistakes

---

[2] This CDSS simulator was a dynamic online application developed in .Net framework, and used MSSQL as the database. This application can be used in other studies by entering clinical scenarios into the database and easily setting different parameters such as the number of questions shown to each user from different categories and the proportion of the questions to be randomly accompanied by correct or incorrect advice. It also retrieves raw data to generate basic reports that can be used in statistical analysis software such as SPSS.

Table 1. Frequency of GP's decision type by category of advice (Correct/Incorrect) in difficult questions PPV: Positive Predictive Value, NPV: Negative Predictive Value.

Difficult questions	Correct Advice	Incorrect Advice	Total	
Right Decision	59	29	88	PPV = 0.67
Wrong Decision	28	29	57	NPV = 0.51
Total	87	58	145	

Table 2. Frequency of GP's decision type by category of questions (Easy/Difficult)

	Correct Decision	Wrong Decision	Total
Easy	113	32	145
Difficult	88	57	145
Total	201	89	290

Table 3. Frequency of GP's decision type by category of questions (Easy/Difficult) when the advice is correct

Correct advice	Correct Decision	Wrong Decision	Total
Easy	113	32	145
Difficult	59	28	87
Total	172	60	232

in GPs' clinical decision making. The Negative Predictive Value (NPV) was 51 and the Positive Predictive Value was equal to 67

Responses to easy and difficult questions (Table2) were also compared to measure the effect of difficulty of the questions on the correctness of the decisions GPs made. The P value from Kendall Tau b test is significant at 0.001, but this result could have a bias as pieces of incorrect advice were only given in the difficult questions. Therefore to evaluate the pure effect of the difficulty, only the responses to the questions with correct advice (Table 3) were compared in a separate test. The result was P=0.112 which shows a considerable difference, but this difference is not statistically significant.

3. Discussion

The significant difference in GPs' decision making accuracy given advice correctness implies that in difficult cases, when doctors are provided with correct advice their decision making is generally much better than when the advice is incorrect. In other words when the case is difficult bad advice from the system could deceive them which makes it appear that (at least in difficult cases) GPs over-rely on the wrong advice. PPV of about 0.67 versus NPV of 0.51 shows GPs identify correct advice better than wrong advice.

The statistically insignificant difference in doctors' decision making accuracy given case difficulty *when only correct advice is provided* (Table 3), shows that the significant difference obtained in overall comparison of the responses (Table 2) cannot be explained by the difficulty of the questions and the main cause of difference was the incorrect advice provided to the participants. This in turn confirms our finding outlined above.

On the other hand the statistically insignificant difference in doctors' decision making accuracy given case difficulty (when correct advice is provided) implies that when the advice is correct, doctors' decision making accuracy is not affected by the difficulty of the cases. In other words if GPs are provided with correct advice the precision of the decision made is the same no matter how difficult the case.

Although a glance at the figures in Table 3 may lead one to expect a significant difference, the calculated P value of 0.112 showed no *statistically* significant difference, however the sizeble difference cannot be ignored and an insufficient sample size could be the reason that the difference did not reach the significant level.

4. Conclusion

In real medical practice, for easy cases, physicians usually are more confident about their decisions so it is less probable they would need to consult a CDSS or even be deceived with a wrong piece of advice. On the other hand these systems are expected to make fewer mistakes in easy cases; it is in difficult cases that more system errors and more consultations are expected, hence a higher level of consideration is needed to reduce the number of mistakes in the final outcome, as this study shows that physicians themselves cannot fully act as a layer of defense against this problem.

Conversely when users are provided with correct advice, no matter how difficult the case, doctors have similar degrees of accuracy in making clinical decisions. Since in real practice physicians need consultation with colleagues or CDSSs in difficult cases but rarely for easy ones, this finding is promising, because in difficult cases when CDSS attains a certain level of accuracy and does not make mistakes, physicians also will make no more mistakes than they do in easy cases. In plain language, the system's correct advice makes difficult cases become easier for GPs.

These two findings together show CDSSs are quite effective provided they are accurate enough, while inaccuracy in the systems can cause medical errors. Besides, by linking system comments to related medical literature (accessible to users via system) CDSSs can provide physicians with the facility to double check their decisions when they don't feel quite confident or they find a case difficult.

References

[1] J. Wyatt and M. Anderson, *Decision Support Systems*, National Institute for Clinical Excellence, 2004.
[2] S. Dreiseitl, M. Binder, Do physicians value decision support? a look at the effect of decision support systems on physician opinion, *Art Intel Med* **33** (2005), 25 – 30.
[3] C.S. Jao, D.B. Hier, W.L. Galanter, Using clinical decision support to maintain medication and problem lists A pilot study to yield higher patient safety," *Systems, Man and Cybernetics*, 2008, 739-743.
[4] L.G. Bergman and U.G.H. Fors, *Decision support in psychiatry – a comparison between the diagnostic outcomes using a computerized decision support system versus manual diagnosis*, BMC Medical Informatics and Decision Making, 2008.
[5] K. Tan, P.R.F. Dear, S.J. Newell, Clinical decision support systems for neonatal care, *Cochran Database of Systematic Reviews* **2** (2005), Art. No.: CD004211D.
[6] A.S. Elstein, Effects of a Decision Support System on the Diagnostic Accuracy of Users: A Preliminary Report, *JAMIA*, (1996), 422-428.
[7] E. Alberd, A.A. Povyakalo, L. Strigini, P. Ayton, M. Hartswood, R. Procter, R. Slack, Use of computer-aided detection (CAD) tools in screening mammography: a multidisciplinary investigation, *Brit J Radiology* **78** (2005), S31-S40.
[8] L. Theodore et al, Computer Decision Support as a Source of Interpretation Error: The Case of Electrocardiograms, *JAMIA* **10** (2003), 478–483.

International Perspectives in Health Informatics
E.M. Borycki et al. (Eds.)
IOS Press, 2011
doi:10.3233/978-1-60750-709-3-17

Automation Bias – A Hidden Issue for Clinical Decision Support System Use

Kate GODDARD [a,1], Abdul ROUDSARI [b], Jeremy C. WYATT [c]

[a] *Centre for Health Informatics, City University, London, UK*
[b] *School of Health Information Science, University of Victoria, Victoria, British Columbia, Canada*
[c] *Institute for Digital Healthcare, University of Warwick, UK*

Abstract. Automation bias – the tendency to over-rely on automation – has been studied in a variety of academic fields. Clinical Decision Support Systems aim to benefit the clinical decision making process. Although most research shows overall improved performance with use, there is often a failure to recognize the new errors that CDSS can introduce, and the healthcare field has a gap in this research. This paper outlines some of the most compelling theoretical factors in the literature involved in automation bias, and builds a simple model to be tested empirically. Ultimately, this will uncover the mechanisms by which this bias operates and help CDSS producers and healthcare practitioners optimize the medical decision making process.

Keywords. automation, human judgment, cognition, reliance

Introduction

Clinical Decision Support Systems (CDSS) aim to provide clinicians and healthcare professionals with intelligently filtered information centered on the patient. This includes the provision of Alerts and Reminders, Image Recognition, Diagnostic Assistance, Therapy Planning and Critiquing.

Although most CDSS are 80-90% accurate, it is known that occasional incorrect advice given may tempt users to reverse a correct decision, and thus introduce new errors. This error can be termed *automation bias*, where users tend to accept computer output without sufficient thought. For example, Friedman et al [1], noticed that in some cases, clinicians would override their own correct decisions in favor of the erroneous advice from the DSS – in 12% of cases the DSS caused the physician to add the correct diagnosis on their list, but in 6% of cases their own correct decisions were dropped in favor of the erroneous computer-generated advice – a net gain of 6% in diagnostic accuracy.

Previous studies have investigated automation bias within the field of medical informatics [2,3]. Further research is required to identify quantify the frequency and severity of automation bias, and the factors involved to mitigate risk and refine the appropriate usage of CDSS to maximize benefits gained from CDSS implementation.

---

[1] Corresponding author: Centre for Health Informatics, City University, Northampton Square, London, EC1V 0HB, UK, Email: kate.goddard.1@city.ac.uk

This review aims to outline some of the most salient factors cited in the literature posited to lead to over-reliance.

1. Decision Making

Faulty decision making in healthcare has been implicated in a wide range of medical errors. There is a tendency to assume that implementation of CDSS will mitigate imperfect human decision making. However these systems may elicit new types of decision errors if flawed, particularly if reliance is not well calibrated. Psychological judgment and decision making literature can help understand the factors and processes which can lead users to over-rely on CDSS and accept imperfect advice.

Dual process theories posit that judgment and thus decisions can be based on either logical Bayesian processing, or faster, rule-of-thumb (heuristic) based processing. For example by using a "confidence heuristic" [4] advisors use their own confidence levels to infer their ability, expertise, task-related knowledge, or accuracy on a given task. Many similar heuristics exist, many are internal and self generated; automation bias may be a case of using automation as the heuristic source for the accurate answer. Particularly if people are less confident of their own opinion by counteracting variance of trust in self or trust in human sources.

Mosier and Skitka [5] coined the term automation bias to refer to "the tendency to use automated cues as a heuristic replacement for vigilant information seeking and processing". It was proposed that insufficient cognitive processing was the cause of over reliance on automation. Rather than carry out more effortful logical processing of information, people often use heuristic-based, effort-saving strategies.

Literature was reviewed using PubMed, Web of Science and more generic search engines such as Google Scholar as sources of studies. Search terms were based on themes of automation and decision support, human-computer interaction, performance and error related to reliance on advice.

2. Individual differences

The socio-technical system formed between a decision aid and the user crucially depends on the human factors involved. There are a number of theories which postulate how human factors affect automation reliance. Riley [6] suggested that reliance, trust and confidence act as the primary cognitive mediators for human-computer interaction. For example, the Theory of Technology Dominance (TTD) [7] posits that DSS and task experience, and task complexity and cognitive fit are important factors when investigating reliance on intelligent decision aids.

2.1. Attitudinal

Trust in automation has perhaps been one of the topics with the most research in terms of investigating properly calibrated reliance, with the assumption that the higher the level of trust placed in automation, the more the user is likely to rely on it [8]. If too much trust is placed on an unreliable system, automation bias may occur.

Trust in automation is often calibrated according to the user's perception of advisor competence [9]. Trust can be significantly reduced by any sign of incompetence in the automation. Distrust in one function of an automatic component can spread to reduce trust in another function of the same component, but not generally to other components in the same system, or to other systems. There is a strong high positive correlation between operators' trust in and use of the automation; operators use automation they trust and reject distrusted automation, tending to prefer manual control. There is an inverse relationship between trust and monitoring of the automation. Trust may also affect, and be a product of a number of other factors such as complacency, situational awareness and mental workload amongst other factors [10].

Working parallel with trust in automation is the confidence the user has in their task-related abilities, or "self efficacy". Less confident users tend to seek greater amounts of advice [11]. Confidence levels are higher when there is a greater amount of information on which advisors can base their recommendations and when users receive recommendations from numerous advisors [12]. Lee and Moray [13] identified self confidence as an important trade off factor with trust in the automation, when trust in the automation exceeded self-confidence, the automation was more likely to be used and over-relied on. Trust and confidence have emerged as the critical factors in investigations into human-automation mismatches in the context of machining [14].

2.2. Non-attitudinal

Many studies have highlighted the impact of clinical task experience on appropriateness of reliance – studies generally imply that the more task experience a user has, the less likely they are to rely on automation, with overreliance tending to be more prevalent in less experienced groups. Berner [15] assessed a group of clinicians working a set of difficult cases using the Quick Medical Reference (QMR) DSS, and suggested that the extent of benefit gained by different users varied with their level of experience, with support benefitting the least experienced most.

Training and DSS experience also have strong positive effects on performance; exposure to rare automation failures sensitizes users to incorrect advice [16].

3. Environmental factors

Psychological research shows that humans tend to change decision strategies based on the amount of time available [17] and information demands [18]. In an aviation study, Mosier et al [19] examined the impact of operational variables on diagnosis and decision-making processes, focusing on information search. Time pressure, a common operational variable, had a strong negative effect on information search and diagnosis accuracy, and the presence of incongruent information heightened these negative effects.

Task complexity has been found to increase reliance on advice [20] and decision aids [21], as work load increases to reach the user's cognitive capacity, aid from external resources is increasingly, and potentially erroneously relied on. Task load has been shown to interact with trust to affect automation reliance [22]; as described, a positive relationship between automation trust and automation use exists and there is a suggestion that task load has a negative effect on this.

4. Cognitive Fit

Cognitive style has direct effects on perceived usefulness, perceived ease of use, and subjective norms of automation [23]. Both perceived usefulness and subjective norms affected actual technology usage significantly. People with innovative cognitive styles are more likely to perceive a new technology as useful and easy to use than are those with adaptive cognitive styles. There may also be a difference in appropriateness of reliance depending on whether the user has a primarily compensatory or non-compensatory style of decision making. Users employing a compensatory strategy may be more likely to take account of all information available; a non-compensatory strategist is more likely to adhere fewer cues on which to base their decision. "Cognitive fit" theory [24] proposes that the correspondence between user, task and information presentation format leads to superior task performance for individual users.

5. Model

Using the above overview of literature pertaining to human reliance in human-computer interaction, principles of the Theory of Technological Dominance (TTD) [7] have been augmented (Figure 1) to create a simple hypothetical view of how some of the most compelling factors in the literature may affect reliance on automated advice.

The most commonly cited drivers of reliance; trust and self-confidence, and the balance between them is hypothesized to be a key driver in automation bias. Over-trust being directly related to over use, as with lower confidence levels in users' own pre-advice decisions. Higher DSS experience (such as through training) may increase DSS use (discouraging disuse), but appropriately so; however low general experience in the field of study may increase tendency to over-rely on external support. External pressures such as time and task complexity may decrease cognitive resources and have a similar effect. Similarly to DSS experience, improved cognitive fit (fit between task requirements, user abilities and system characteristics) may increase appropriate use.

It is noted that these factors may be interlinked. Self confidence may increase with general experience, for example. Trust in the DSS can be better calibrated on increased DSS experience. Cognitive fit may be related to personality types and inherent tendency to trust automation. This is subject for further investigation.

6. Conclusion

The factors involved in the phenomenon of automation bias are complex and this overview is by no means exhaustive (this limitation is being diminished by a systematic review being completed by the authors). However despite the high risk associated with medication error there is little direct research into overreliance on technology within the healthcare and CDSS field. The model generated as a result of reviewing the most salient potential contributing factors will be tested empirically by the Centre for Health Informatics at City University, London. This model represents a theoretical starting point for more research into drivers of automation bias, in addition to its existence. Through this type of research it is hoped that clinical DSS can be built with evidence-based designs to reduce over-reliance while concurrently encouraging users to utilize correct advice.

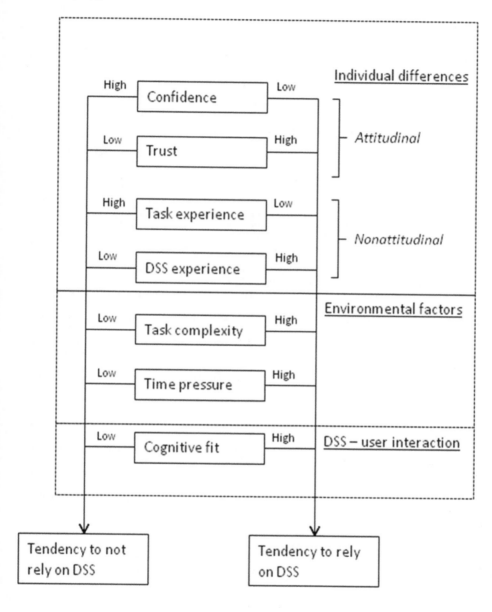

Factors are assumed to be independent but interactive.

Figure 1. Model for factors leading to automation bias (adapted from TTD [7])

References

[1] C.P. Friedman, A.S. Estein, F.M. Wolf, G.C. Murphy, T.M. Franz, P.S. Heckerling, P.L. Fine, T.M. Miller, V. Abraham, Enhancement of clinicians' diagnostic reasoning by computer-based consultation: a multisite study of 2 systems, *JAMA* **282** (1999), 1851-1956.

[2] J.I. Westbrook, E.W. Coiera, A.S. Gosling, Do online information retrieval systems help experienced clinicians answer clinical questions? *JAMIA* **12** (2005), 315-321.

[3] W.N. Southern, J.H. Arnsten, The effect of erroneous computer interpretation of ECGs on resident decision making, *Med Decision Making* **29** (2009), 372-376.

[4] P.C. Price, E.R. Stone, Intuitive evaluation of likelihood judgment producers: evidence for a confidence heuristic, *J Behav Decision Making* **17** (2004), 39–57.

[5] K.L. Mosier, L.J. Skitka, Human decision makers and automated decision aids: made for each other? in: R. Parasuraman, M. Mouloua, editors, *Automation and Human Performance: Theory and Application.* Erlbaum, Mahwah, NJ, (1996), 201–220.

[6] V. Riley, A general model of mixed-initiative human-machine systems, in *Proceedings of the Human Factors Society. 33rd Annual Meeting,* Santa Monica, CA (1989), 124-128.

[7] V. Arnold, S.G. Sutton, The theory of technology dominance: understanding the impact of intelligent decision aids on decision makers' judgments, *Adv Account Behav Res* **1** (1998), 175-194.

[8] P. de Vries, C. Midden, D Bouwhuis, The effects of errors on system trust, self-confidence, and the allocation of control in route planning, *Int J Human-Computer Stud* **58** (2003), 719-735.

[9] B.M. Muir, Trust in automation: 1. Theoretical issues in the study of trust and human intervention in automated systems, *Ergonomics* **37** (1994), 1905–1922.

[10] J.D. Lee, K.A. See, Trust in Automation: Designing for Appropriate Reliance, *Human Factors* **46** (2004), 50-80.

[11] R.S. Cooper, *Information processing in the judge–adviser system of group decision-making,* unpublished master's thesis, University of Illinois, Urbana-Champaign, 1991.

[12] D.V. Budescu, A.K. Rantilla, Confidence in aggregation of expert opinions, *Acta Psychologica* **104** (2000), 371–398.

[13] J.D. Lee, N Moray, Trust, control strategies and allocation of function in human-machine systems, *Ergonomics* **35** (1992), 1243-1270 .

[14] K. Case, M.A. Sinclair, M.R.A. Rani, An experimental investigation of human mismatches in machining, *Proceedings of the Institution of Mechanical Engineers Part B – Journal of Engineering Manufacture* **213** (1999), 197–201.

[15] E.S. Berner, R.S. Maisiak, Influence of case and physician characteristics on perceptions of decision support systems, *JAMIA* **6** (1999), 428-34.

[16] J.E. Bahner, A.D. Huper, D Manzey, Misuse of automated decision aids: Complacency, automation bias and impact of training experience, *Int J Human-Computer Stud* **66** (2008), 688-699.

[17] P. Wright, The harassed decision maker: time pressures, distractions, and the use of evidence, *J Applied Psych* **59** (1974), 555-561.

[18] J.W. Payne, Task complexity and contingent processing in decision making: an information search and protocol analysis, *Org Behav Human Perf* **16** (1976), 366-387.

[19] K.L. Mosier, N Sethi, S McCauley, L Khoo, J.M. Orasanu, What you don't know can hurt you: factors impacting diagnosis in the automated cockpit, *Human Factors,* **49** (2007), 300-10.

[20] F, Gino, D.A. Moore, Effects of task difficulty on use of advice, *J Behav Decision Making* **20** (2007), 21–35.

[21] G. Bin, Moderating effects of task characteristics on information source use: An individual level analysis of R&D professionals in new product development, *J Inform Sci* **35** (2009), 1-21.

[22] M.A. Daly, *Task load and automation use in an uncertain environment*, Masters Thesis, from: https://research.maxwell.af.mil/papers/ay2002/afit/afit-gaq-env-02m-05.pdf, 2002.

[23] I. Chakraborty, P.J. Hu, D. Cui, Examining the effects of cognitive style in individuals' technology use decision making. *Decision Supp Sys* **45** (2008), 228-241.

[24] I. Vessey. The theory of cognitive fit: One aspect of a general theory of problem solving?, in P. Zhang, D. Galletta, editors, *Human-computer Interaction and Management Information Systems: Foundations, Advances in Management Information Systems Series,* Sharpe, Armonk, NY:M.E., 2006.

Clinical Informatics

International Perspectives in Health Informatics
E.M. Borycki et al. (Eds.)
IOS Press, 2011

doi:10.3233/978-1-60750-709-3-25

The SignOut Discharge Summary System: Using Workflow Byproducts to Pre-Populate and Assemble Discharge Summaries

Joseph KANNRY [a,1], Preetham BILUMANE [a]
Jill GOLDENBERG [a]
[a] *Department of Information Technology, Mount Sinai Medical Center, NY, NY*

Abstract. At the time of hospital discharge, communication between inpatient and outpatient physicians is poor. Multiple studies demonstrate that discharge summaries, a means of improving information exchange between inpatient and outpatient providers, are frequently not available to the outpatient provider at the time of the post discharge visit. We have constructed a web-based solution for generating discharge summaries, SignOut Discharge Summary System (SDSS) which uses the workflow byproduct of SignOut data to pre-populate summaries, a post-discharge preparation module to ensure quality, a discharge edit module to designate accurate discharge summary assignment, and integration with HIM. SDSS had 1130 unique users in a recent period and captured signout information for 75% of hospitalized patients. The system has generated 78740 D/C summaries for 17 specialties since going live July 2005. Overall SDSS is responsible for 69% of all hospital discharge summaries and SDSS discharge summaries on average are available 1.91 days after discharge.

Keywords. electronic discharge summary, timely completion, Signout System, housestaff, workflow byproduct

Introduction

Deficits in communication and the transfer of information between inpatient physicians and outpatient providers is well documented [9]. A logical vehicle for this type of information is the discharge summary, yet multiple studies demonstrate that discharge summaries are frequently not available to the provider at the time of the post discharge visit [11, 18, 19]. Studies demonstrate that less than half of all providers receive information concerning discharge medications and recommended plans of care for their recently hospitalized patients [12, 18,19]. Van Walraven and colleagues found that discharge summaries were available only 8.2% of the time at the post discharge visit and 68.2% at any visit. Similarly, in a study by Wilson and colleagues[19], only 27.1% of outpatient providers ever received their patients' discharge summary. Another study

---

[1] Corresponding Author: Joseph Kannry, joseph.kannry@mountsinai.org

by Van Walraven and colleagues, established that patients assessed by providers with access to the discharge summary had a decreased trend toward rehospitalization (relative risk 0.74, 95% confidence interval 0.50 to 1.11) [17]. In the same study, discharge summaries were only available for 12.2% of post-discharge visits.

The two biggest barriers to reviewing the discharge summary are availability (i.e., generation at the time of follow-up visit) and accessibility[18]. Summaries were most commonly unavailable because they were not generated in time for the follow-up visit (20.0%) or they were not sent to the follow-up provider (50.8%). Even when available, discharge summaries may not always contain the information outpatient providers require[12, 15]. Discharge summary systems can significantly address accessibility and availability by ensuring that the discharge summary is electronically available at the time of the follow-up visit[4, 8, 9]. We have constructed a web-based solution; the SignOut-Discharge Summary System (SDSS) to provide providers with information about hospitalization immediately available upon discharge. We hypothesize that pre-populating and incrementally generating discharge summaries will significantly improve the timeliness of summary completion. This paper describes our solution the SignOut Discharge Summary System (SDSS).

1. Background

Mount Sinai hospital is a 1,171 bed hospital staffed by 689 residents and fellows with over 2,000 attendings. The SignOut system was originally developed in 1997 as a handoff tool for housestaff to electronically update patient status daily to facilitate sign out between providers. In 2005, the system was modified so that housestaff could convert a compilation of these "signouts" into a discharge summary. Prior to these modifications to the SignOut system, the timeliness of discharge summary completion by dictation was slow estimated at 17 days. It was hypothesized that giving housestaff the ability to generate a summary from a document already in use might better align with their workflow and thus lead to more timely summary completion. Currently 75% of all admissions appear in SDSS. The front end of the SignOut Discharge Summary System is written in Java and JSP and resides on a Solaris web server. The backend database is an Oracle 8I database residing on a R6000 AIX machine. Integration of the SignOut System with our clinical repository, "Enterprise Data Repository" (EDR), ensures automated transfer of patient demographics and continuous updating of patient location (i.e., bed and floor) from EDR. Summaries are produced when patients are discharged from the SignOut System. The concept of integrated SignOut Discharge System has been mentioned once in the peer reviewed literature and anecdotally one other time [14]. General practitioners have stated that electronic discharges summaries would be preferred over any manual process [1]. We have developed a web based Discharge Summary generator, the SignOut Discharge Summary System (SDSS). SDSS generates discharge summaries, as a byproduct of a daily workflow process and iterative completion involving the following steps: Step 1 - Admission, Step 2 - Hospitalization, Step 3 - Peridischarge, Step 4 - Post Discharge Prep, Step 5 - Post Discharge. In this paper we describe how SDSS has resulted in a more timely completion of summaries.

2. Methods

Discharge summaries are assembled and generated by capturing information at the 5 points in the workflow process. This capture is accomplished by the SignOut module, Post Discharge Preparation Module, Discharge Edit Module, and integration with HIM (Health Information Management System). Workflow integration is stressed so that information capture is part of daily workflow and not an artifact.

The bulk of information is captured as a workflow byproduct in Steps 1 and 2 in the SignOut module. Patients are added to SignOut upon admission - Step 1. At our institution, at the end of every working day, inpatient housestaff must signout to the on-call team - Step 2. Residents generate patient lists and include information that the on-call team needs to be aware of for the night or the weekend. Information that the residents supply for signout is entered directly into the SignOut System module upon admission and updated at the end of each day by house staff using computer terminals located throughout the hospital. To edit an individual patient, providers click on a name and are taken to the patient edit screen. Information from the daily SignOut that is used to populate the discharge summary includes attending and housestaff physician names and pager numbers, name and pager of discharging physician (author of summary), admitting diagnosis, discharge diagnosis, code status, history of present illness, past medical history, hospital course, problem list, medications, allergies, relevant test results, and consultant names.

The peri-discharge period (i.e. Step 3) defined by this paper as the period in which discharge is imminent (i.e. from impending discharge to actual discharge). The best time to capture information about plans for the post-discharge period is during the peri-discharge period. Prescriptions are written, follow-up appointments made, tests are scheduled etc. The post discharge preparation button takes the user to tabs for discharge examination, discharge medications, follow-up appointments, testing, and discharge instructions.

Once the patient is ready to be discharged the patient is in the discharge to post discharge period - Step 4. It is at this point in the workflow that provider is taken to the discharge edit screen. Provider Assignment in SDSS is built on the principal of provider designation and assignment of patient responsibility [6, 7, 10]. At the time of discharge, the final step in generating a discharge summary in SDSS is to identify and designate the discharge attending. Due to coverage schemes, rotations etc the identification of the discharge attending is frequently different from that of the attending of record during the hospital stay. At our institution, the discharge attending is responsible for content and completion of the final discharge summary so the identity of this attending determines HIM assignment. The rest of the information on the discharge edit screen is designed to collect information known only at the time of discharge. Once the provider is satisfied with the summary, the provider presses a button complete discharge summary which signs the preliminary version of the summary. In housestaff based services the housestaff complete the summary, create a preliminary version which must be reviewed and electronically signed by the attending.

Step 5 occurs in the post-discharge period when attendings need to review and finalize discharges summaries. To ensure that medical records can track the status of discharge summaries, SDSS summaries are sent to Softmed, Sinai's HIM system. Upon receipt of a SignOut discharge summary the status in Softmed changes from not done to awaiting attending signature. In Softmed, attendings can review, edit, and sign discharge summaries making them final. Further changes to the discharge summary require amendments. Softmed is available onsite and remotely via our Extranet. Discharge Summaries are immediately accessible in both their preliminary and final form in the clinical repository as well as our Electronic Medical Record(EMR). Both preliminary and final versions of summaries are accessible via EDR (i.e., the clinical repository) to all physicians in training and/or have admitting privileges.

3. Results

Three services accounted for the vast majority (69%) of discharge summaries in the system. Medicine accounted for 34%, pediatrics 17%, and surgery 18% of all discharge summaries were live since discharge Summaries were introduced when the system went live July 11, 2005. Table 1 looks at the percentage of SDSS generated discharges summaries. All discharge summaries at Mount Sinai fall into one of two categories, SDSS or dictated as handwritten discharges summaries are no longer accepted. SDSS by 2008 accounts for 69% of the discharge summaries. An earlier analysis of SDSS and hospital admissions has consistently shown that 75% of patients admitted to Mount Sinai are in SDSS. Table 2 looks at the average number of days after discharge that discharge summaries were completed In Table 2 the average # days post-discharge that summaries were available after discharge was 1.91 days. The limited data that we have prior to SDSS is that discharge summaries were on average available at 17 days. SDSS resulted in a 15 days reduction when compared to pre-SDSS. The average number of days available after discharge is stable for over 2.5 years and then in 2008 increases by 1 day. Numbers in the table are for preliminary discharge summaries and data for 2005 is from the July go-live to year's end.

Table 1. Percentage SDSS Discharges Summaries/All Discharge Summaries

Year	SDSS D/C Summaries	Dictated D/C Summaries	% SDSS
2007	22424	14420	61%
2008	26932	12269	69%

Table 2. Average Availability of Discharge Summaries

Year	# Days post-discharge
2005	1.5
2006	1.2
2007	1.3
2008	2.7
Average	1.91

4. Discussion

The goal of SDSS was to improve the availability and accessibility of discharge summaries. At the time SDSS was being developed, because discharge summaries were not being completed in a timely manner. This system was thought to better align with housestaff workflow and capture work already done. SDSS is certainly being used as 69% of discharges summaries are generated by SDSS. The availability of discharges summaries without delay is critical, as patients discharged from Mount Sinai Hospital are required to have a follow-up outpatient appointment within 2 weeks. SDSS summaries were on average available 1.91 days after discharge over the 3.5 year period. The hospital reports an average of 3-5 days for all discharge summaries which includes the 31% dictated. In contrast nationally, discharge summaries are unavailable or not completed at the time of the post discharge visit over 50% of the time[12, 18, 19]. Prior to SDSS, Mount Sinai Discharge Summaries were on average available at 17-18 days. We were not able to obtain further details on pre-SDSS on timely completion due to changes in leadership, record-keeping, and methodology. Discharge summaries are accessible immediately upon completion from any terminal at the medical center and securely via a remote access. In 2008 there was a spike in the number of discharge summaries generated as well as an increase of over a day in the availability of discharges summaries. Both numbers had been stable from July 11, 2005 till the end of 2007. An analysis is underway as well as monitoring for changes in 2009.

A limitation of our analysis was table 2 addresses discharges summaries that are comprehensive and complete but with a status of preliminary because the summaries must be signed by an attending before being legally final. However, the institution reports that final summaries are on average available at 3-5 days which would mean that there is only a brief delay (i.e., few days) going from preliminary to final. The word preliminary is used in the same context of a preliminary pathology or radiology report meaning these reports are complete and actionable but are subject to final attending signoff. If these preliminary reports were not available there would be no discharge summary information. It should also be noted that at some institutions including those of the author, housestaff signed summaries were or are final summaries. The discharge summaries provide information that discharge summaries traditionally are not required to provide. This information includes both admitting and discharge diagnosis, and code status during admission.

A consistent complaint by providers regarding discharge summary quality is information on the post-discharge plan is frequently missing and it is difficult to communicate with inpatient providers [9]. This was addressed in large part with the post-discharge preparations section and discharge edit screen of SDSS. The communication issues were addressed for the post-discharge period by at least providing contact information such as provider names and pagers to enable communication. Studies looking at different formats of discharge summary quality have found no difference between dictated and discharge summary [16] or handwritten and electronic discharge summaries [3]. A study well underway by the authors is examining the quality of SDSS Discharge Summaries [5].

A unique feature of our study is the discharges summaries are pre-populated data from SignOut System. However, this is also a limitation of this study as there are few examples of the approach [14]. As a result findings from this study may not be generalizable to electronic discharges summaries as a whole. Another limitation is the study was conducted at only one institution, Mount Sinai. While there seems to be institutional consensus that both the timeliness of discharge summaries has significantly improved, it is unclear how much of this can be attributed to SDSS. While studies suggest that electronic discharge summaries contribute to improved timeliness[8, 13], there is little data institutionally available to separate out confounding variables that occurred during the implementation and use of SDSS. These variables include changing the suspension policy for discharge summaries incomplete at 21 days, making attendings solely responsible for final summaries, and changes in methodology determining delinquency rates.

5. Conclusions

Discharge summaries, the major source of information about hospitalization are frequently unavailable [2, 12, 18, 19]. The SignOut Discharge Summary System successfully made discharges summaries available on average 1.91 days after discharge and accessible on campus at all terminals and off campus using the standard remote access solution. The system is innovative in that it uses the workflow byproduct of SignOut data to pre-populate discharge summaries, a post-discharge preparation module to ensure quality discharge summaries at the point physicians are capturing the information, verification of the discharge attending name at the time of discharge, and integration with HIM for medical records tracking and final signature. SDSS discharge summary documents are readily accessible and available via API links to the clinical repository and EMR. In summary, we have successfully developed the web-based SignOut Discharge Summary System that provides timely information about hospitalizations .In little over 3.5 years and as of 2008 accounts for 69 per cent of all completed discharge summaries at Mount Sinai Medical Center. SDSS to date has 78740 discharge summaries. These discharge summaries are immediately available upon completion and accessible in a secure HIPAA compliant mechanism by any offsite or onsite physicians affiliated with Mount Sinai Hospital[2].

References

[1] M. Alderton and J. Callen, Are general practitioners satisfied with electronic discharge summaries?, *Him J* **36** (2007), 7-12.
[2] J.I. Balla and W.E. Jamieson, Improving the continuity of care between general practitioners and public hospitals, *Med J Aust* **161** (1994), 656-659.
[3] J.L. Callen, M. Alderton, and J. McIntosh, Evaluation of electronic discharge summaries: a comparison of documentation in electronic and handwritten discharge summaries, *Int J Med Inform* **77** (2008), 613-620.
[4] J. Craig, J. Callen, A. Marks, B. Saddik, and M. Bramley, Electronic discharge summaries: the current state of play, *Him J* **36** (2007), 30-36.
[5] J. Goldenberg, J.J. Mermelstein, Ramiro Markoff, Brian, A. Dinescu, B. Korc, J. Kannry, A. Dunn, A. Federman, and N. Kathuria, Speed or Accuracy? Seeking Both in an Electronic Standardardized Discharge Summary Tool, in: *Society of Hospital Medicine 2009 Annual Conference*, Chicago, Ill, 2009.
[6] J. Kannry and C. Moore, DocFind: A Web-Based Application that Facilitates Attending and Housestaff Provider Communication, In Process.
[7] J. Kannry and C. Moore, MediSign: using a web-based SignOut System to improve provider identification, *Proc AMIA Symp* (1999), 550-554.

---

[2] Acknowledgements to Deborah Redmond, Nava Birnberg and Dr. Joel Forman for leadership and support Babu Manam for programming, Dianne McLaughlin and Elizabeth Roman from Medical Records for hospital data.

[8]   J. Kirby, B. Barker, D.J. Fernando, M. Jose, C. Curtis, A. Goodchild, C. Dickens, E. Olla, R. Cooke, I. Idris, and G.A. Thomson, A prospective case control study of the benefits of electronic discharge summaries, *J Telemed Telecare* **12 Suppl 1** (2006), 20-21.

[9]   S. Kripalani, F. LeFevre, C.O. Phillips, M.V. Williams, P. Basaviah, and D.W. Baker, Deficits in Communication and Information Transfer Between Hospital-Based and Primary Care Physicians: Implications for Patient Safety and Continuity of Care, *Jama* **297** (2007), 831-841.

[10] A. Kushniruk, T. Karson, C. Moore, and J. Kannry, From prototype to production system: lessons learned from the evolution of the SignOut System at Mount Sinai Medical Center, *AMIA Annu Symp Proc* (2003), 381-385.

[11] R.J. Mageean, Study of "discharge communications" from hospital, *Br Med J (Clin Res Ed)* **293** (1986), 1283-1284.

[12] R.J. Mageean, Study of "discharge communications" from hospital, *Br Med J (Clin Res Ed)* **293** (1986), 1283-1284.

[13] K.J. O'Leary, D.M. Liebovitz, J. Feinglass, D.T. Liss, D.B. Evans, N. Kulkarni, M.P. Landler, and D.W. Baker, Creating a better discharge summary: improvement in quality and timeliness using an electronic discharge summary, *J Hosp Med* **4** (2009), 219-225.

[14] S. Quan and O. Tsai, Signing on to sign out, part 2: describing the success of a web-based patient sign-out application and how it will serve as a platform for an electronic discharge summary program, *Healthc Q* **10** (2007), 120-124.

[15] D. Tsilimingras and D.W. Bates, Addressing Postdischarge Adverse Events: A Neglected Area, *Joint Commission Journal on Quality and Patient Safety* **34** (2008), 85-97.

[16] C. van Walraven, A. Laupacis, R. Seth, and G. Wells, Dictated versus database-generated discharge summaries: a randomized clinical trial, *Cmaj* **160** (1999), 319-326.

[17] C. van Walraven, R. Seth, P.C. Austin, and A. Laupacis, Effect of discharge summary availability during post-discharge visits on hospital readmission, *J Gen Intern Med* **17** (2002), 186-192.

[18] C. van Walraven, R. Seth, and A. Laupacis, Dissemination of discharge summaries. Not reaching follow-up physicians, *Can Fam Physician* **48** (2002), 737-742.

[19] S. Wilson, W. Ruscoe, M. Chapman, and R. Miller, General practitioner-hospital communications: a review of discharge summaries, *J Qual Clin Pract* **21** (2001), 104-108.

International Perspectives in Health Informatics
E.M. Borycki et al. (Eds.)
IOS Press, 2011
doi:10.3233/978-1-60750-709-3-32

Delivery of Psychosocial Care for Cancer Patients: A Pilot Investigation

Kathleen ABRAHAMSON[1], Morgan DURHAM[1],
Kelli NORTON[2], James G. ANDERSON[3]

[1] *Western Kentucky University, Department of Public Health, Bowling Green, KY, USA*
[2] *Regenstrief Institute, Indianapolis, IN, USA*
[3] *Purdue University, Department of Sociology, West Lafayette, IN, USA*

Abstract. Psychosocial distress is common in cancer patients. Although common, psychosocial distress is frequently under-diagnosed and poorly managed in the U.S. health system. This paper describes 25 in-depth telephone interviews with health care professionals working within cancer care centers. Interview questions address perception of the psychosocial services offered within their cancer care organizations. Results indicate that access to psychosocial care is frequently dependent upon the subjective judgment of busy clinicians. Information technology could improve the delivery of psychosocial care by easing the administration of psychosocial assessments and increasing clinician contact with research evidence regarding distress management.

Keywords. cancer, positive deviance, psychosocial distress

Introduction

Psychosocial distress, defined as "an emotional experience of a psychological, social, and/or spiritual nature that may interfere with the ability to cope effectively with cancer, its' symptoms and treatment" [1] is a significant problem for cancer patients, their family members, and caregivers. Psychosocial distress ranges from normal feelings of apprehension regarding a cancer diagnosis to levels of depression and anxiety that interfere with treatment and daily living. Approximately 35-45% of U.S. cancer patients report significant emotional distress [2,3], though this number likely underestimates the number of cancer patients who experience some level of psychosocial distress during the course of their treatment. Unresolved psychosocial distress negatively influences treatment selection, compliance with recommended treatment, quality of life, and disease progression. Although common, psychosocial distress is frequently under-diagnosed and poorly managed in the U.S. health system. Clinical practice guidelines for the management of psychosocial distress have been established, but they are rarely fully implemented [4,5]. Only 5-10% of cancer patients receive formal psychosocial services [6].

Corresponding Author: Kathleen Abrahamson, Western Kentucky University, Department of Public Health, 127A Academic Complex, Bowling Green, KY 42101; Email: Kathleen.abrahamson@wku.edu; Phone: (270) 745-6973

Cancer patients are a heterogeneous population possessing a wide range of ages, disease sites, prognoses, beliefs, social supports/demands, and reactions to the disease process. Past research has demonstrated that some psychosocial interventions are successful for sub-samples of the cancer population. What remains unknown is a mechanism to provide effective psychosocial care to a diverse population of cancer patients in a manner which is cost effective for resource constrained clinical environments. For this pilot project we interviewed 25 cancer care providers (health care administrators, oncologists, nurses, social workers) working within cancer centers in the state of Indiana, U.S.A. Questions were created, and data was analyzed, using a positive deviance perspective. Positive deviance as defined by Spreitzer and Sonenshein [7] is, "intentional behavior that departs from the norms of a referent group in honorable ways." Through in-depth interviews with cancer care providers we identified mechanisms of providing psychosocial care which deviate from the current clinical norm in a positive manner, are potentially transferable to other organizations, and thus warrant further examination [5].

1. Methods

In-depth telephone interviews were conducted with of 25 cancer care providers working within 10 cancer care organizations in the state of Indiana, U.S.A. Respondents were selected based upon response to an initial query letter sent to comprehensive cancer centers in the central region of Indiana indicating they would be willing to participate in a 30 minute structured interview. Both urban and rural cancer care organizations were represented, as well as organizations which serve primarily inpatients, primarily outpatients, and those that serve both. See Table 1 for a description of survey respondents and organization characteristics.

Table 1. Characteristics of Survey Respondents

Job Title:	
Social Worker	7
Nursing	7
Administration	8
Physician	2
Counselor	1
Total	25
Years in Job:	
0-5	14
6-10	5
>10	5
No Answer	1
Total	25
Location:	
Urban Facility	7
Rural Facility	3
Total	10
Patient type:	
Inpatient only	1
Outpatient only	4
Both	5
Total	10

Institutional Review Board approval was obtained prior to contacting respondents, and telephone interviews were taped and transcribed in a manner that did not identify the respondent or the respondent's organization. Because of the exploratory nature of these initial interviews, the survey instrument was created specifically for this pilot investigation. Survey questions addressed the current processes of psychosocial distress management within respondent organizations; respondent perspectives on the efficiency and effectiveness of these processes; barriers to the management of psychosocial distress; resources available to assist in the management of psychosocial distress; inter-organizational communication in regards to interdisciplinary teamwork, time spent with supervisors/ subordinates, and decision making processes; and respondent suggestions for process improvement.

The organizational behavior that defined positive deviance in this project was the ability to address cancer related distress in manner at least partially consistent with NCCN practice guidelines [1]. If centers identified as positive deviants noted barriers and resources that were similar to other organizations, but differed in terms of organizational innovation and processes, it would be likely that non-positive deviant centers could adapt similar processes which would enable improved management of psychosocial distress.

1.1. Analysis

Reponses to interview questions were first coded according to content by the second author. Initial codes were reviewed by the first author and discrepancies were discussed and resolved. The first goal of research designed from a positive deviance approach is to identify the organizations which meet the criteria for positive deviant behavior, in this case by at least partially following guidelines for the management of psychosocial distress. Therefore, these initial analyses are descriptive with a focus on provider perceptions of how psychosocial distress is managed and the organizational barriers, resources, and processes that support management of distress.

2. Results

All respondents noted the availability of mental health professionals, either within their organizations or through outside referrals, that dealt specifically with cancer related psychosocial distress. Providers from all but 3 organizations said their patients had access to mental health professionals within their organization. The 3 organizations relying solely on outside referrals were located in rural areas. Only 4 respondents representing 3 organizations noted the presence of psychosocial services directly related to colon or rectal cancer. Each of these 3 organizations offering specialized colorectal cancer services was located in an urban area. Twenty-two respondents (88%) felt their facility encouraged interdisciplinary communication in regards to cancer care, and only 1 respondent felt their cancer care facility had difficulty with staff turnover. Importantly, 8 respondents (32%) representing 5 organizations (50%) said their organization did not assess all cancer patients for psychosocial distress upon admission, and 13 (52%) respondents representing 6 organizations (60%) said their organization did have a systematic assessment tool available to determine the level of patient distress. Only 4 respondents (16%) representing 2 organizations (20%) said their facility had established an objective definition of psychosocial distress that would guide further treatment, and respondents from 8 of the 10 organizations were not aware of an established clinical pathway for the treatment of psychosocial distress. Only 8 respondents had frequent contact with research findings regarding psychosocial distress.

During the interview respondents were asked directly if they felt their organization paid adequate attention to psychosocial distress in cancer patients. Though these questions address organizational issues, they deal with provider perceptions and therefore are reported on an individual level. Thirteen respondents (52%) felt their facilities paid adequate attention to psychosocial distress, 10 (40%) did not, 2 had no comment. When asked what could be done to improve the amount of attention paid to psychosocial distress, responses included increasing the number of staff (6), adopting a systematic assessment tool (4), increasing staff participation in the process (3), improving staff education (1), and assessing all patients upon admission (1). Respondents were also asked if they felt their organizations dealt with psychosocial issues in a manner which was efficient. Results were similar, with 13 (52%) stating that psychosocial care within their organization was efficient, and 10 (40%) stating that psychosocial care was not dealt with in an efficient manner, and 2 having no comment. When asked what could be done to improve efficiency, responses included the adoption of a systematic assessment tool (7), increasing the number of staff (4), improving staff communication (2), and assessing all patients upon admission (1).

3. Discussion

Psychosocial distress in cancer patients is common and often not well managed within the US health care system [4,5]. We conducted in-depth interviews with cancer care providers using a positive deviance perspective, which seeks to identify those organizations that are providing high levels of care within resource constrained environments. Analyses thus far are descriptive, providing information regarding the resources available to manage psychosocial distress directly from those working within cancer care organizations. Two primary themes have emerged. First, mental health professionals are widely available to cancer patients, but less geographically accessible to cancer patients being served in rural settings. Second, although mental health professionals may be available, lack of a systematic assessment and universal use of an accepted assessment instrument limits who receives a referral for such services. Objective assessment of patients using an established assessment tool is a corner stone of clinical practice guidelines regarding the management of cancer related distress [1]. Many respondents noted an over-reliance on subjective clinician judgment to determine who receives psychosocial services. We found psychosocial services are often available, but not accessible to those who for a variety of reasons fail to be identified as distressed by busy clinicians.

Respondents noted that the delivery of psychosocial services could be improved through the use of a systematic assessment tool upon admission, as well the addition of more staff members to provide patients with time and attention. It is our belief that implementation of innovative information technology could greatly assist cancer providers with the provision of psychosocial care. Well established assessment tools such as the distress thermometer are available in computerized forms, increasing the ease of administration in busy clinical settings [8]. Interdisciplinary communication could be facilitated when assessments are computerized and thus accessible to a variety of staff/departments. The low numbers of staff who have frequent contact with research evidence would be improved through the addition of computerized, evidence-based clinical practice guidelines, directing patients identified as highly distressed in the assessment process through an established pathway to treatment and referral. However, the success of psychosocial interventions with cancer patients depends not only on the quality of the interventional design or technology, but on organizational culture and processes of implementation. Due to the sensitive nature of many psychosocial issues, care must be taken to implement systems in a manner that does not interfere with patient/provider communication. Further analyses of this pilot data are needed to identify innovative mechanisms by which organizations deliver psychosocial care within resource constrained environments.

3.1. Limitations

This project was designed to collect preliminary or pilot data, and is limited by a low number of respondents. Respondents are nested within organizations, and thus any analysis must acknowledge that respondents working within the same organizational settings will have answers which are likely correlated. Also, though both urban and rural organizations are represented, respondents are from a single state and thus may be influenced by geographic customs or policies.

Acknowledgement. The Cancer Care Engineering project is supported by the Regenstrief Foundation and the Walther Cancer Institute in Indianapolis, Indiana and the Department of Defense, Congressionally Directed Medical Research Program, Fort Detrick, MD (W81-XWH-08-1-0065 and W81XWH-10-0540) administered jointly through the Oncological Sciences Center at Purdue University and the Indiana University Simon Cancer Center.

References

[1]   NCCN Clinical Practice Guidelines in Oncology: Distress Management. (2008), Accessed on November 20, 2008 at www.nccn.org.
[2]   Carlson, L. & Bultz, B. Cancer Distress Screening: Needs, Models and Methods. *Journal of Psychosomatic Res* **55** (2003a), 403-409.
[3]   Carlson, L. & Bultz, B. Benefits of Psychosocial Oncology Care: Improved Quality of Life and Medical Cost Offset. *Health Quality of Life Outcomes* **1** (2003b), (article available: http://www.hqlo.com/content/1/1/8).
[4]   Jacobsen, P.B. Screening of Psychosocial Distress in Cancer Patients: Challenges and Opportunities. *J Clin Oncology* **29** (2007), 4526-4527.
[5]   Jacobsen, P.B. & Ransom, S. Implementation of NCCN Distress Management Guidelines by Member Institutions. *J Nat Comprehen Cancer Network* **5** (2007), 66-98.
[6]   Clark, P.M. Treating Distress:Working Toward Psychosocial Standards for Oncology Care. *Proceedings of the 26th Conference of the Oncology Nursing Society* (2001).
[7]   Spreitzer, G. & Sonenshein, S. Toward a Construct Definition of Positvive Deviance. *Amer Behav Sci* **47** (2004), 828-847.
[8]   Abrahamson, K. Dealing with Cancer Related Distress. *Amer J Nurs* **110** (2010), 67-69.

International Perspectives in Health Informatics
E.M. Borycki et al. (Eds.)
IOS Press, 2011
doi:10.3233/978-1-60750-709-3-37

Critical Care Providers Refer to Information Tools Less During Communication Tasks After a Critical Care Clinical Information System Introduction

Mark BALLERMANN[a], Nicola T. SHAW[b,1], Damon C. MAYES[c],
R. T. Noel GIBNEY[d]

[a]Department of Family Medicine, University of Alberta, Edmonton, AB, Canada
[b]Health Informatics Institute, Algoma University, Sault Ste. Marie, ON
[c]Alberta Health Services, Edmonton, AB, Canada
[d]Division of Critical Care Medicine, University of Alberta, Edmonton, AB, Canada

Abstract. Electronic documentation methods may assist critical care providers with information management tasks in Intensive Care Units (ICUs). We conducted a quasi-experimental observational study to investigate patterns of information tool use by ICU physicians, nurses, and respiratory therapists during verbal communication tasks. Critical care providers used tools less at 3 months after the CCIS introduction. At 12 months, care providers referred to paper and permanent records, especially during shift changes. The results suggest potential areas of improvement for clinical information systems in assisting critical care providers in ensuring informational continuity around their patients.

Keywords. clinical information system, intensive care, nursing, respiratory therapists, critical care

Introduction

Critical Care Providers (CCPs) manage massive quantities of information while providing care for highly complex patients in Intensive Care Units (ICUs) [1]. Coordinated care depends on CCPs understanding patient care plans [2]. CCPs verbally communicate while referring to different information tools to achieve this understanding [3]. Verbal communication is especially prevalent during "verbal report" when Registered Nurses (RNs) and Respiratory Therapists (RTs) change shifts [4,5].

Electronic charting tools such as a Critical Care clinical Information System (CCIS) may improve information management in ICUs [6] if the system is accepted by front-line care providers [7]. For a complex multi-user system such as a CCIS, the chances of acceptance are better if users who are required to do more work after a system implementation also perceive direct benefits of the system [8].

A CCIS was introduced to two ICUs at the University of Alberta and Stollery Children's Hospital in Edmonton, Alberta, Canada in March 2009. To investigate

---

[1] Corresponding Author.

whether CCP communication is impacted by the CCIS, we analyzed time-and-motion observational data to calculate the percentages of time ICU physicians, RNs, and RTs spent referring to different information tools while verbally communicating with colleagues before, 3, and 12 months after implementation. Similar values were derived for the first 20 minutes of RN and RT shifts (i.e., verbal report). We find role-specific changes in information tool use after a CCIS introduction that may be suggestive of areas for improvement in electronic documentation systems to fit CCP work.

1. Methods

1.1. Setting and participants

University of Alberta research ethics (File:B-241107) and site approvals (File:6035) were obtained prior to data collection. The study was conducted in the General Systems ICU (GSICU) at University Hospital, and Pediatric ICU (PICU) at the Stollery Children's Hospital. Both ICUs are busy academic referral centres. At the time of study, GSICU had 24 beds, and PICU had 17 beds. Posters and presentations informed staff members about the nature of the study, and CCPs were approached by observers. Physicians (40 of 41 individuals working as attending physicians, chief residents, or fellows at year 5 or higher after MD training), nurses (131 of 263 working in the ICUs), and 62 respiratory therapists of 84 provided informed consent during the study. Baseline data were collected between September 2008 and February 2009. The CCIS was introduced in March 2009. The CCIS is an electronic charting tool designed to capture data from various sources. Vital signs monitor data was connected at the outset. Ventilator data was connected in June 2009. Laboratory data was connected to the system in October 2009. Medication orders remain recorded on paper. During the H1N1 pandemic in November 2009, the GSICU briefly returned to paper charting due to the need to increase their capacity and the difficulty of training additional staff members to use the system. GSICU returned to computerized charting December 2009.

1.2. Observations

Trainee observers were each paired with experienced observers and scored activities of a participant simultaneously for calculations of interrater reliability. When percentage agreement was above 85%, trainees conducted solo observations. Observations lasted 90 minutes with no prior notice. Observations were suspended if the participant left the ICU or went on a break. For RTs and RNs, shift change observations started at 30 minutes before and ended 60 minutes after shifts started (07:00 or 19:00). Equal numbers of observations were conducted at shift change and at mid-shift. Observation numbers were balanced between day shifts and night shifts. Observations were balanced across different day types including weekends, mid-weeks, Mondays, and Fridays. Physician observations were similarly conducted, with the exception that morning and evening shift changes were replaced by observations conducted during morning rounds starting at 09:00, and afternoon sign-out rounds, starting at 16:00. We conducted 163 hours of physician observations, 159 hours of nurse observations, and 158 hours of respiratory therapist observations.

1.3. Data Collection Tools

Observers recorded tasks of CCPs using PDAs (HP iPaQ hx2490 or 110) running WOMBAT software [9]. Observers referred to work definitions to consistently score activities. Professional communication tasks were recorded if CCPs verbally communicated with colleagues regarding patient information. Information tools used were recorded. These included permanent records (paper records kept for archival purposes), paper (not part of the long term record), and the CCIS (the electronic chart application running on computer). Computer use aside from the CCIS was separately recorded, and is not reported here.

1.4. Statistics

Percentages of time spent on professional communication tasks using information tools were calculated in Microsoft Excel and compared using R[10]. Kruskal-Wallis tests were used to compare usage patterns across the 3 time points. Mann-Whitney U-Tests were used to determine whether usage of information tools during verbal report significantly differed from overall usage.

2. Results

The mean percentages of time RNs spent on professional communication tasks while referring to paper or permanent records during the baseline time point were 5% and 8%, respectively (Figure 1A). RNs referred to permanent records during significantly higher percentages of time during verbal report (p<0.05). At 3 months after the CCIS was introduced, the mean percentages of time RNs referred to paper and permanent records were 0.6% and 4%. RNs also referred to the CCIS during 0.7% of the time spent on professional communication. By 12 months the mean percentages of time RNs referred to paper, permanent records, and the CCIS were 6%, 10%, and 5%, respectively. The amount of time permanent records, and the CCIS were referred to significantly varied over time (p<0.01). At 12 months, RNs referred to permanent records significantly more during verbal report than during all observation times, and spent significantly less time not referring to information tools during verbal report (Figure 1A; solid symbols).

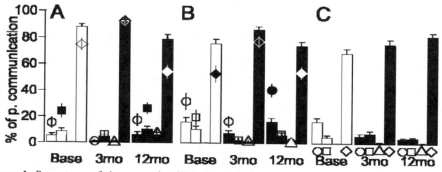

Figure 1. Percentages of time spent by CCPs on professional communication tasks while referring to information tools after a CCIS introduction. A=ICU RNs. Base (white bars)=baseline data, 3mo (black)=3 month data, 12mo=12 month data. B= RTs, C=Physicians. Circle=paper, Square=permanent paper records, Triangle=CCIS, Diamond=No tool. B= RTs, C=Physicians. Symbols overlaid on bars represent percentages in the first 20 minutes of Nurse and RT shifts. Solid symbols represent statistically significant differences in tool use when compared with overall percentages (bars). Means (+/- S.E.M.).

RTs were recorded spending mean percentages of 16%, and 10% of their professional communication time referring to paper, and permanent records, respectively at baseline (Figure 1B). During report, RTs referred to information tools significantly more often (solid symbols). At 3 months, RTs referred to paper and permanent records for 7% and 1%, and referred to the CCIS 0.6% of the time spent on professional communication tasks. There was no significant difference between the percentages of time information tools were referred to during verbal report and overall. By 12 months the percentages of time spent referring to paper and permanent records had returned to 16% and 6% respectively. RTs spent 2% of the time on communication tasks referring to the CCIS at 12 months. At 12 months, RTs spent significantly more time referring to paper during report than during all observation times ($p<0.05$), and significantly less time referring to the CCIS than overall ($p<0.05$).

Physicians spent increasing proportions of time performing professional communication tasks without referring to information tools at 3 and 12 months, when compared with baseline observations (Figure 1C). During the baseline time point, the mean percentages of time physicians spent referring to paper and permanent records were 16% and 4%. At 3 months the use of paper and permanent records decreased to 7% and 1%, and by 12 months these mean percentages were 16% and 6%. Physicians spent small percentages of time communicating while referring to the CCIS at the 3 and 12 month time points (0.6% and 0.3%). Comparable verbal report data was not available for physicians as they spent longer communicating when handing off patients to colleagues, and these times were not as clearly delineated from other kinds of work.

3. Discussion

We report the percentages of time RNs, RTs, and physicians were recorded referring to information tools while communicating with other CCPs before and after the introduction of a CCIS to two ICUs. CCPs did not spend as much time referring to the CCIS while communicating with colleagues as they did with paper and permanent records. RTs and RNs used paper and permanent records more during baseline observations suggesting these tools assist in planning care at the beginning of shifts. CCPs observed at 12 months did not appear to depend on the CCIS as much as permanent records and paper. The findings are vitally important for high quality care in ICUs as they suggest potential unmet needs for CCPs in coordinating care.

Several explanations for these results exist. RNs and RTs interviewed in the month after the CCIS introduction mentioned possible explanatory factors. CCPs could at times encounter difficulty rapidly finding needed information in the CCIS. After the CCIS introduction some information was kept in paper charts, but other information is stored in the CCIS, an information environment that has been referred to as "hybrid" [11]. In "hybrid" environments, single information sources would be less likely to contain all the information CCPs may need, and the use of paper may permit the easier aggregation of all information needed for complete reports. Finally, CCPs may find it difficult to collaborate around CCIS workstations when planning care. A qualitative study of physician communication patterns during ward rounds reported that the introduction of a computerized patient record introduced potential difficulties with effective communication that could be partially resolved by orienting the display such that it was more easily visible for round participants [12]. Our findings may generalize to other settings where electronic charting is introduced, but this will depend on many factors. Results from the WOMBAT method have not been published in ICU settings by other groups, and thus have only been partially validated.

After a CCIS introduction CCPs communicating referred to the CCIS less when compared with paper information sources. The acceptance of the CCIS could be enhanced if future changes to the system better support CCPs' information access needs, especially around times when continuity of information is challenged such as shift change.

Acknowledgements

We gratefully acknowledge the assistance of the staff and management of the University of Alberta GSICU, and Stollery Children's Hospital PICU, research observers Tineke Chattargoon, Sara Belton, Kelly Speer, Deb Jandura, Sally Ho, Aireen Wingert, Kelly Arbeau, and Ashwini Kulkarni. Funding was provided by Alberta Health Services and the Canadian Institutes of Health Research (CIHR PHE 91423). Michela Brown, Johanna Westbrook, and Krish Thiru contributed to early versions of the research work plan. Donna Manca served as nominated principle applicant following NTS' move to Algoma University.

References

[1] O.Manor-Shulman, J.Beyene, H.Frndova, C.S.Parshuram Quantifying the volume of documented clinical information in critical illness. *J Crit Care* **23** (2008), 245-50.
[2] G.Alvarez, E.Coiera Interdisciplinary communication: an uncharted source of medical error? *J Crit Care* **21** (2006), 236-42.
[3] T.W.Reader, R.Flin, K.Mearns, B.H.Cuthbertson Interdisciplinary communication in the intensive care unit. *Br J Anaesth* **98** (2007), 347-52.
[4] R.Sidlow, R.J.Katz-Sidlow Using a computerized sign-out system to improve physician-nurse communication. *Jt Comm J Qual Patient Saf* **32** (2006), 32-6.
[5] N.T.Shaw, M.Ballermann, R.Hagtvedt, S.Ho, D.C.Mayes, R.T.N.Gibney Intensive care unit nurse workflow during shift change prior to the introduction of a critical care clinical information system. *electronic Journal Health Informatics* (2010), Forthcoming.
[6] N.T.Shaw, R.L.Mador, S.Ho, D.Mayes, J.I.Westbrook, N.Creswick, K.Thiru, M.Brown Understanding the impact on intensive care staff workflow due to the introduction of a critical care information system: a mixed methods research methodology. *Stud Health Technol Inform* **143** (2009), 186-91.
[7] D.F.Sittig, M.Krall, J.Kaalaas-Sittig, J.S.Ash Emotional aspects of computer-based provider order entry: a qualitative study. *J Am Med Inform Assoc* **12** (2005), 561-7.
[8] J. Grudin, Why CSCW applications fail: problems in the design and evaluation of organizational interfaces. CSCW 88. *Proceedings of the 1988 ACM conference on Computer-supported cooperative work* , 85-93. 1988. New York, NY, ACM. 9-26-1988.
[9] J.I.Westbrook, A.Ampt Design, application and testing of the Work Observation Method by Activity Timing (WOMBAT) to measure clinicians' patterns of work and communication. *Int J Med Inform* **78** (2009), S25-S33.
[10] R Development Core Team. (2009). *R: A Language and Environment for Statistical Computing.*
[11] W.T.Hamilton, A.P.Round, D.Sharp, T.J.Peters The quality of record keeping in primary care: a comparison of computerised, paper and hybrid systems. *Br J Gen Pract* **53** (2003), 929-33.
[12] C.Morrison, M.Jones, A.Blackwell, A.Vuylsteke Electronic patient record use during ward rounds: a qualitative study of interaction between medical staff. *Crit Care* **12** (2008), R148.

E-Learning and Education

International Perspectives in Health Informatics
E.M. Borycki et al. (Eds.)
IOS Press, 2011
doi:10.3233/978-1-60750-709-3-45

Harmonizing the Competency Cacophony

H. Dominic COVVEY[a], Shirley L. FENTON[a],
Sandra SABARATNAM[b], Noemi CHANDA[b]
[a]*National Institutes of Health Informatics,*
[b]*University of Waterloo, Waterloo, Ontario, Canada*

Abstract. Many have addressed the challenge of defining Health Informatics (HI) competencies, and eleven efforts have produced detailed lists of competencies. Although there are commonalities among these lists, several aspects of this work frustrate our using it to define a consensus view of HI competencies. This project has involved the documentation and comparison of the competencies produced by key authors and an effort to suggest competency terminology that derives from and harmonizes these efforts, but does not emphasize any one contribution. It is our hope that this will enable us to use what has gone before with a minimum of reinvention.

Keywords. health informatics competencies, health informatics education

Introduction

Many efforts have addressed the issue of defining Health Informatics competencies, and eleven of these have produced detailed lists of competencies [1-11]. Each individual or group has elected to approach the challenge in its own way and to arrive at its own unique list of competencies. Although there are commonalities among these lists, several aspects of this work frustrate our using it to define a consensus view of HI competencies.

One of the things that stands in the way of our using previous work is the fact that each group has used different definitions of what a competency is. Some, e.g., Staggers, et al. and COACH, define a competency as the ability to do a task. We have called these 'Task-Level Competency Definitions', one example being: "Is able to participate in or lead strategic planning processes". Others (e.g., Covvey, et al.) define a competency as the skills, knowledge, experience, (and sometimes) attitudes and values (SKEAVs) that enable the person to do a task. We have called these latter competencies 'SKEAV-Level Competencies Definitions', one example being: "Has <u>knowledge</u> of the theories, concepts and nature of strategic planning", or "Has served on a team involved in strategic planning" (an experience element) while another might be "Has mastered one or more strategic planning methodologies" (a skill element). From this comparison it is clear that Task-Level Competencies are at a higher level of abstraction than SKEAV-Level Competencies, as, typically, several SKEAV-Level Competencies will be required to fully enable a person to perform a task.

Another challenge is that each competency definer has used unique descriptors for each competency – at either level – and sometimes these descriptors are ambiguous. No one has developed a detailed description of each competency to a level where it would be sufficient to guide curriculum or syllabus development; a great deal is left up to interpretation. Finally, each group's work has become identified with the group and its biases, real or imagined, leading to a 'not-invented-here' reaction by some and the ignoring of what could be a valuable contribution.

We undertook the Competency Harmonization Project (CHP) to propose a consensus definition of HI competencies that takes account of all the major efforts.

As a special note: although we used our own competency framework to organize all competency statements, we have not favored our own work in any way in our attempt to harmonize competencies.

1. Methodology

Our approach to this challenge has involved several interventions:
1. We limited our initial work to the competencies associated with Applied Health Informaticians[3] – those professionals who apply the concepts, methods and tools developed by Research and Development Health Informaticians[3] (e.g., teachers, researchers and systems development innovators). Applied Health Informaticians typically serve as CIOs, CMIOs, Clinical Informaticians, and other roles in areas that run from defining needs to implementing and managing systems and personnel. Later work will target the roles of the Research and Development Health Informaticians.
2. We searched the world literature on competency definitions and identified key detailed competency definition projects.
3. We used, the set of 27 **Challenges** (Table 1) faced by an Applied Health Informatician and the **Tasks** (micro-roles) that need to be performed in order to address these challenges, to organize other authors' competencies into consistent groups, each of which having like competency elements. These terms are only used for organization and are not included in the harmonization of terms. These concepts are documented in "Pointing the Way:…"[3, 12] Please note that the **Tasks** are too detailed for inclusion here. This organization also enables us to relate the work of others to our structured derivation of competencies.
4. We documented the competencies developed by various groups in a table called the Harmonization Matrix that aligns competencies from these efforts under our Challenges and Tasks framework. This table is about 100 pages in length and cannot be included here.
5. We have proposed competency descriptors that subsume all definers' terms, minimizing association with a particular source unless particularly appropriate descriptor was used.
6. We have identified and suggested corrections to gaps in each project's definitions, the entire set serving as a comparator for critiquing the products of each effort.
7. We are subjecting the Competency Matrix with the set of proposed descriptors, including gap-fillers to a consultation process for critique, comments and suggestions. The results of this work will ultimately be published in the form of a web-based system that makes all of the components accessible.

Health Informatics Challenges

The following are the challenges faced by the Applied Health Informaticians in the identified macro-roles:

1. *Collaboration*

2. *Understanding of the Nature of the Health System and Desired Outputs*

3. *Formulation of IT/IM Components of the Strategic Plan*

4. *IT/IM Strategic Business Planning, IT/IM Strategic Market Planning*

5. *IT/IM Needs Analysis*

6. *Determination of the Organization's IT/IM Situation (IT/IM Audit)*

7. *Definition and Implementation of Organizational Approach to IT/IM*

8. *Determination of the State of the Industry and Analysis of Vendors and Solutions*

9. *IT/IM Technology Assessment*

10. *Evaluation, Adoption, and Implementation of Standards*

11. *IT/IM-Related Policy Development*

12. *Development of the Justification For and the Value of Systems*

13. *Obtaining Consensus on Solutions, Budget, Plan*

14. *Procurement of Solutions (Products and Services)*

15. *Re-engineering of Work and Information Management Processes*

16. *Implementation of Solutions*

17. *Planning and Day-to-Day Management of IT/IM Resources*

18. *Management of Other's Data*

19. *Integration of Multiple Systems*

20. *Maintenance and Support of Solutions*

21. *Evaluation of Solution Outcomes*

22. *Management of Change (Acting as Change Agent)*

23. *User, Customer, Inter-Departmental and Public Liaison, Relations, Communications, and Publication*

24. *Continuing Education*

25. *System and Methods Customization and Ad Hoc Development*

26. *Utilization of Technology (Personal Productivity, Specific Tools)*

27. *General Day-to-Day Issues*

Table 1. Health Informatics Challenges

2. Observations

In reviewing each of the competency efforts and attempting to align them, we have come to a number of realizations, which have presented us with significant challenges.

Firstly, the formal definition of competency involves the determination of the entire set of skills, knowledge, experience, attitudes and values, or a subset of these (typically at least skills, knowledge and experience) a person must master to be deemed 'competent'. However, many of the efforts to define competencies in Health Informatics (note that we include biomedical, medical, nursing, etc. informatics under this term) have elected to define competency as the set of tasks one must be able to perform in order to be considered competent. This creates a challenge when one attempts to compare the competencies produced by various authors. It also provides a less-than-optimally-desirable outcome, as describing tasks does not provide the curriculum developer with useful guidance as to what a person must master – it only describes the outcome state to be achieved. This is certainly a more easily achieved goal in competency definition, but not as useful a goal, leaving much up to imagination and interpretation. In the case of Task-Level Competency definition, further work would need to be done, in addition to a careful definition of the task, to define the skills, knowledge, etc. that competently carrying out such a task would require.

Next, a variety of techniques can be used to identify competencies, including: reviewing existing programs to see what they teach, interviewing individuals in the field regarding what they believe the competencies should be, or deriving the competencies in a more structured way. Our own work used the latter approach. We have reason to be concerned regarding the other approaches, as we found that our competency definition was generally more complete than others, with the other efforts having many gaps compared to ours. Of course there are areas, albeit fewer, where other efforts defined competencies that we missed or with which we do not agree, at least as to emphasis. Nonetheless, we treated all efforts equally and based the set of harmonized competencies on the union of the competency sets of all efforts.

A final point is that each group defined its competencies at different levels of detail. For example, some defined one competency at a very granular level, while other competencies were only described at a high level and others not at all. It appeared that different groups had chosen certain areas on which they wished to focus or that they wanted to emphasize, while minimizing their focus on other areas.

3. Results

We have developed the Competency Harmonization Matrix that compares and aligns the competencies identified by the 11 key efforts. We have augmented this with the results of our literature search, listing most publications in this area up to the summer of 2009. We have suggested initial Harmonized Competency Terms that would best, in our minds, communicate the meaning various contributors wished to convey, but using terms that do not favor one or other effort. In addition to this, we have launched a refinement process that adds definitions to all terms and then opens these definitions to improvement.

These documents are very large and unable to be presented in a paper of this length, but will be demonstrated in our presentation and made available in their final form. However, we have included here, in Table 2, an example that shows data used to produce the Competency Harmonization Matrix.

Authors	Capabilities or Competencies
Staggers, et al.	*n/a*
COACH	*4.6 - Understands and applies knowledge of the roles and relationships of health providers and managers along with the organizational and regulatory structure in which they work*
	6.2 - Works collaboratively and contributes to project planning, implementation, monitoring and evaluation
AMIA	*5.11 Demonstrate Internet/Intranet communication skills*
	5.13 Demonstrate use of email, addressing, forwarding, attachments, netiquette
IMIA	*1.4 - Use of application software for documentation, personal communication including Internet access, for publication and basic statistics*
	3.3 - Ability to communicate electronically, including electronic data exchange, with other health care professionals
Schleyer	*n/a*
Garde, Harrison & Hovenga	*Social Competency (Collaboration, Communication etc.)*
Storey, et al.	*Communications Technologies*
	Electronic Data Interchange: Links to Other Organisations, Voice Communications Systems
	Strategic Planning: Working with Partners
Covvey	*1.1.3. Human Networking Skills*
	2.2.5. Virtual Conferencing and Collaboration
	8.1.6. Facilitation Skills
	8.1.4. Consensus Mapping Technique
Hersh	*(11) Organization and management issues in informatics:*
	(11.1) Organization behavior
	(11.2) Organizational issues in failure and success of informatics projects
	(11.3) Change management
	(11.4) Project management
	(11.5) Business issues in informatics
Huang	*Team and interpersonal skills*
Health informatics National Occupational Standards	*A3 Develop your personal networks*
	F402 Develop, sustain and evaluate collaborative work with others
	F403 Develop and sustain effective working relationships with staff in other departments/organisations
	F403 Develop and sustain effective working relationships with staff in other departments/organisations

Table 2. Competencies Related to a Challenge

We are now preparing a number of documents that will allow open review of the harmonized terms and suggestions for improvement. This review will take two forms, a workshop to get expert critique of the products of the work to-date, a Delphi process to get the broadest possible input on the document that results from the workshop, and publication via the web using a Wiki approach that allows continuing critique and improvement.

In line with our orientation to avoid leaving a perception of ownership of this work in our hands, we intend to seek a national body, e.g., AMIA, through the AMIA Education Committee or another like body, to adopt it with the objective of carrying it through an appropriate review process and then forward through time.

4. Lessons Learned and Next Steps

It is clear from this work that we have a great deal to gain from the integration and harmonization of competency definition efforts. Much excellent work has been done by highly capable groups. However, this work is locked up to some degree in being associated with these groups, leading to repeated re-invention. The work reported here attempts a systematic review of what has gone before, but then takes this a step further by 'de-identifying' that work and producing generic statements of competency from it.

Once this has been accomplished, there is the need to correlate the Task-Level Competency Definitions with the more detailed and useful SKEAV-Level Competency Definitions to get the greatest value from the work already done in this area.

We believe that we have to move away from definitions identified with a particular person or group, so that the content becomes depersonalized and potentially more influential. Finally, we have to learn from each other recognizing gaps in our thinking, and homing in on a comprehensive definition of HI competencies.

5. Recommendations and Conclusion

We believe that this work will ultimately provide a consensus definition of HI competencies that all our Health Informatics organizations should adopt and, as required, adapt to their own purposes.

Acknowledgements

The idea of pursuing this effort came from discussions with the AMIA Education Committee during the time that the first author was a member. Thanks go particularly to John Holmes and Paul Gorman for their comments at the time. This work was supported by a research grant provided by the University of Waterloo.

References

[1]   American Medical Informatics Association (AMIA) and American Health Information Management Association (AHIMA). *Joint Work Force Task Force: Health Information Management and Informatics Core Competencies for Individuals Working With Electronic Health Records*, October 2008.
[2]   Canada's Health Informatics Association (COACH). *Health Informatics Professional Core Competencies version 2.0.* Toronto March 2009. See: http://coachorg.com/career_development/ professionalism/core_competencies.htm.

[3]   H.D. Covvey, D. Zitner, R. Bernstein, Pointing the Way: Competencies and Curricula in Health Informatics. University of Waterloo 2001. See: http://hi.uwaterloo.ca/hi/Resources.htm.

[4]   S. Garde, D. Harrison, E.J. Hovenga, Skill Needs for Nurses in their Role as Health Informatics Professionals: A Survey in the context of Global Health Informatics Education. *Int J Med Inf* **74 (11)** (2005), 899-907.

[5]   W. Hersh, AMIA-OHSU 10x10 Program: Course Description. Oregon Health & Science University. 2009. See: https://www.amia.org/10x10/partners/ohsu/description.asp.

[6]   HISA. Health Informatics Education, A Joint Project by the Health Informatics Society of Australia and the Commonwealth Department of Health and Aging. Commonwealth of Australia 2002. See: http://www.health.gov.au/internet/hconnect/publishing.nsf/content/7746b10691fa666cca257128007b7e af/$file/hiefrept.pdf.

[7]   Q. Huang, Competencies for graduate curricula in health, medical and biomedical informatics: a framework. *Health Informatics Journal* **13 (2)**, (2007),89-103. [See: 'An overview of some curricula in graduate health, medical and biomedical informatics programs around the world' document at http://www.fhs.usyd.edu.au/health_informatics/Docs/HMInformatics_curricula.pdf.]

[8]   IMIA. Recommendations of the International Medical Informatics Association (IMIA) on Education in Health and Medical Informatics. *Meth Inf Med* **39 (3)**, (2000), 267-277. See: http://www.imia.org/pubdocs/rec_english.pdf.

[9]   NHS. NSH Quality Scheme for Health Informatics Learning and Development: Evidence Matrix for HI NOS (Health Informatics National Occupational Standards 2008. See: http://www.connectingforhealth.nhs.uk/systemsandservices/capability/phi/hottopics/hiqs/guidance.zip.

[10] T.K. Schleyer, Competencies for Dental Informatics V 1.0. University of Pittsburgh Center for Dental Informatics 1999. See: http://www.dental.pitt.edu/informatics/competencies.php.

[11] N. Staggers, C. Gassert, C. Curran, Delphi Study to Determine Informatics Competencies for Nurses at Four Levels of Practice. *Nurs Res* **51 (6)**, (2002),383-90.

[12] H.D. Covvey, S. Fenton, D. Mulholland, K. Young, Making Health Informatics Competencies Useful: An Applied Health Informatics Competency Self-Assessment System, *Stud Health Tech Inform.* **129(Pt 2)** (2007),1357-61

International Perspectives in Health Informatics
E.M. Borycki et al. (Eds.)
IOS Press, 2011
© 2011 ITCH 2011 Steering Committee and IOS Press. All rights reserved.
doi:10.3233/978-1-60750-709-3-52

The National Student Forum and the Emergence of Health Informatics Clubs

Shirley L. FENTON[a], H. Dominic COVVEY [a]

[a] *National Institutes of Health Informatics, Waterloo, Ontario, Canada*

Abstract. Our greatest hope for the future of eHealth and the enabling of our health system is today's students. However, we face a challenge: few students are aware of careers in Health Informatics and other aspects of eHealth. This paper describes an initiative to engage our future workforce in HI. The National Student Forum for Health Informatics was established, in collaboration between the National Institutes of Health Informatics and COACH, to provide much needed opportunities for students to become involved in HI educational programs, research and student-student interaction. A key activity of NSF is the instantiation of Health Informatics Clubs at Canadian colleges and universities. We describe the rationale for NSF, its goals and objectives, its leadership and organization, and the development of the first HI Club at the University of Waterloo. Initiatives such as NSF are essential if we are to resolve the human resources crisis in HI.

Keywords. health informatics education, student participation, social networking, health informatics workforce.

Introduction

Students represent the future and the actualization of the promised value of Health Informatics (HI) and eHealth for our health system. Students will be tomorrow's leaders and practioners and the first generation with the potential to deliver on the promises of the past. Both the National Institutes of Health Informatics (NIHI) and COACH saw the creation of the National Student Forum for Health Informatics (NSF) as an important means of enhancing opportunities for students to pursue their education in HI, participate in HI research and better understand the array of options they have in pursuing a career in the eHealth domain.

NSF was established in the summer of 2009. It is managed by students for students. Julie Kim, a Ph.D. student at the University of Toronto and practicing HI professional, served as the inaugural leader of NSF with the assistance of other students and with the facilitation of NIHI and COACH. The role of the leader is to develop NSF capabilities and resources, to engage students in NSF activities, to identify student needs and to work with NIHI and COACH to address these needs.

NSF is a vehicle for connecting students who are involved in the increasing number of HI educational programs across Canada. The primary objective of NSF is to enhance students' educational experience and provide opportunities for them to be involved in research and dialogue about new and emerging issues. Through active student involvement, NSF is a vehicle to foster discussion, collaboration and learning among students, regardless of their academic discipline, level of study or location.

Some of the initial activities of NSF have been the creation of a Student Registry (a part of NIHI's National Community of Scholars system), the development of a Student Track in the biannual Advances in Health Informatics Conference (AHIC), the introduction of students to resources including a repository of recorded presentations on HI topics created by NIHI, the co-ordination of regular interactive discussion sessions among students, and the facilitation of the creation of student clubs at colleges and universities. Initiatives like these leverage existing resources in the community and to minimize the cost to students in participating.

1. Goals and Objectives

Pursuant to our recognition of the importance of students to the future of HI, we have committed ourselves to the goals of assisting the recruitment of students into the HI field, and fostering and facilitating their education and participation in research, as they take part in the academic programs that have emerged or are emerging throughout Canada. We have developed the NSF as the primary means of delivering opportunities for students.

2. Objectives and Importance

The objectives of the NIHI National Student Forum are:
1. To motivate the involvement of students in HI education and research.
2. To provide a national locus for networking, discussion, collaboration and academic exchange for HI students regardless of their primary academic affiliation, level of study or geography.
3. To facilitate productive exchange among HI students through co-ordination and the provision of an enabling infrastructure and resources.
4. To work with HI students to identify their needs and priorities related to education and research, and then to work with students, academics and programs to satisfy these needs.
5. To identify and provide opportunities for students to participate in educational programs, research projects, meetings, workshops, and conferences and symposia.
6. To help expose students to the expertise and experience of individuals with long histories in HI and to assist in arranging relationships with potential mentors.

3. Leadership

The NIHI National Student Forum is chaired by one or more students and co-chaired by a member of the Board or a Founding Member of NIHI – the latter to ensure NIHI's co-ordination and continuing support.

The student chair(s) serve for 2 years and will be elected by a majority vote of participating student members, after the inaugural chair's term.

4. Participation Opportunities

Student members in the NIHI National Student Forum will have a number of initial opportunities for participation, a set that will be expanded on by its membership.

1. Regular, facilitated and supported virtual meetings of the entire NSF membership or of sub-groups thereof, the latter determined by the NSF members. An example of a sub-group might be students interested in improving their co-op placement experiences.
2. Regular opportunities to present student research project plans, designs and results. This is planned to be realized as a monthly, virtual student research seminar.
3. A regular opportunity to develop and participate in a student track in our biennial Advances in Health Informatics Conference – AHIC (first occurrence in 2010) or in other conferences (e.g., Information Technology and Communications in Health – ITCH 2011) co-ordinated with it.
4. A student HI blog or Wiki dedicated to topics of interest to students.
5. A mentorship program that will pair students with senior HI professionals in both academia and industry.
6. A website providing access to co-op placement and employment opportunities, where hiring organizations and students can identify themselves to each other.
7. A website that allows students to register their research interests and expertise (existing or desired), research projects, etc. to facilitate interactions among them and with faculty members and others.

5. NIHI National Student Forum Membership

Students wishing to join NSF submit the following information via the NIHI website: (1) contact information, (2) a statement of interests (with associated keywords), (3) a statement of expertise (with associated keywords), (4) a 1-page resume, (5) a list of publications and funded research projects (if any). No fee is associated with membership. No student satisfying the above requirements will be refused membership. Students may have any primary discipline, but must be or have been registered within the last 2 years in a recognized academic program at any level.

6. Organizational Framework

NIHI is a non-directive organization that follows the principles of management based on complexity theory and the concepts of emerging behaviors (sometimes called "chaordic" management). It is dedicated to catalyzing, fostering and facilitating initiatives in the areas of HI research and education. It is a "bottom-up" organization built on the absolute belief in the potential of individuals to self-organize and accomplish great things if given the opportunity. NIHI works with all its members to achieve the common purpose of realizing the full potential of our health system though the development and application of the concepts, methods and tools of Health Informatics. The National Student Forum is an instantiation of these ideas placed in the able hands of students.

7. The Creation of HI Clubs by NSF

One of the initial activities of the NSF has been the facilitation of the creation of HI Clubs, the first of which was established at the University of Waterloo. Table 1 lists a description of the materials we have provided that are required to create an HI Club. In addition, a template for a club's constitution is available from the NIHI website. This constitution was based on an example constitution provided by the University of Waterloo's Federation of Students [1].

Table 1. Materials Required to Create a Health Informatics Club

Materials to Create A Health Informatics Club	
Note: This will vary from school to school. Enquire at your school for details on forming a club.	
Item	Comments
Cover Letter	This will state your club's desire to be considered for membership by the Federation of Students Internal Admissions Committee or other appropriate body at your college or university.
Candidate Members' List	This is a typed list of names, student numbers (where applicable) or alternate status (alumni/ae, grad students, associate members, etc.). There will usually be a requirement of having some minimum number of members.
Executive Officers' Contact List	This typed list must contain: names, student numbers, telephone numbers, and email addresses of proposed executives (those organizing the club). Many schools require a majority of the executive team to be undergrad students from the base college/university.
Governing Structure	This will specify the governing structure and the responsibilities of each executive officer. This is also incorporated into the club's constitution.
Constitution	An example of a constitution is attached to this checklist.
Acknowledgement Form	This will vary from school to school, but is usually available as a form. The intention of this form is to indicate that all executive officials have read and understand the policies and procedures of the school's federation of clubs organization. It usually must be signed by the club's President and at least one other executive member.
Member Fees	There must be an account of the fees that members will be charged and on what renewal basis (e.g., term, year, one-time).
Refund Policy	This describes the club's refund policy for membership fees.

8. Results

Although the NSF is still in its early phases, an HI Club was established by staff and University of Waterloo students in September 2009. This concept has proved to ignite student interest and the UW Health Informatics Club (UWHIC) already has over 280 members. We are in the process of promoting this concept across Canada and developing other components of NSF. Given the interest of students at the initial site, and the number of students across Canada that have registered in NSF (over 100 as of June 2010), we harbor significant hope that the NSF will flourish.

9. Discussion

Research has documented the value of student clubs [2-5]. Clubs are seen as mechanisms to increase student engagement, to build a sense of community, to foster student-student and student-program interactions and to improve their performance in a variety of programs. Disciplines, such as Computer Science and Electrical Engineering, have well established networks of student clubs and student chapters. For example, a recent web search found that the IEEE has student chapters in over 1800 institutions around the world with over fifty in Canada alone. A similar search produced very little evidence of the existence of Health Informatics or Biomedical Informatics clubs.

In the area of healthcare, a network of university rural health clubs consisting of medical, nursing and allied health students members is thriving in Australia [6]. Established in the early 1990s, it now has over 9,000 student members who belong to twenty-nine clubs. The clubs are part of a national strategy to address the rural health workforce shortage. The National Rural Health Network (NRHN) and its constituent clubs aim to increase the rural health workforce and health outcomes for rural and remote Australians and receive government funding.

With the establishment of NSF and UWHIC, Canada is in the forefront in the creation of HI clubs. Learning from the success of the NRHN, fostering a strong network of HI clubs across Canada is an important part of a national strategy to build our HI workforce.

10. Conclusions

NSF is engaging students across Canada and the concept of HI clubs already has had a significant outcome. Based on our experience with NSF and the interest in its activities, we believe that it is an idea whose time has come. NSF provides a self-directed opportunity that complements what happens in the class room and does so in a social environment that encourages the development of the human skills so important in collaboration, a key aspect of HI. If we are to succeed in increasing the numbers of entrants into education in eHealth-related disciplines, we must reach out to and engage students in ways that work.

Acknowledgements

The authors would like to thank COACH and its representatives Alison Gardner, Neil Gardner, Julie Kim and Derek Ritz for collaborating in this effort. We would also like to acknowledge Julie Kim, who so ably has taken on the leadership of NSF as its inaugural Chair, and also University of Waterloo students, Sandra Sabaratnam and Emilia Bakaic, who enthusiastically undertook to form the first HI Club in Canada at the University of Waterloo and became its first co-presidents.

References

[1] University of Waterloo Federation of Students, Student Club Constitution Example, available from: http://clubsandsocieties.feds.ca/system/files/Constitution+Example.pdf, cited October 18, 2010.

[2] J.D. Foubert, L.U. Grainger, Effects of involvement in clubs and organizations on the psychosocial development of first-year and senior college Students, *NASPA Journal* **43:1** (2006), available from: http://okstate.academia.edu/documents/0011/1822/foubert_graingerpub.pdf, cited October 18, 2010.

[3] J. L. Gersting, F.H. Young, Service Learning via the Computer Science Club, *SIGCSE Bulletin* **30:4,** December 1998.

[4] C.E. Sanders, M.E. Basham, P.I. Ansburg, Building a sense of community in undergraduate psychology departments, *Observer* **19:5** (2006), 291-300.

[5] N. Zepke, L. Leach, Integration and adaptation: Approaches to the student retention and achievement puzzle, *Active Learning in Higher Education* **6:1** (2005), available from: http://alh.sagepub.com/content/6/1/46, cited October 18, 2010.

[6] J.V. Turner, L.M. Scott, University rural health clubs: nurturing the future Australian rural workforce. *Rural and Remote Health* **7:649,** 2007.

58

International Perspectives in Health Informatics
E.M. Borycki et al. (Eds.)
IOS Press, 2011
© 2011 ITCH 2011 Steering Committee and IOS Press. All rights reserved.
doi:10.3233/978-1-60750-709-3-58

Clinical Informatics in Undergraduate Teaching of Health Informatics

Stefan V. PANTAZI [a,1], Felicia PANTAZI [b], Karen DALY [a]

[a] *Conestoga College, Kitchener, Ontario, Canada*
[b] *University of Victoria, Victoria, British Columbia, Canada*

Abstract. We are reporting on a recent experience with Health Informatics (HI) teaching at undergraduate degree level to an audience of HI and Pharmacy students. The important insight is that effective teaching of clinical informatics must involve highly interactive, applied components in addition to the traditional theoretical material. This is in agreement with general literature underlining the importance of simulations and role playing in teaching and is well supported by our student evaluation results. However, the viability and sustainability of such approaches to teaching hinges on significant course preparation efforts. These efforts consist of time-consuming investigations of informatics technologies, applications and systems followed by the implementation of workable solutions to a wide range of technical problems. In effect, this approach to course development is an involved process that relies on a special form of applied research whose technical complexity could explain the dearth of published reports on similar approaches in HI education. Despite its difficulties, we argue that this approach can be used to set a baseline for clinical informatics training at undergraduate level and that its implications for HI education in Canada are of importance.

Keywords. undergraduate HI education, simulation, clinical informatics

Introduction

Our vision of the field [1] places clinical informatics at the core of HI education. The insight that effective teaching of clinical informatics at undergraduate level should involve highly interactive applied components (e.g., hands-on training on actual systems) in addition to theoretical concepts (e.g., lecturing) has theoretical foundations grounded in theoretical HI research [2] as well as in general learning theory.

A recent literature review [3] indicates that interactive, visualization and simulation environments enable experiential learning and engage students and underlines that "simulations and case-based scenarios build upon well-defined educational theories, such as constructivism, experiential learning, adult learning theory, social presence, and situated learning". In [2] the notion of knowledge spectrum was defined as the span between a complex reality represented by experimental data and information gathered from observations and physical measurements to the high-level abstractions

---

[1] Corresponding Author: Professor, Health Informatics, School of Health & Life Sciences and Community Services, Conestoga College Institute of Technology and Advanced Learning, 299 Doon Valley Drive, Kitchener, ON, Canada, N2G 4M4; email: spantazi@conestogac.on.ca; web: http://hi.conestogac.on.ca/spantazi/

(e.g., theories, hypotheses, beliefs, concepts, formulae). The knowledge spectrum concept can help characterize our observation of what appears to be an effective way to teach informatics. According to this view, no one part of the spectrum, by itself alone, can lead to effective teaching. What appears to matter is the frequent conceptual movement across the spectrum and the ability to enable this movement during the limited lifetime of a course[2]. This conceptual movement can be linked to the frequent switching between theoretical and applied concepts. The idea resembles a very early model known as "Dale's Cone of Experience" [4] which also supports the idea that no single teaching methodology is appropriate and advocates the use of various types of media in teaching[3]. In order to confirm and act on this observation, a project consisting in the evaluation, installation and maintenance of a hospital information system (HIS) was initiated in summer 2009 in order to serve as a clinical simulation medium for undergraduate HI courses delivered in the 2009 Fall term.

1. Methods

Our experience with Health Informatics (HI) teaching at undergraduate level involved a heterogeneous audience of undergraduate students in Health Informatics (Conestoga College, "Health Informatics II" course) and Pharmacy (University of Waterloo, "Foundation of Application of Health Informatics" course). Both courses have benefited from a course delivery methodology involving distinct theoretical and applied components (i.e., 2 hours/week traditional frontal lecturing and discussions plus 2 hours/week labs and tutorials). This setup enabled well the frequent switching between theoretical and applied but has also made it necessary to use and manage the installation and troubleshooting of computer and software applications. A Hospital Information System (HIS) solution was deemed necessary in order to enhance this experiential learning component. After evaluating a multitude of existing options the research has focused on existing open source solutions such as Veteran's Affairs (VA) VistA Hospital Information System (HIS). This has led to the installation of a local, College-wide HIS that was completely under the control of the course instructor.

While experimenting with the original US FOIA (Freedom of Information Act) distribution of VA VistA HIS, we have encountered a significant number of installation and configuration issues, despite the availability of a very rich documentation resource [5]. The installation and maintenance of a complex HIS cannot be completely separated from context of its application and, in our situation, has become a form of applied research. Choices have been made to install the Medsphere OpenVistA GT.M integration package and to provide VistA terminal access on and off campus, from any platform, including Mac and PC laptops. The technical complexities and specific aim of the approach may explain the complete lack of literature describing similar educational setups. As a consequence, the complete set of instructions (text, screen recordings + audio voice over) for the Medsphere OpenVistA HIS installation procedure have been made available to HI degree students during the labs. Two examples of well-defined problems for which solutions had to be found were the set up

---

[2] This observation forms the basis of Dr. F. Pantazi's Master's thesis research in the School of Health Information Science at Univ. of Victoria
[3] See last paragraph on page 133

of virtual printing and enabling health care professional role playing for clinical workflow simulation.

1.1. Virtual Printing

Printing is an important function of any HIS (e.g. printing of patient wristbands, reports, etc.). In addition, in a teaching and simulation environment, the deliverables of practical work done by students and which form the basis of course work evaluation, are often obtained through printing (e.g., printing an activity log). However, the distributed and virtualized nature of our VistA installation prevents the efficient and economical use of a set of physical printers where over a hundred students can print and retrieve their printing output at the same time. The viable option was to install and define a virtual (software-based) printer (e.g., PDF printer) queue with sequentially named files, automatically accessible through a web server, at a central location. This approach has made it possible to evaluate efficiently the hands-on applied work results of individual students through individualized reports (Figure 1) and activity logs printouts that demonstrate the completion of assigned tasks.

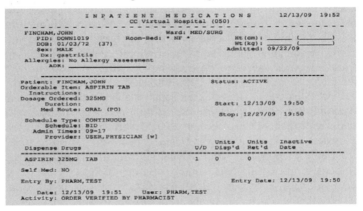

Figure 1. Example of printed (PDF) medication profile

1.2. Healthcare Professional Role Playing

The applied component of the two HI courses also involved lab work which had to be completed, concurrently, by over a hundred individual students. Therefore it was necessary that every student is provided with a fully functional individual account which allowed them to simulate various clinical workflows, including playing the role of a pretend VA pharmacist with the ability to write, review and approve inpatient medication orders. The medication orders had to be written for simulated patients that were registered, admitted and managed by students as well, using a set of predefined but non-individual roles (e.g., Admission-Discharge-Transfer (ADT) clerk, physician, nurse). The typical, simplified workflow involved a sequence of views in VA VistA HIS. The workflow starts with the ADT clerk menu, continued with the clinical chart view (physician and nurse interface) was followed by the Unit Dose pharmacist menu and the inpatient medication and activity log report (pharmacist views) and ended with the barcoded medication administration (BCMA) application (nurse view). The workflow steps and instructions have been documented by the instructor in form of tutorials using screen recording technology combined with a voice-over that explained the tasks and provided the necessary context for the lab work. Students work was done in pairs or in groups of up to five members.

1.3. Practical Examinations

A practical component was introduced for the first time, in both informatics courses, during the final exam. The practical exam aimed at testing individual student ability to complete a clinical workflow.

For the Pharmacy students, the examination had a clinical and administrative focus and consisted of add, accepting and verifying new inpatient medication ordered for an existing patient of their choice using their individual VA pharmacist account. Task completion was demonstrated by medication profiles and activity logs to be printed and submitted using an electronic drop-box. In addition, students have been asked to complete a novel task which they were never trained on. The task was related to inpatient pharmacy management consisting in printing and interpreting administrative reports (e.g., Unit Dose AMIS - cost per ward).

Conestoga College course examination had both a clinical and IT focus. Students have been asked to complete clinical workflows which included new patient registration and admission, inpatient management, medication orders and pharmacy order verification. In addition, informatics degree students have been tested in their ability to function as a system manager that creates user accounts for newly hired ADT managers and VA pharmacists. Finally, informatics degree students have been offered the opportunity to demonstrate their proficiency with installing the Medsphere OpenVistA GT.M-based distribution of the VistA HIS, from scratch on a clean virtual machine.

2. Results

A large majority of Conestoga HI students, working in pairs, have been successful in replicating, multiple times, the installation and system management (e.g., user account registration, modification, deletion) procedures of Open VistA HIS during labs. With very few exceptions, most HI degree and pharmacy students have been able to follow lab and tutorial instructions and have succeeded to complete the role playing tutorials. Anonymous student feedback was sought on a weekly basis from students. An important anonymous pharmacy student comment and which may have reflected the opinion of more than one individual, was about difficulties with VistA textual interface. It challenged the importance of learning the VA VistA system, especially since it is not being used in any Canadian hospital. This prompted the immediate introduction of a group assignment to explore relevant literature and which was aimed at answering questions such as: "Why do you think VA VistA is considered one of the most successful systems of its kind? What is the VA VistA system modeling? What is it supposed to represent?" Many student answers were surprisingly convergent on the idea that VA VistA HIS aims at modeling the flow of work within VA facilities.

In both, the HI degree and pharmacy informatics courses, the results for the practical components of the final exam involving role playing and completion of clinical workflow tasks have been positive. Nearly all students have been able to complete the required tasks. In addition, during the final exam, six out of twenty-four Conestoga degree students have demonstrated their ability to install completely from scratch and unaided, the GT.M-based OpenVistA HIS.

3. Discussion

While many factors may explain the good student performance, an important result of this experience is that it establishes a base line for clinical informatics training at undergraduate level. The experience also supports the idea that a HIS installation can function as an effective simulation environment for clinical tasks and workflows that can be used to enhance student learning and experimentation with existing clinical information systems. Finally – and this is the major focus of this discussion – this positive experience gives us hopes and confidence in the possibilities to address an important area in HI education that is currently lacking: clinical informatics. The attempt to explain the current situation in this area hinges on the perception of an apparent duality of existing informatics approaches and systems that tend to be either clinical or administrative in nature but never both. The importance of this dual perspective on informatics becomes clear in light of a simple observation: most often than not, data collected by clinical applications has high administrative value. Clinical data can be often abstracted and analyzed for policy-making and administrative decision making purposes (e.g., case costing, case-mix analysis, public health studies). On the other hand, data collected solely for administrative purposes (e.g., administrative reporting, policy making) is often of very little use for clinical decisions concerning individual patients as it usually does not capture the necessary clinical context. However, existing definitions of the capabilities of HI professionals in Canada consistently favor the management and administrative aspects of Health Informatics [6]. This may also be partially due to the perception of the challenge to train clinical-informatics professionals who, ideally, would need to cover as well as possible three major roles [1]:

- *clinician* with the ability to understand and operate with complex clinical concepts,
- *software engineer* with the ability to design, implement prototypes, test and maintain domain-specific (e.g., clinical informatics) applications, and
- *behavioral scientist* with the ability to analyze medical decision making, human factors, social and organizational issues related to clinical system implementation.

The grand challenge of creating this kind of HI professional is educating technically strong professionals who possess enough clinical domain knowledge allowing them to design, implement, evaluate, maintain and evolve clinical information systems. Currently, training existing clinicians as software engineers for a short period of time (e.g., 1-2 years) is a difficult proposition. Alternatively, training existing software engineers to function well in clinical environments may also be difficult due to the high complexity of the application domain. The only alternative appears to be a 4-year long, comprehensive undergraduate degree that includes coursework related to clinical medicine and clinical informatics complemented by a significant clinical internship component. This approach would yield graduates with a unique combination of technical expertise and medical domain knowledge. From a computer science perspective [7], this approach aims at a true domain-specific (e.g., clinical domain) application developer with the ability to function efficiently at the interface between professional programmers (e.g., system programmers, professional application programmers) and the end users with limited technical background (e.g., clinicians). In terms of existing undergraduate HI education, aiming to create such graduates would address the administrative-clinical duality by correcting for the lack of clinical concepts and clinical informatics in existing HI curricula.

4. Limitations and Future Work

VA VistA HIS has over 9,000 different menu functions in its menu driven interface. Currently, our workflow simulations involve less than 100 distinct functions. We envision increasing the number of professional roles to include lab technicians, nurses and other allied health professions in order to create more complex and plausible hospital workflow simulations. We intend to enable the simulation of additional pharmacy processes (e.g., packaging, dispensing, administration) and simulated the functionality of the 24-hour medication cart exchange. Other future plans are related to the creation of a multitude of clinically plausible simulations of variable difficulty. This could challenge students and allow them insights into clinical workflows and medical thinking that can reveal common sources of medical error. Current limitations are related to the technical difficulties of simulating lab sample collection workflows followed by simulated real-time lab test analyses and HL7 messaging with lab information systems. Once these limitations are overcome, we envision the extension of simulation to enhance the case-based teaching in nursing programs and local medical schools. This experience also gives us hope for advancing towards the vision of a healthcare professional role playing game, involving a virtual hospital simulation environment capable of recording, playback and annotation of clinically plausible simulation runs that are integrated with real or simulated physical devices (e.g., vital signs measurement devices, medication dispensing robots, tele-presence, simulated lab test equipment). It is our belief that setting up and managing high fidelity simulations of clinical environments is a necessary effort to educate highly sought-after HI professionals that can relate well to clinical environments.

References

[1] S.V. Pantazi, Pantazi F., Moehr J.R., *Health Informatics (HI): An introduction and overview, in Fundamentals of Health Information Management. Canadian Healthcare Association*, Ottawa, 1995. p. 457.
[2] S.V. Pantazi, J.F. Arocha, J.R. Moehr, Case-based Medical Informatics. *BMC J Med Inf Decision Making* **4(1)** (2004).
[3] M.M. Hansen, Versatile, Immersive, Creative and Dynamic Virtual 3-D Healthcare Learning Environments: A Review of the Literature, *JMIR* **10(3)** (2008); p. e26.
[4] E. Dale, *Audio-visual methods in teaching,* Third ed, The Dryden Press, New York, 1969.
[5] US Veteran's Affairs VISTA, [cited March 14, 2010], Available from: http://www4.va.gov/vdl.
[6] The Health Informatics Professional Role Profiles, [cited March 14, 2010]; Available from: http://www.coachorg.com/career_development/professionalism/role_profiles.htm.
[7] N. Dale, J. Lewis, *Computer Science Illuminated.* Jones & Bartlett, USA, 3rd ed, 2007.

International Perspectives in Health Informatics
E.M. Borycki et al. (Eds.)
IOS Press, 2011
© *2011 ITCH 2011 Steering Committee and IOS Press. All rights reserved.*
doi:10.3233/978-1-60750-709-3-64

Critical Success Factors for Implementing Healthcare e-Learning

Te-Shu LEE[a] , Mu-Hsing KUO[a], Elizabeth M. BORYCKI[a] , David YUNYONG [a]

[a] *School of Health Information Science, The University of Victoria,*
Victoria, British Columbia, Canada

Abstract. The use of e-Learning in educational institutes has rapidly increased along with the development of information and communication technology (ICT). In healthcare, more medical educators are using e-Learning to support their curriculum design, delivery and evaluation. However, no systematic work exists on characterizing a collective set of Critical Success Factors (CSFs) for implementing e-Learning in the healthcare education institutions. The aim of this paper is to study the CSFs of implementing healthcare e-Learning

Keywords. critical success factors, e-learning, healthcare education

Introduction

The purpose of e-Learning, like any other learning approach, is to achieve learning objectives. Many organizations have successfully introduced it to improve education. For example, a 12-year meta-analysis of research by the U.S. Department of Education found that higher education students using e-Learning generally performed better than those in face-to-face courses [1]. The MIT OpenCourseWare is designed to put all of the educational materials from its undergraduate- and graduate-level courses online, partly free and available to anyone, anywhere. This program allows students to attend 'classes' across physical, political, and economic boundaries at minimum costs [2]. The Medical College of Wisconsin, uses the course-management platform called ANGEL to teach cardiopulmonary and physical-exam psychomotor skills, physical-exam findings and relationship to pathophysiology. Its tutorial features hyperlinks to physical-exam skills, videos and clinical-skills websites. Subsequently, case-based lessons with video interviews, audio of normal and abnormal cardiac and pulmonary auscultatory sounds, pictures of abnormal physical exam findings and X-rays for individual cases is introduced. This e-Learning module has improved the knowledge and skills of medical students in cardiopulmonary testing, and assesses their ability to accurately identify cardiac and pulmonary auscultatory sounds by using interactive e-modules in the setting of limited teacher and patient resources [3].

Other successful examples show that e-Learning deploys knowledge quickly and efficiently to a large number of dispersed learners. However, no systematic work exists on characterizing a collective set of CSFs for implementing e-Learning in the education institutions. An appropriate set of CSFs will help them to keep in mind the important issues that should be dealt with when designing and implementing an e-Learning initiative. Therefore, the aim of this paper is to study the CSFs that are part of implementing healthcare e-Learning so that health organizations can adopt them in their systems.

1. Prior Studies on e-Learning Critical Success Factors

Critical Success Factors can be defined as key areas of performance that are essential for the organization to accomplish its mission. A broad range of factors that can influence the success of e-Learning have been mentioned in the literature. For example, Papp [4] explored distance learning from a macro perspective and suggested some factors such as suitability of the course, content, maintenance, platform and measuring the success of e-Learning that can assist faculty and universities in e-Learning environment development. He suggested studying each one of these factors in isolation and also as a composite should be done to determine which factor(s) influence and impact e-Learning success. Benigno and Trentin [5] suggested a framework for the evaluation of e-Learning-based courses, focusing on two aspects: (1) evaluating the learning, and (2) evaluating the students' performance. They considered factors such as student characteristics, student–student interaction, effective support, learning materials, the learning environment and the IT. Soong et al. [6] using a multiple case study approach, verified that there are factors that affect e-Learning: human characteristics, technical competency and the e-Learning mindset of both instructor and student, level of collaboration and perceived IT infrastructure. They recommended that all these factors should be considered holistically. Govindasamy [7] considered seven quality benchmarks for successful e-Learning: institutional support, course development, teaching and learning, course structure, student support, faculty support, and evaluation and assessment. Based on an extensive study by Baylor and Ritchie [8], the impact of seven independent elements related to educational technology (planning, leadership, curriculum alignment, professional development, technology use, instructor openness to change, and instructor computer use outside school) on five dependent measures (instructor's technology competency and integration, morale, impact on student content acquisition, and higher order thinking skills acquisition) were studied using stepwise regression. Wagner and Flannery [9] pointed to organizational, work and individual support as important in influencing a learners' acceptance of computer-based learning. Childs et al. [10] indicated that librarians are important, as they can provide support material, teach information skills, organize online information sources, as well as generate their own e-learning packages. Selim [11] suggested e-Learning critical factors within a university environment can be grouped into four categories: instructor, student, IT and university support. He used confirmatory factor models to test them; however, the results were inconclusive.

2. Healthcare e-Learning Critical Success Factor (CSF) Aspects

Based on the above, this paper narrows healthcare e-Learning CSFs into the learners' aspects, instructor's aspects and technological aspects. Student access to lecture notes in advance did not, however, decrease their attendance at lectures; instead they came better prepared and were more engaged, and teachers thought they could concentrate more on important concepts or issues within the content they were covering. Students' initial perceived satisfaction with technology-based e-Learning will determine whether they will use the system continually. An unsatisfactory perception will hamper students' motivation to continue their distance education. Furthermore, e-Learning depends mainly on the use of computers as assisting tools. Therefore, a fundamental IT course could be a requirement to students. Much research indicates that learners' attitude towards computers or IT is an important factor in e-Learning satisfaction. A more positive attitude toward IT, for example, in an e-Learning environment when students are not afraid of the complexity of using computers, will result in more satisfied and effective learners [12]. Prior IT experience and attitude towards e-Learning are critical to e-Learning success. As stated before, research concludes that e-Learning-based courses compare favorably with traditional learning and e-Learning students perform as well or better than traditional-learning students. Therefore students like to use e-Learning if it facilitates their learning and allows them to learn anytime and anywhere in their own way [4].

E-Learning needs to take place in learner-centered environment. Hase and Ellis [13] observed that many of the early programs were very teacher-centered, and pointed out that it is not easy for teachers to move from entrenched models of pedagogy to allow learning to become more self-directed. One challenge for making e-Learning more learner-centered is deciding how to tailor courses to local needs, cultures, and contexts. This requires teachers to have a good understanding of their students' needs [14].

Students in Internet distance-learning courses often face technical problems, requiring timely assistance from the instructor. Previous research indicated that instructors' timely response significantly influenced learners' satisfaction. Soon et al. [15] emphasized that instructors' failing to respond to students' problems in time had a negative impact on learning. On the other hand, if an instructor is capable of handling e-Learning activities and responding to students' needs and problems promptly, learning satisfaction will improve [16, 17]. In addition, instructors' attitudes toward e-Learning may positively influence students' satisfaction [10]. When instructors are committed to e-Learning and exhibit active and positive attitudes, their enthusiasm helps to motivate students. In light of this, school administrators must be very careful in selecting instructors for e-Learning courses.

Focused instructor training might be very helpful. It is so important that instructors have good control over IT and are capable of performing basic troubleshooting tasks. Due to e-Learning courses' flexibility in time, location, and methods, participation and satisfaction of e-Learning learners are speeded up [18]. Therefore, course content should be carefully designed and presented carefully. As for all educational effort, the instructor plays a central role in the effectiveness and success of e-Learning-based courses. Webster and Hackley [19] proposed three instructor characteristics that affect e-Learning success: attitude towards technology, teaching style and control of the technology.

In a distributed learning environment, students often feel isolated since they do not have the classroom environment in which to interact with instructors. Teaching styles, especially interactions between teachers and students, play a decisive role in learning activities. Without interactions between teachers and students, learners are more prone to distractions and may have difficulty concentrating on the course materials. To overcome this, Volery and Lord [20] suggested that instructors need to provide various forms of office hours, contact methods with students and should exhibit interactive teaching styles. In a virtual learning environment, interactions between learners and others can help solve problems and improve progress. There are three kinds of interactions in learning activities: students with teachers, students with materials and students with students. Arbaugh [18] proposed that the more learners perceive interaction with others, the higher the e-Learning satisfaction. Piccoli et al. [12] further recommended interacting electronically could improve learning effects.

The success e-Learning depends on the quality of the teaching process and the effectiveness of online access. Lecturers constantly need to upgrade their technical skills. How to use IT to deliver e-Learning courses efficiently and effectively is important. So ensuring that the university IT infrastructure is rich, reliable and capable of providing the courses with the necessary tools to make the delivery process as smooth as possible is critical to the success of e-Learning. IT tools include network bandwidth, network security, network accessibility, audio and video plug-ins, courseware authoring applications, Internet availability, instructional multimedia services, videoconferencing, course management systems and user interface.

Technological design plays an important role in students' perceived usefulness and eases of use of a course and will have an impact on their satisfaction. Technology quality and Internet quality significantly affect satisfaction in e-Learning [12, 19, 21]. If the technical advice and support are lacking, the projects will not succeed [6]. A software tool with user-friendly characteristics, such as learning and memorizing few simple ideas and meaningful keywords, demands little effort from its users. Users will be willing to adopt such a tool with few barriers and their satisfaction will be improved. Therefore, the higher the quality and reliability in IT, the better the learning effects will be. E-Learning may also involve learning and discussion using other equipment such as video conferencing. Thus, both technology and Internet quality are important factors in e-Learning.

In developing fully online programs, it is critical that institutions make sufficient investment in their technology and services infrastructure. The efficient operation of a fully online program rests upon the strength of its technology and services architecture, as the core business of the institution is now being delivered entirely via the web. The right systems, processes, and practices to meet students and faculty needs will provide the institution with the foundation for a successful program. An array of servers, databases, and software applications is required to power the e-Learning platform, as well as a network service infrastructure and hosting environment to ensure a high degree of reliability and uptime. However, maintaining this infrastructure to ensure the utmost reliability and uptime can be immensely complex and challenging.

3. Conclusion

E-Learning integration into university courses is the product of the IT explosion. It is basically a web-based system that makes information or knowledge available to users or learners and without regard to time or geographic constraints. The Internet is a major technological advancement reshaping not only our society but also that of universities worldwide. There is no doubt that e-Learning plays an important role across all business sectors and education settings. As technology is now available and relatively user-friendly, those universities which do not embrace it will be left behind in the race for globalization and technological development. In the light of this, universities have to capitalize on the Internet for teaching, using advanced online delivery methods. Since the learning environment becomes more complicated, it needs to evaluate related critical factors carefully before, during and after any adoption.

This paper reviews the existing CSFs proposed by various authors in the literature. By combining these factors, a set of CSFs for e-Learning implementation is identified. We believe that the study result can help healthcare educational settings to deepen the theoretical and practical understanding of e-Learning implementation and to recognize mandatory aspects to be considered in implementation process. This, in turn, will lessen failure rates and help make e-Learning more effective, efficient and successful.

References

[1] B. Means, Y. Toyama, R. Murphy, M. Bakia, K. Jones, *Evaluation of Evidence-Based Practices in Online Learning: A Meta-Analysis and Review of Online Learning Studies,* 2009, accessed on December 4, 2009 from http://www.ed.gov/rschstat/eval/tech/evidence-based-practices/finalreport.pdf

[2] MIT OpenCourseWare (MIT OCW), 2009, accessed on December 4, 2009 from http://ocw.mit.edu/OcwWeb/web/home/home/index.htm

[3] J. Jevtic, D. Torre, J. Sebastian, *Cardiopulmonary Cases - A Clinical Exam Skills E-Learning Module,* MedEdPORTAL, 2007, accessed on December 6, 2009 from http://services.aamc.org/30/mededportal/servlet/s/segment/mededportal/?subid=454

[4] R. Papp, *Critical Success Factors for Distance Learning,* Americas Conference on Information Systems, Long Beach, CA, USA, 2000.

[5] V. Benigno, G. Trentin. The Evaluation of Online Courses, *J Comp Assist Learn* **16** (2000), 259–270.

[6] B. M. H. Soong, H. C. Chan, B. C. Chua, K. F. Loh, Critical Success Factors for On-line Course Resources, *Comp Educ* **36**(2) (2001), 101–120.

[7] T. Govindasamy, Successful Implementation of e-Learning; Pedagogical Considerations, *Internet Higher Educ* **4**(3–4) (2002), 287–299.

[8] L. Baylor, D. Ritchie, What factors facilitate teacher skill, teacher morale, and perceived student learning in technology-using classrooms? *Comp Educ* **39** (2002), 395–414.

[9] D. Wagner, D. Flannery, A quantitative study of factors affecting learner acceptance of a computer-based training support tool, *J Euro Indust Train* **28**(5) (2004), 383–399.

[10] S. Childs, E. Blenkinsopp, A. Hall, G. Walton, Effective e-learning for health professionals and students—barriers and their solutions. A systematic review of the literature—findings from the HeXL project, *Health Inf Lib J* **22** (Suppl. 2) (2005), 20–32.

[11] H.M. Selim, Critical success factors for e-learning acceptance: Confirmatory factor models, *Comp Educ* **49**(2) (2007), 396-413.

[12] G. Piccoli, R. Ahmad, B. Ives, Web-based virtual learning environments: a research framework and a preliminary assessment of effectiveness in basic IT skill training, *MIS Quarterly* **25**(4) (2001), 401–426.

[13] S. Hase, A. Ellis, *Problems with online learning are systemic, not technical,* in J. Stephenson (Ed.), Teaching and learning online: Pedagogies for new technologies. London: Kogan Page, 2001.

[14] J. Eklund, M. Kay, H. Lynch, E-learning: emerging issues and key trends: Australian Flexible Learning Network, 2003. http://www.flexiblelearning.net.au/research/2003/elearning250903final.pdf

[15] K. H. Soon, K. I.. Sook, C. W. Jung, K. M. Im, The effects of Internet-based distance learning in nursing. *Comp Nurs* **18**(1) (2000), 19–25.

[16] J. B. Arbaugh, Managing the on-line classroom: a study of technological and behavioral characteristics of web-based MBA courses, *J High Tech Manage Res* **13** (2002), 203–223.

[17] V. A. Thurmond, K. Wambach, H. R. Connors, Evaluation of student satisfaction: determining the impact of a web-based environment by controlling for student characteristics, *Amer J Dist Educ* **16**(3) (2002), 169–189.

[18] J. B. Arbaugh, R. Duray, Technological and structural characteristics, student learning and satisfaction with web-based courses – An exploratory study of two on-line MBA programs, *Manage Learn* **33**(3) (2002), 331–347.

[19] J. Webster, P. Hackley, Teaching effectiveness in technology-mediated distance learning, *Acad Manage J* **40**(6) (1997), 1282–1309.

[20] T. Volery, D. Lord, Critical success factors in online education, *Int J Educ Manage* **14**(5) (2000), 216–223.

[21] J. P. Wu, R. J. Tsai, C. C. Chen, Y. C. Wu, An integrative model to predict the continuance use of electronic learning systems: hints for teaching, *International Journal on E-Learning* **5**(2) (2006), 287-302.

International Perspectives in Health Informatics
E.M. Borycki et al. (Eds.)
IOS Press, 2011
doi:10.3233/978-1-60750-709-3-69

Development of a Graduate Level Course in e-Health and Emerging Technology in Saudi Arabia

Mowafa Said HOUSEH [a,1] , Basema SADDIK[a], Bakheet AL-DOSARI [a]

[a] *College of Public Health and Health Informatics, King Saud Bin Abdul Aziz University for Health Science, Riyadh, Kingdom of Saudi Arabia*

Abstract. This paper provides an overview of a newly developed course in E-health and Emerging Technology for King Saud Bin Abdul Aziz University for Health Sciences (KSAU-HS) Masters of Health Informatics program. The paper provides an overview of the program, description on the course development process, instructional methods, and course evaluation. The paper also describes the faculty's experience in the development of the course. Future evaluation will focus on students' learning experience and content used in the course.

Keywords. health informatics, education, e-health, emerging technology

Introduction

Creating content for any course can be a challenging task. In January 2010, a graduate course in *E-health and Emerging Technology* was created for graduate students at King Saud Bin Abdul Aziz University for Health Sciences (KSAU-HS), Graduate Program in Health Informatics. This is the only university within the region that provides a graduate level course in health informatics and to date it has 53 graduates from various health and technical backgrounds successfully working within the field [1].

This paper discusses the creation of an e-health and emerging technology course within the program. The paper provides information on the university and the program, objectives of the course, course content, and methods used to instruct.

1. Program Objectives

Little is known about the field of health informatics within the Kingdom of Saudi Arabia. In 2002, a key meeting with leading health informatics professionals led to the development of a national e-health strategy which recommended the creation of a college for health informatics education [2]. In 2004 KSAU-HS, the only health sciences university in the Middle East, was created. A year later the college of Public

---

[1] Dr. Mowafa Househ, King Saud Bin Abdul Aziz University for Health Sciences, College of Public Health and Health Informatics, Riyadh, Kingdom of Saudi Arabia; Email: househmo@ngha.med.sa

Health and Health Informatics was established. The goal of the health informatics program at KSAU-HS is to:

> ...overcome the severe shortage of qualified capabilities in the field of health informatics technology. Graduates of the program shall contribute to the management, development, and application of health informatics technology at hospitals and health centers, and solve the problems that may impede the advancement of health informatics and its utilization[3].

The program is two years in length and covers topics from medical terminology and statistical analysis to ethics in health informatics and project management. All courses are taught in English. Students are required to take 10 courses over the two year period and complete a health informatics project. The program is primarily course based and plans for a thesis based stream are currently being discussed.

To be admitted into the college, students need to have:

- Obtained a bachelors degree in medicine, dentistry, nursing, pharmacy, radiography, laboratory medicine, medical engineering, and management of health information technology.
- Gained two years of relevant work experience.
- Achieved a minimum of 550 in TOEFL Exam.
- Two recommendation letters.
- To scored favorably on an interview.
- Pass an entrance exam [3].

The requirements are rigorous, especially for a new program, but are needed to ensure academic rigor and quality of the program. A group of 20 students are accepted twice a year into the program.

2. Course Development

In April of 2009, an independent review of the program found that, among many other recommendations, a course on e-health and emerging technologies was needed. Faculty members began discussions to create such a course but found it difficult to find standardized material that would cover such a large domain topic. Faculty members decided to create something unique: a new course that was based on scientific literature defining the role of e-health, evaluation methods used, as well as providing examples of how e-health was used internationally. Furthermore, the course was developed based on national curriculum standards and the Commission on Accreditation for Health Informatics and Information Management Education (CAHIIM).

3. Course Objectives

The purpose of the course was to provide students with practical knowledge of e-health and emerging technologies within the field. The course was 15 weeks long and organized around three themes: 1) defining e-health and domain areas; 2) methodologies used in e-health evaluation; 3) international application of e-health. These three themes comprised the focus of the course.

The first theme of the course focused on defining e-health and relevant domain areas. The duration for this part of the course was 9 weeks and it provided a definition of e-health and a study of four relevant domain areas: telehealth, human computer interaction, consumer informatics, and emerging technologies. A module on electronic health records was omitted because there was a dedicated course focusing on the topic. These topics were viewed by faculty as relevant topics and important to the study of e-health.

Faculty also decided that it was important for students to understand the various qualitative, quantitative, and mixed methods studies that are used in e-health evaluation. Students had already taken a research methods course. However, the students had little knowledge on how such methodologies were implemented within the e-health domain. Two weeks of the course was dedicated to studying e-health evaluation methods. The first week focused qualitative methods and the second week focused on quantitative and mixed methods.

The third theme of the course focused on international e-health applications. The duration of this part of the course was for three weeks. The first week focused on national strategies in Australia, Canada, South Africa, and England around e-health. The second and third week focused on studies around e-health conducted in these countries. Students were expected to learn from the experiences of e-health use and implementation from around the world and learn from their successes and failures. The last week of the course was a review of what had been taught in the course. Table 1 provides a scheduled breakdown of the course by week.

4. Course Content

Content for each of the first two course themes (Table 1, Parts 1 and 2,) was retrieved based on several relevant journals within the health informatics community. Four journals were used for supplying content material to the course: 1) Journal of American Medical Informatics Association; 2) Journal of Medical Internet Research; 3) Methods of Information in Medicine; 4) International Journal of Medical Informatics. Several articles for each domain area were part of the required readings for the students.

Table 1. E-health and emerging technology weekly lecture schedule

Date	Topic
Part 1: Domain Areas of E-health	
Week 1	Defining E-health
Week 2 & 3	Telehealth
Week 4 & 5	Human Computer Interaction
Week 6 & 7	Consumer Informatics
Week 8 & 9	Emerging E-health Technologies
Part 2: Evaluation Methods	
Week 10	Qualitative E-health Cases
Week 11	Quantitative E-health Cases
Part 3: International E-health	
Week 12	National Strategies
Week 13 & 14	International Case Studies
Week 15	Review

Sample papers included in the course were: E-Health Definition: [4]; Telehealth: [5]; Human Computer Interaction: [6], [7]; and Consumer Informatics: [8], [9].

As for the third part of the course, international e-health applications, a Google search was made on the various e-health initiatives occurring in several countries around the world. Sample content used in the course included references [10], [11] and [12].

5. Students and Instructional Methods

Thirteen female and three male students were enrolled in the class. Five female students participated via video conferencing because they could not attend face-to-face classes, which were 500kms away. The remaining eleven students attended class in a face-to-face session with the instructor. Each student in the face-to-face session had access to a computer with secured internet access. Distant students had access to laptops with secure access to an internet connection. There was a video conferencing monitor in the class for the instructor to view distant students, and distant students also had a screen where they could view the instructor. Also, a screen and projector were present in the face-to-face room, as well as the distant room. Both students could see the instructor's power-point slides. Students were also given access to blackboard, an online course management system, where they could access their grades, links to reading material, and a discussion forum. Figure 1 shows the classroom setup.

The course was designed to be taught in both lectures and in-class group work and discussions. During each class, a lecture would be given around each topic, and sample articles would be discussed within the class.

6. Evaluation

Individually, students were required to complete a literature review around a specific topic related to e-health. Also, they were required to work as a group to develop a business case for the implementation of an e-health strategy within their work environment. Each student was required to present their business case findings. Students were also given marks for participating in class and online through the blackboard discussion forum. A final exam was also included in the evaluation. Table 2 provides a summary of the evaluation.

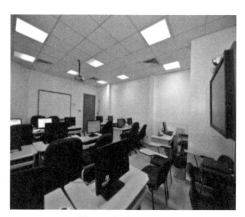

Figure 1: Classroom

Table 2. Student Evaluation

Components	Date	Weight
Literature Review	Week 5	25%
Group Project	Week 10	25%
Group Presentation	Week 12	10%
Participation	Continuous	20%
Final Exam	Subsequent to Week 15	20%

7. Conclusions

This paper provided an overview of a course developed in e-health and emerging technology for KSAU-HS health informatics graduate program. The paper discussed the steps used to create a course on e-health and emerging technologies. Background on the program, the development process, topics taught, instruction methods, and evaluation were discussed in this paper. Future evaluation plans will focus on students' learning experience and content used in the course

References

[1] RiyadhNews. Suadi 2010 E-Health Conference [Internet], 2010, available from: http://www.alriyadh.com/2010/04/17/article517301.html
[2] M. Altuwaijri, Electronic-health in Saudi Arabia: Just around the corner. *Saudi Medical Journal*, **29(2)** (2008), 171-178.
[3] KSAU-HS. KSAU-HS Health Informatics Program [Internet], 2010, available from: http://eapps.ksau-hs.edu.sa/en/colleges_departments/ph_hi/index.html.
[4] H. Oh, C. Rizo, M. Enkin, A. Jadad, What is eHealth (3): A systematic review of published definitions [Internet], *JMIR* **7(1)** (2005), available from: http://www.jmir.org/2005/1/e1
[5] P.A. Jennett, K. Andruchuk, Telehealth: 'real life' implementation issues, *Computer Methods and Programs in Biomedicine* **64** (2001), 169 - 174.
[6] V. Patel, J. Arocha, D. Kaufman, A Primer on Aspects of Cognition for Medical Informatics, *J Am Med Info Assoc* **8(4)** (2001), 324-343.
[7] V. Patel, A. Kushniruk, S. Yang, Impact of a Computer-based Patient Record System on Data Collection, Knowledge Organization, and Reasoning, *J Am Med Info Assoc* (2000).
[8] L.O. Grady, *Future directions for depicting credibility in health care web sites*, 2006, 58-65.
[9] K.M. Akesson, B. Saveman, G. Nilsson, *Health care consumers ' experiences of information communication technology — A summary of literature*, 2006, 633-645.
[10] *British Columbia. eHealth Strategic Framework. 2005*; Ministry of Health. (November), available from: http://www.health.gov.bc.ca/library/publications/year/2005/ehealth_framework.pdf.
[11] *Australia. National Strategy* [Internet], Australian Health Ministers' Conference, 2008, available from: www.ahmac.gov.au
[12] M. Mars, C. Seebregts, *Country Case Study for e-Health South Africa*, South Africa, 2006, 1-46.

Evaluation

International Perspectives in Health Informatics
E.M. Borycki et al. (Eds.)
IOS Press, 2011
© 2011 ITCH 2011 Steering Committee and IOS Press. All rights reserved.
doi:10.3233/978-1-60750-709-3-77

Clinical and Economic Results from a Randomized Trial of Clinical Decision Support in a Rural Health Network

Eric L. EISENSTEIN [a,b], Kensaku KAWAMOTO [a],
Kevin J. ANSTROM[b], Janese M. WILLIS [a], Garry M. SILVEY [a], Fred S. JOHNSON[c],
Rex EDWARDS [b], Jean MISE [d],
Susan D. YAGGY [e], David F. LOBACH[a]

[a] Division of Clinical Informatics, Department of Community and Family Medicine,
Duke University Medical Center, Durham, NC
[b] Duke Clinical Research Institute, Durham, NC
[c] Division of Community Health, Department of Community and Family Medicine,
Duke University Medical Center, Durham, NC
[d] Community Care Partners of Northern Piedmont Community Care, Henderson, NC
[e] North Carolina Foundation for Advanced Health Programs, Raleigh, NC

Abstract. Background: Replication studies evaluate technologies in usual use settings. Methods: We conducted a clinical trial to determine whether reductions in clinical and economic results observed in a previous study could be replicated in a larger setting. Subjects were randomized to receive intervention (email notifications for sentinel health events sent to their care managers) or control. Main Outcome Measures: The primary outcome was the rate of emergency department visits for low severity conditions. Secondary outcomes included: medical costs and other clinical event rates. Results: We randomized 13,454 individuals (intervention, 6740; control, 6714). Subjects in both groups had similar rates of clinical events and medical costs. Conclusion: The use of email notifications to care managers was associated with no reductions in clinical events or medical costs.

Keywords. clinical decision support, randomized clinical trial, clinical outcomes, economic outcomes, population health management

Introduction

Replication is an essential element in health information technology (IT) evaluation. Replication builds upon the recognition that practice-based studies are needed to test health IT in usual use settings and is particularly important when factors other than the health IT itself may influence overall system performance [1-5].

1. Research Objectives

The objective of the Five County Community Care Program (5CCP) study was to determine whether use of a clinical decision support (CDS) system in a rural setting would be associated with reductions in clinical and economic outcomes.

2. Methods

2.1. Study Setting and Population

The 5CCP health network was established in 2004 to serve as a care management organization for Medicaid managed care patients in a five county area of North Carolina [6]. As a part of this effort, the regional health information exchange and data repository serving Durham County was expanded to support 35 5CCP healthcare partners (3 community hospitals, 6 health centers, 16 primary care practices, 5 county social service departments, 4 county health departments and the 5CCP organization). Key elements of this health information exchange are the Community-Oriented Approach to Coordinated Healthcare (COACH) system through which care managers record and share client information and the COACH population health management system (COACH PHMS), which evaluates patient information on a weekly basis [7,8]. Medicaid Carolina Access beneficiaries in 5CCP counties were randomized by family unit to the intervention and control groups using a 1:1 allocation ratio.

2.2. Study Interventions

The COACH PHMS triggers notifications based upon the occurrence of a set of sentinel health events detected by a CDS engine known as SEBASTIAN [7]. A complete listing of the 5CCP notification conditions has been reported [6]. Notifications were generated for all study subjects. However, the study protocol stipulated that notifications for the intervention group would be sent via electronic mail to care managers; whereas those for the control group were withheld.

2.3. Study Measurements, Data Sources and Analyses

Four types of study measurements were assessed: (1) baseline characteristics, (2) notifications generated, (3) clinical events, and (4) medical costs.

All information used in this study's evaluations came from COACH, which serves as a repository for enrollment, notification, missed appointment and North Carolina Medicaid claims data for the 5CCP subjects. Claims data billing codes were used to identify all evaluated clinical events excepting missed appointments. Reimbursement amounts were used as estimates of medical costs [9].

All study analyses were performed for subjects in the intervention vs. control groups. Baseline characteristics and notification results were summarized as percents for categorical data and as median (25th, 75th) for continuous data. Outcome estimates and between-group treatment comparisons were derived using general estimating equations with a working correlation matrix to account for subject clustering within families. A two-sided alpha was used to determine statistical significance (p ≤ .01) without correction for multiple comparisons.

3. Results

On September 1, 2007, 13,454 individuals were randomized to have their care managers receive CDS generated email notifications of sentinel events (n = 6740) or control (n = 6714) (Table 1). Patients in both groups were matched with respect to demographic and clinical characteristics.

Table 1. Baseline characteristics

Patient Characteristics	Control (n=6714)	Intervention (n=6740)
Age <18 years (%)	67.5	65.8
African-American race (%)	61.2	62.4
Male gender (%)	43.2	42.6
Family size, Median (25th, 75th)	2 (1, 2)	2 (1, 2)
Diabetes (%)	4.5	4.8
Asthma (%)	9.6	10.0

Email notifications averaged 27.6 and 25.9 per 100 subjects in the control and intervention groups, respectively. Nearly 90% of notifications in both groups were ED-related, with low-severity ED visits accounting for more than half of all notifications.

Subjects in the control and intervention groups had similar ED, outpatient event, and missed appointment rates through 12 months of follow-up (Table 2). These results were associated with no significant differences in ED, outpatient and total medical costs. Treatment-related differences in hospital events and costs were not significant.

Table 2. Clinical event rates and patient medical costs by treatment group

	Control (n=6714)	Intervention (n=6740)	P-value
Clinical Event Rates*			
Emergency Department*			
Low Severity	13.7	13.2	0.52
>3 in 90 Days	5.2	5.2	0.95
Total	38.9	37.3	0.30
Hospitalization	2.9	3.7	0.03
Outpatient Encounters	1154.5	1163.7	0.87
Missed Appointments	4.2	4.9	0.19
Medical Costs Per Patient ($)			
Emergency	136	117	0.12
Hospitalization	163	246	0.04
Outpatient	1460	1450	0.89
Total	1766	1821	0.56

* rates are shown as events per 100 patients

4. Discussion

Our evaluation found no significant reductions in clinical events or medical costs for subjects in the information intervention vs. control groups. The inability to replicate the positive emergency department-related clinical and economic results associated with email notifications to care managers in the HIT Value study conducted in Durham County, North Carolina raises questions as to whether this was an issue of differences in study populations or of differences in the interventions as delivered.

Although the 5CCP study had a longer follow-up period than the HIT Value study (12 vs. 9 months), fewer intervention subjects triggered a notification (13% vs. 18%). However, this difference largely was due to the generation of fewer outpatient notifications in 5CCP and not to differences in the rates of ED visits, which were 28% higher than in HIT Value. These findings suggest that differences in study results were not due to differences in the underlying ED event rates for subjects in the two populations.

Since HIT Value and 5CCP used the same computer systems (COACH and COACH PHMS), we suspected that differences in study results were caused by differences in how care managers used these systems. A post-hoc review verified that 5CCP care managers had not fully integrated the email notifications into their work flow. They had not consistently updated COACH with actions taken and did not fully understand how to use email alerts. The 5CCP study team then implemented a productivity reporting system that links email notification generation to the actions care managers report in COACH. Implementation of this feedback reporting and monitoring system was coupled with protocol retraining for care managers. It is anticipated that these steps to increase implementation fidelity will be associated with improved effectiveness of the 5CCP intervention in subsequent phases of this study [10].

5. Conclusion

In contrast to a previous study, the use of an asynchronous decision support system to notify care managers of sentinel health events was not associated with significant reductions in clinical and economic outcomes compared with controls. The difference between study results appears to arise from the degree to which the notices were used by the recipient care managers. These results highlight the importance of implementation fidelity and the need for replication of health IT interventions to test their utility in practice-based settings.

Acknowledgements

The work described in this manuscript was funded by Grant Number H2ATH07753 of the Office for the Advancement of Telehealth (OAT) of the Health Resources and Services Administration of the U.S. Department of Health and Human Services. The authors thank Allyn Meredith, MA and Denise Masters for their expert editorial assistance.

References

[1] J. Aarts, M. Berg, Same systems, different outcomes--comparing the implementation of computerized physician order entry in two Dutch hospitals, *Methods Inf Med* **45** (2006), 53-61.
[2] M. Campbell, R. Fitzpatrick, A. Haines, A.L. Kinmonth, P. Sandercock, D. Spiegelhalter, P. Tyler, Framework for design and evaluation of complex interventions to improve health, *BMJ* **321** (2000), 694-696.
[3] L.W. Green, R.E. Glasgow, Evaluating the relevance, generalization, and applicability of research: issues in external validation and translation methodology, *Eval Health Prof* **29** (2006), 126-153.
[4] B. Haynes, Can it work? Does it work? Is it worth it? The testing of healthcare interventions is evolving, *BMJ* **319** (1999), 652-653.
[5] S.R. Tunis, D.B. Stryer, C.M. Clancy, Practical clinical trials: increasing the value of clinical research for decision making in clinical and health policy, *JAMA* **290** (2003), 1624-1632.
[6] E.L. Eisenstein, D.F. Lobach, K. Kawamoto, et al. A Randomized Clinical Trial of Clinical Decision Support in a Rural Community Health Network Serving Lower Income Individuals: Study Design and Baseline Characteristics, in J.G. McDaniels, editor, *Advances in Information Technology and Communication in Health*, 1 ed., IOS Press, (2009), 220-226.
[7] K. Kawamoto, D.F. Lobach, Design, implementation, use, and preliminary evaluation of SEBASTIAN, a standards-based web service for clinical decision support, *AMIA Symposium 2005*, 380-384.
[8] D.F. Lobach R. Low, J.A. Arbanas, J.S. Rabold, J.L. Tatum, S.D. Epstein, Defining and supporting the diverse information needs of community-based care using the web and hand-held devices, *Proc AMIA Symp* (2001), 398-402.
[9] E.L. Eisenstein, M. Ortiz, K.J. Anstrom, D.F. Lobach, Health information technology economic evaluation, in: A.W. Kushniruk, E. Borycki, editors, *The Human and Social Side of Health Information Systems*, 1st ed., Hershey, PA: Idea Group Publishing (2008), 240-58.
[10] E.L. Eisenstein, D.F. Lobach, P. Montgomery, K. Kawamoto, K.J. Anstrom, Evaluating implementation fidelity in health information technology interventions, *AMIA Annu Symp Proc.* (2007), 211-215.

82

International Perspectives in Health Informatics
E.M. Borycki et al. (Eds.)
IOS Press, 2011
© 2011 ITCH 2011 Steering Committee and IOS Press. All rights reserved.
doi:10.3233/978-1-60750-709-3-82

Economic Analysis of Centralized vs. Decentralized Electronic Data Capture in Multi-Center Clinical Studies

Anita WALDEN [a], Meredith NAHM [a], M. Edwina BARNETT [b], Jose G. CONDE [c],
Andrew DENT [b], Ahmed FADIEL [d], Theresa PERRY [b], Chris TOLK [e],
James E. TCHENG [a], Eric L. EISENSTEIN [a]

[a] *Duke University, Durham, North Carolina;*
[b] *Jackson State University, Jackson, Mississippi;*
[c] *University of Puerto Rico, San Juan, Puerto Rico;*
[d] *Meharry Medical School, Nashville, Tennessee;*
[e] *Clinical Data Interchange Standards Consortium*

Abstract. Background: New data management models are emerging in multi-center clinical studies. We evaluated the incremental costs associated with decentralized vs. centralized models. Methods: We developed clinical research network economic models to evaluate three data management models: centralized, decentralized with local software, and decentralized with shared database. Descriptive information from three clinical research studies served as inputs for these models. Main Outcome Measures: The primary outcome was total data management costs. Secondary outcomes included: data management costs for sites, local data centers, and central coordinating centers. Results: Both decentralized models were more costly than the centralized model for each clinical research study: the decentralized with local software model was the most expensive. Decreasing the number of local data centers and case book pages reduced cost differentials between models. Conclusion: Decentralized vs. centralized data management in multi-center clinical research studies is associated with increases in data management costs.

Keywords. cost analysis, clinical research network, clinical trial, data management

Introduction

Through its Clinical and Translational Science Award (CTSA) and other clinical research programs, the National Institutes of Health (NIH) has sought to increase clinical research capacity and the secondary use of clinical data. Although many NIH-funded clinical research programs use a traditional multi-center clinical research network (CRN) model in which a single data coordinating center provides electronic data capture (EDC) services for all study sites, other, more complex, CRN data management models have arisen in which more than one organization provides data management services [1]. This arrangement necessitates the designation of a 'central coordinating center' whose function is to consolidate data captured by the study's local data centers. While the intent of policy makers to expand clinical research capabilities is clear, the relative economic attractiveness of decentralized vs. centralized data management models for CTSA and NIH clinical research networks has not been evaluated. This consideration is particularly important in an era during which the costs of conducting clinical research have escalated while research productivity has decreased [2-4]. We evaluated the incremental costs associated with decentralized vs. centralized data management models for the types of multi-center clinical research studies typically conducted by CTSA and NIH clinical research networks.

1. Methods

1.1. Study Design

Economic analyses typically evaluate the incremental costs and non-monetary benefits associated with the use of a new technology versus the standard of care [5]. However, as the benefits from an investment in EDC capabilities are not well defined, we focused our analysis on the incremental costs associated with different data management models for multi-center clinical research studies. We assumed that personnel costs would be a reasonable proxy for the marginal costs of conducting those studies.

1.2. Data Management Models

Three data management models were evaluated: centralized, decentralized-local software and decentralized-shared database. The centralized model represents traditional practice and includes a central coordinating center that develops and controls the clinical research study's EDC system. This EDC system is then used by all of the sites to enter study data and resolve errors. We also considered two decentralized models. In the decentralized-local software model, two or more local data centers independently develop EDC systems for a single clinical research study and provide data entry and error resolution services for one or more study sites. A central coordinating center then collects study data sets from each local data center and merges them to create a single study database. In the decentralized-shared database model, the study's central coordinating center develops a single data dictionary and database for the clinical research study that are shared with local data centers that then use this software to provide EDC data entry and error resolution services for the study's sites. At the conclusion of the study, local data centers provide copies of their database to the central coordinating center for consolidation into a single study database.

1.3. Study Outcomes

This study's primary outcome was total data management costs for a clinical research study. Secondary outcomes included total data management costs for sites, local data centers and central coordinating centers, and per-patient data management costs for the same clinical research study.

1.4. Data Management Economic Model

1.4.1. Economic Model Components

Economic models are frequently used to evaluate problems for which it is not feasible to collect empirical data and have previously been used in studies of clinical research methods and practices [3, 6-8]. We developed three clinical research network economic models to estimate the data management costs for conducting clinical research studies using one centralized and two decentralized EDC data management strategies, as described above. All models shared a common component that estimated data management costs for study sites with separate components for central coordinating and local data centers. Total trial data management costs for each model were computed as the sum of each model's component costs.

1.4.2. Economic Model Construction:

This study's economic models were constructed using the following procedures. First, we identified a set of 43 data management tasks required by one or more economic model component. We assumed that data management begins when a clinical study's case book is finalized and ends with the creation of the study's final analytic data set. For each task, we assigned a task description, described the work to be accomplished, and assigned a primary work unit to measure the amount of activity that occurs when the task is performed (for example: unique case book pages, repeated case book pages, query rules, users at a site, EDC system training sessions, and analytic files created). We also identified a job level that was responsible for the completion of the task and the per-unit duration for the task in hours (for example: time required to program a single query rule, conduct a training session, or grant database access to one user). We also created a table of standard job levels and their associated hourly rates of pay. For each job level, we assigned an hourly rate based upon pay scales in an academic research organization (assuming 1450 billable hours per year) (statistician, $78; clinical data manager, $65; technical, $47; clerical, $29; and coordinator, $43). Lastly, we mapped each of the 43 data management tasks to one or more of the economic model components in which they would be performed. This step completed the development of our multi-center clinical research economic models.

1.4.3. Clinical Study Descriptions

A set of clinical research study descriptors served as inputs for our economic models. These descriptors defined the number of times individual model tasks were performed in specific clinical studies (Table 1). For the initial models, we assumed that all sites in the two decentralized models would have local data centers.

Table 1. Clinical Study Cost Driver Summaries

Clinical Study Cost Drivers	CRN-1	CRN-2	CRN-3
Patients	1000	135	130
Sites	9	3	2
Users per site	2	2	2
Duration (Yrs)	5	1	1
Case Report Form			
Unique pages	99	80	21
Total Pages	217	128	21
Query rules	384	45	35

1.5. Sensitivity Analyses

Two sensitivity analyses were conducted. First, we estimated the incremental costs associated with mapping a study's unique data elements to an international data standard. Second, we simultaneously varied the number of local data centers (2 and 8) and the total number of case book pages (120, 220, and 320), assuming 75% unique pages and 1 query rule per total page) to assess the relative economic importance of the number of local data centers and trial complexity.

2. Results

In all data management models, the CRN-1 study was more costly than the CRN-2 study and the CRN-2 study was more costly than the CRN-3 study (Table 2). Within each clinical study, decentralized data management models were more costly than the centralized model. While the decentralized-shared database model was less costly than the decentralized-local software model, it never approached the lower cost of the centralized model in any of the three studies. Interestingly, the relative cost differential between the centralized and decentralized modalities was less in the CRN-3 than in the CRN-2 study and less in the CRN-2 than in the CRN-1 study, denoting that cost differences between models are in part related to the size and complexity of their associated clinical research studies.

Table 2. Clinical Study Data Management Costs

Study Trials	Data Management Models		
	Clinical Research Organization Costs		
	Centralized	Decentralized	
		Local Software	Shared Database
CRN-1			
Trial Costs ($)			
Study sites	1,174,457	1,174,457	1,174,457
Local data centers	0	3,944,232	1,677,623
Central coordinating center	777,769	230,360	602,762
Total	1,952,226	5,349,048	3,454,842
CRN-2			
Trial Costs ($)			
Study sites	91,384	91,384	91,384
Local data centers	0	389,035	130,662
Central coordinating center	161,861	48,945	134,705
Total	253,244	529,364	356,751
CRN-3			
Trial Costs ($)			
Study sites	27,122	27,122	27,122
Local data centers	0	174,128	72,824
Central coordinating center	102,674	33,053	71,560
Total	129,796	234,303	171,507

2.1. Sensitivity Analyses

In all data management models for the three clinical research studies, mapping a study's unique data elements to an international data standard was associated with modest cost increases. However, in no instance were the overall study effects altered—centralized is less costly than decentralized and decentralized shared-database is less costly than decentralized-local software.

Per-patient data management costs for the CRN-1 study were similar in both decentralized models with two local data centers across all case book page assumptions. However, with eight local data centers, the decentralized-local software model was more costly than the decentralized-shared database model, and this difference increased with the number of case book pages. There were no scenarios in which the centralized model was more costly than either of the decentralized models.

3. Discussion

Our work suggests that decentralized data management will be more costly than centralized data management for the same clinical research study. Although the cost differential between data management models decreases as the number of local data centers and case book pages are reduced, there is no scenario in which either of the decentralized models is less costly than the centralized model. While the decentralized-shared database model tended to be somewhat less costly than the decentralized-local software model, it remained far more expensive than the centralized model in all scenarios evaluated. Of note, mapping a study's unique data elements to an international data standard at the conclusion of a study was associated with only a modest cost increment in all data management models.

Inefficiencies necessitated by both decentralized models account for their higher data management costs when compared with the centralized model. These inefficiencies are caused by the introduction of a new organization (local data center) that is interposed between the study site and the central coordinating center, by the duplication of activities when more than one organization is responsible for data management, and by the need to impose new controls as study data is passed through an additional organizational level. In the decentralized-local software model, local data centers are responsible for implementing and operating a data management system for their sites. With 9 local data centers, these activities are performed 9 times instead of once in the centralized model. Although local data centers do not develop data management systems in the decentralized-shared database model, they still are responsible for duplicate operations.

3.1. Previous Work by the Clinical Data Interchange

Standards Consortium (CDISC) and others suggests that mapping clinical research study data to industry standards 'at the back end' will most likely lead to increased costs as was demonstrated in the present study [9]. However, CDISC advocates an alternative data management strategy by which standards are implemented during protocol and case book design for one study and then reused in similar studies [10]. By creating knowledge components that can be reused across multiple clinical research studies, it is anticipated that there will be significant reductions in the time required to perform tasks such as developing case books and databases, programming edit checks and cleaning study data, statistical programming and analysis, and performing data exchange [11]. Applying benchmarks from other industries that implemented standards, it has been estimated that as much as 60% of non-subject participation time and cost could be saved through the use of standards and the creation of reusable data management components [9]. Research in this and other studies suggests that application of the CDISC Study Data Tabulation Model (SDTM) increases development time the first time the standard is applied; however, when the standard is reapplied on a similar study, there is a net decrease in effort [12]. This implies that the ability to achieve data management cost savings within NIH research networks through the creation of standards-based knowledge components will be in part a function of the extent to which these components can be reused across multiple studies.

Our study is limited in that we only included personnel costs. Had we included the full costs of clinical data management (investments in software, hardware, facilities, and training) the cost advantage for the centralized model would have been magnified. While it is clear that non-monetary benefits accrue from increasing clinical research capabilities, work is needed to identify those benefits in more detail so that the cost vs. benefits of decentralized vs. centralized data management models may be evaluated more fully.

4. Conclusion

The use of decentralized vs. centralized data management models in the types of multi-center clinical studies conducted by CTSA and NIH research networks is associated with an increase in total and per-patient data management costs. Innovations in clinical data management should be encouraged, and there are non-monetary benefits related to the implementation of decentralized data management models in specific scenarios. However, findings from the present study should be factored into any decisions related to data management models in clinical research studies in order to improve the efficiency of funding allocation.

5. Acknowledgements

The project entitled, "Feasibility and Economic Evaluation of Standards-Based Interoperability between Investigational Sites and Clinical Research Network Data Centers" is funded by the Clinical Research Network Feasibility Award (#8059-S06).

References

[1] L. Freidman, C.D. Furberg, D.L. DeMets, *Fundamentals of Clinical Trials, 3rd edition,* Mosby-Year Book, St. Louis, 1996.
[2] E.R. Dorsey, J. de Roulet, J.P. Thompson, J.I. Reminick, A. Thai, Z. White-Stellato, C.A. Beck, B.P. George, H. Moses III, Funding of US biomedical research, 2003-2008, *JAMA* **303** (2010), 137-143.

[3] E.L. Eisenstein, R. Collins, B.S. Cracknell, O. Podesta, E.E. Reid, P. Sandercock, Y. Shakhov, M.L. Terrin, M.A. Sellers, R.M. Califf, C.B. Granger, R. Diaz, Sensible approaches for reducing clinical trial costs, *Clin Trials* **5** (2008), 75-84.

[4] H. Moses III, E.R. Dorsey, D.H. Matheson, S.O. Thier, Financial anatomy of biomedical research, *JAMA* **294** (2005), 1333-1342.

[5] E.L. Eisenstein, M. Ortiz, K.J. Anstrom, D.F. Lobach, Health information technology economic evaluation, in: A.W. Kushniruk, E. Borcycki, editors, *The Human and Social Side of Health Information Systems, 1st ed.*, Idea Group Publishing, Hershey, PA, 2008, 240-58.

[6] M. Campbell, R. Fitzpatrick, A. Haines, A.L. Kinmouth, P. Sandercock, D. Spiegelhalter, Framework for design and evaluation of complex interventions to improve health, *BMJ* **321** (2000), 694-696.

[7] E.L. Eisenstein, P.W. Lemons, B.E. Tardiff, K.A. Schulman, M.K. Jolly, R.M. Califf, Reducing the costs of phase III cardiovascular clinical trials, *Am Heart J* **149** (2005), 482-488.

[8] J.S. Li, E.L. Eisenstein, H.G. Grabowski, E.D. Reid, B. Mangum, K.A. Schulman, J.V. Goldsmith, M.D. Murphy, R.M. Califf, D.K. Benjamin, Economic return of clinical trials performed under the pediatric exclusivity program, *JAMA* **297** (2007), 480-488.

[9] C. Rozwell, R.D. Kush, E. Helton, F. Newby, T. Mason, *Business Case for CDISC Standards: Summary 2006*, PhRMA-Gartner-CDISC Project, 2006.

[10] C. Rozwell, R.D. Kush, E. Helton, Saving Time and Money*, Applied Clinical Trials*, 2007.

[11] C. Rozwell, R.D. Kush, E. Helton, CDISC Standards: Enabling Reuse without Rework, *Applied Clinical Trials*, 2006.

[12] N. Hayes, P. Warfel, O. Oladapo, et al. CDISC Implementation Mostly in Clintrial™ at Duke Clinical Research Institute. 2004.

International Perspectives in Health Informatics
E.M. Borycki et al. (Eds.)
IOS Press, 2011
doi:10.3233/978-1-60750-709-3-89

Sociotechnical Evaluation of a Clinical Transformation Project in a Specialized Cancer Care Centre

Margaret BISHOP[a,b,1], Jeff BARNETT[a,b], Maria T. VLACHAKI[b], Howard PAI[b]

[a] *University of Victoria, Victoria, British Columbia, Canada,*
[b] *British Columbia Cancer Agency- Vancouver Island Centre,
Victoria, British Columbia, Canada*

Abstract. The radiation therapy (RT) department at the British Columbia Cancer Agency - Vancouver Island Centre (VIC) is responsible for delivering radiation treatments to cancer patients from Vancouver Island, which has a population base of approximately 750,000. The purpose of this analysis is to examine a process transformation project undertaken by a VIC clinical champion using a sociotechnical approach and identify factors that influenced the project outcome. Beginning in January 2009, a radiation oncologist at VIC initiated a project to transform the clinical process of generating prescriptions for radiation therapy. The project objective was to replace the paper-based process for radiation therapy (RT) prescriptions with an electronic process to achieve benefits such as increased legibility, accuracy, and accessibility of prescriptions. The electronic prescription (e-Rx) process was designed and developed by health informatics students from the University of Victoria, and the new process was trialed and implemented for approximately half of the new patients seen by the VIC RT department. This pilot implementation was brought to a halt two weeks later, due to concerns raised by the RT department. Using a sociotechnical approach, the authors identify several factors that negatively impacted the project's successful implementation: lack of leadership endorsement and organizational strategy, insufficient formal and informal organizational power of the clinical champion, underestimation of complexity, and inadequate management of the implementation process. Although these factors have been well documented in the literature for large-scale system implementation projects, understanding the way by which they influence smaller-scale process transformation projects in highly specialized clinical settings may help future project managers and coordinators to set such projects up for success.

Keywords. case study, clinical transformation, sociotechnical evaluation

1. Introduction

The BC Cancer Agency – Vancouver Island Centre (VIC) provides specialized cancer care to residents of Vancouver Island, British Columbia, which has a population of approximately 750,000. Radiation Therapy (RT) involves the use of ionizing radiation to treat cancer. The VIC RT department treats approximately 150 patients per day, and uses Varian Medical Systems[TM] software tools for managing patient demographic information, information on radiation treatment planning and delivery, and radiation

---

[1] Corresponding Author: Margaret Bishop, email: mbishop@uvic.ca

quality assurance processes [6]. The sociotechnical approach to information technology (IT) applications in health care views work practices as interrelated networks, emphasizes the need to understand the cooperative work processes that exist in health care settings, and suggests user involvement and qualitative research methods as the most appropriate ways to analyze practice changes [2]. The sociotechnical challenges of IT implementation in health care settings have been well documented for large-scale system implementation projects. We have applied the same principles to a smaller-scale process transformation project in a highly specialized clinical setting. The project we examined aimed to replace the paper-based RT prescription with an electronic prescription (e-Rx) process at VIC. This project was motivated by workflow inefficiencies and problems with the legibility and accessibility of paper-based RT prescriptions. Identifying and understanding the barriers encountered in this case study may assist project managers and coordinators in the successful design and implementation of similar IT-based clinical transformation processes and projects.

2. Electronic Radiation Therapy Prescription Project (e-Radiate Rx)

The Electronic Radiation Therapy Information and Telecommunications Enhancement Project (e-Radiate) was created to improve the quality and effectiveness of health information in the VIC RT Department, including booking, planning, treatment and quality assurance activities, through the implementation of information technology. The project was led by a radiation oncologist with special interest in health informatics. Development of the e-Rx for radiation therapy was to represent the first major step in streamlining the planning, treatment, communication and workflow processes in the VIC RT department. Over the course of sixteen months, the new process was designed, developed, and piloted in the VIC RT department.

2.1. Objectives

The objectives of e-Radiate Rx project were to develop and evaluate an e-Rx form and process that could be implemented in the VIC RT department. The new process should allow for improved legibility, accuracy, and accessibility of RT prescriptions, and should enhance RT prescription workflows.

2.2. e-Rx Development Methodology

The e-Radiate Rx project was a grassroots-type project, initiated and led by an end user and clinical champion. Funding and support for the project were provided by the Health Informatics Theme of the Vancouver Island Research and Development Unit (VIRAD), and the bulk of the work on the project was done by health informatics students from the University of Victoria. Three students worked on the project in succession, each for a four month term. No formal project management was done due to limited resources. The following steps were completed:

- Selection of e-Rx software: Dynamic Documents, an add-on feature to Varian oncology information system software called ARIA^{TM} [1] available for use at VIC, was chosen for the creation of electronic prescriptions.

- Development of e-Rx templates by students through collaboration with radiation therapists and oncologists.
- Development of modified workflows and processes to integrate use of the e-Rx form within the VIC RT department
- Piloting of the e-Rx form and process

2.3. e-Rx Evaluation Methodology

An evaluation methodology was developed in order to define the challenges with the paper-based prescription process using the following methods:

- Issue Logs: Radiation therapists experience several common problems with the paper-based RT prescription process. These relate to timeliness of prescription completion, incorrect or missing information on prescription form, and prescription illegibility. Issue Logs were generated and placed in over 100 patient charts to be used by radiation therapists to record the occurrence of these issues.
- Online questionnaires were developed using Survey Monkey™ [3] to gather data on the perceptions and experiences of the RT staff involved with the RT prescription process. Questionnaire links were sent to approximately 70 individuals at VIC, including therapists, physicists, and radiation oncologists.

2.4. Results

Evaluation of the paper-based RT prescription indicated a need for a revised RT prescribing process. Issues were recorded by radiation therapists in nearly 30% of the cases. In addition, over 60% of the 36 online survey respondents indicated that moving towards an electronic prescription would improve the process for prescribing RT. In April, 2010, six out of twelve VIC radiation oncologists began exclusively prescribing RT electronically using the new e-Rx form and process. This corresponded to approximately half of the new patients treated at the VIC RT department. Fourteen days later, the VIC RT Leadership group halted the pilot study in order to review patient safety and clinical workflow concerns raised by RT staff. These concerns included inadequate access of the e-Rx by RT staff due to limited numbers of computer monitors in the treatment suites, unsatisfactory layout of the e-Rx forms, inefficient process of communication of e-Rx changes to RT staff, and high volume of pilot patients.

3. Sociotechnical Evaluation

The intertwinement of technology and the organization in medical informatics and the implications for large-scale IT implementation projects in health care settings has been addressed by many different authors. Lorenzi and Riley have categorized the most common reasons for system implementation failure in health care organizations into: communication, culture, underestimation of complexity, organizational processes, technology, training, and leadership issues [4]. Berg introduced the sociotechnical approach to the development and evaluation of health information systems, whereby a clinical department is seen as an interrelated assembly of people, processes, tools, and documents whose functioning is primarily geared to the delivery of patient care. This approach allows us to examine the challenges of introducing IT applications into the dynamic yet pragmatic nature of healthcare work [2]. Four factors were identified as having critical importance in the ability of the e-Rx project to succeed.

3.1. Absence of Leadership Endorsement and Lack of Organizational Strategy

The sociotechnical approach emphasizes the importance of seeing information system implementation as a strategic transformation, whereby both the technology and the organization are mutually affected. This process can only get off the ground when properly supported by both central management and future users - "A top down vision and framework for the implementation is crucial; only with such a framework can user needs be articulated that transcend individual wish-lists" [7]. Although this project was supported by some of the practice leaders in the department, the RT practice leadership committee was not approached for formal endorsement at the project outset. As a result, an organizational strategy for the implementation of the e-Rx process was not established. This factor was perhaps the most influential in the failure of the e-Rx pilot implementation. Leadership involvement earlier in the process may have enabled concerns from key user groups to be identified and effectively addressed before issues related to patient safety and work efficiency emerged.

3.2. Insufficient Formal and Informal Organizational Power of Clinical Champion

Lorenzi and Riley highlight the importance of both personal intra-organizational respect and formal organizational power of the change leader in order to successfully manage technological change [5]. Successful systems implementations tend to be led by local champions who make major and personal commitments to the projects, and whose enthusiasm is readily transmitted to the people with whom they work [6]. Although the clinical champion was keenly interested and enthusiastic about the project, he lacked both the formal power to mandate its progress and the informal power to transmit his vision and enthusiasm to the radiation therapists who were critical to the success of the project.

3.3. Underestimation of Complexity

The sociotechnical approach argues that information systems implementation projects should be managed as the politically textured, organizational change processes that they inevitably are [2]. Despite an in-depth analysis of RT prescription workflows, the impact of the e-Rx on the workflow of the radiation therapists who worked on the treatment machines was underestimated. It was ultimately this group of users whose concerns about patient safety stalled the implementation. To obtain the support of all involved user groups and to generate departmental commitment, users need to be involved early, thoroughly and systematically [2].

3.4. Inadequate Management of the Implementation Process

As a result of insufficient formal leadership and strategy and inadequate engagement of the treatment therapists, the VIC RT department was unprepared for the pilot implementation of the e-Rx form and process. Key process decisions such as whether and when a print-out of the e-Rx form would be provided, were not formally agreed upon, and were not adequately communicated to the therapists that worked on the treatment units. The new process was implemented for a large number of patients, spanning all disease sites without installation of additional computer monitors in the treatment units. This resulted in delays in accessing the e-Rx information by the therapists and had a negative impact on treatment workflow. Patient safety issues were raised due to the lack of easy and timely access and verification of radiation prescription specifications.

4. Discussion and Conclusions

The e-Rx process using Dynamic Documents has been successfully implemented in other, similar settings, and the organizational culture at VIC is one that embraces change and has a history of technological leadership. The failed pilot implementation of the e-Rx at VIC was multi-factorial and consisted of a combination of lack of leadership endorsement and organizational strategy, inadequate formal and informal organizational power of the project lead, underestimation of complexity, and inadequate management of the implementation process. We describe a snowball effect where one limitation led to another, with the absence of key leadership endorsement identified as the most important cause of project failure.

As of May, 2010, the project has regained footing with enhanced user engagement and the formal support by RT leadership. The e-Rx form and process have been reviewed and amended by the project team, and the modified process will be piloted for a single disease-site group. Through a sociotechnical evaluation of the e-Rx case study, we are able to better understand how some of the concepts of change management in medical informatics can be applied even to smaller-scale clinical transformation projects in highly specialized health care settings. This case study provides some important insight that can benefit future project managers. Even in small, seemingly simple IT implementation projects, it is important to acquire the formal support and endorsement of leadership, and to continually re-assess the organizational impact of the project. By analyzing the factors that influenced the pilot e-Rx implementation, the VIC RT department was able to garner departmental ownership and momentum needed for the future success of the e-Radiate Rx projects.

References

[1]   Varian Medical Systems, Inc. (2010). [cited 2010 June 6]. Available from: http://www.varian.com/us/oncology/radiation_oncology/
[2]   M. Berg, Patient care information systems and health care work: a sociotechnical approach, *Int J Med Inf* **55** (1999), 87-101.
[3]   Survey Monkey, Inc. [Cited 2010 June 6]. Available from: http://www.surveymonkey.com/.
[4]   A. N. Lorenzi, R. T. Riley, *Managing technological change: Organizational aspects of health informatics*, (2nd ed) New York: Springer, 2004.
[5]   N. Lorenzi, R. T. Riley, Organizational issues = Change, *Int J Med Inf* **69** (2003), 197-203.
[6]   N. Lorenzi, R. T. Riley, Managing change: An overview, *JAMIA* **7** (2000), 116-124.
[7]   M. Berg, Implementing information systems in health care organizations: Myths and challenges, *Int J Med Inf* **64** (2001), 143-156.

94

International Perspectives in Health Informatics
E.M. Borycki et al. (Eds.)
IOS Press, 2011
© 2011 ITCH 2011 Steering Committee and IOS Press. All rights reserved.
doi:10.3233/978-1-60750-709-3-94

Defining a Framework for Health Information Technology Evaluation

Eric L. EISENSTEIN[a], Don JUZWISHIN[b],
Andre W. KUSHNIRUK[c], Meredith NAHM[a]

[a] Duke Center for Health Informatics, Duke University Medical Center, Durham, NC
[b] Health Technology Assessment and Innovation, Alberta Health Services,
Edmonton, Alberta,
[c] School of Health Information Science, University of Victoria,
Victoria, British Columbia

Abstract. Governments and providers are investing in health information technologies with little evidence as to their ultimate value. We present a conceptual framework that can be used by hospitals, clinics, and health care systems to evaluate their health information technologies. The framework contains three dimensions that collectively define generic evaluation types. When these types are combined with contextual considerations, they define specific evaluation problems. The first dimension, domain, determines whether the evaluation will address the information intervention or its outcomes. The second dimension, mechanism, identifies the specific components of the new information technology and/or its health care system that will be the subject of the evaluation study. And, the third dimension, timing, determines whether the evaluation occurs before or after the health information technology is implemented. Answers to these questions define a set of evaluation types each with generic sets of evaluation questions, study designs, data collection requirements, and analytic methods. When these types are combined with details of the evaluation context, they define specific evaluation problems.

Keywords. evaluation framework, health information technology

Introduction

In 2009, Charles Friedman proposed a fundamental theorem of biomedical informatics that delineated the boundaries for this discipline [1]. Friedman depicted his theorem as an inequality positing that, "a person working in partnership with an information resource is in some way(s) "better" than that same person unassisted (Figure 1)."

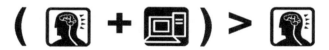

Figure 1. Fundamental Theorem of Informatics

Friedman also proposed two tasks for biomedical informatics. The first task is to develop and sustain information resources seeking to add to the inequality presented in his theorem (increase the imbalance). The second task is to assess whether the inequality is true (people are better with the information resource) and if not, determine why that is the case and revise the information resource so as to increase the likelihood that the inequality will be true. Friedman's second task can be interpreted as assigning to biomedical informatics evaluation the responsibilities of testing the fundamental theorem of biomedical informatics and of determining why people are/are not better off with the use of an information resource. We describe a framework for structuring the field of biomedical informatics evaluation so as to accomplish Friedman's second task.

1. Framework Overview

Our framework for biomedical informatics evaluation contains three dimensions that define generic evaluation types. When these types are combined with contextual considerations, they define specific evaluation problems. The first dimension, domain, determines whether the evaluation will address the information intervention or its outcomes. The second dimension, mechanism, identifies the specific components of the new information technology and/or its health care system that will be the subject of the evaluation study. And, the third dimension, timing, determines whether the evaluation occurs before or after the biomedical informatics system is implemented. Answers to these questions define evaluation types each with generic sets of evaluation questions, study designs, data collection requirements, and analytic methods.

2. Evaluation Domain

Michael Scriven developed a useful formalism that divides evaluation into the fields of formative and summative evaluation [2]. Although Scriven and others have provided formal definitions for these terms, Robert Stake's short-hand version includes the important elements. "When the chef tastes the soup, that's formative evaluation; and when the guest tastes it, that's summative evaluation [3]." Using this distinction, we define formative biomedical informatics evaluation as those aspects of evaluation that seek to optimize the production of information interventions by manipulating person-information resource partnerships. Similarly, we define summative biomedical informatics evaluation as those aspects of evaluation that seek to determine whether people (in the socio-technical system or the wider health care environment) really are 'better' when those information interventions are created. In applying Scriven's distinction to biomedical informatics evaluation, we have separated those aspects of evaluation that are engineering-based from those that more closely resemble heath technology assessment and we have identified distinct areas of evaluation inquiry (Table 1).

For most medical technologies, the roles of developers and evaluators are clearly defined. As an example, pacemaker manufacturers perform rigorous formative evaluations of their devices before they are used in first-in-human studies and they continue to perform formative evaluations throughout the life of their products. These evaluations seek to determine whether a specific pacemaker technology is performing as expected, and are performed according to exacting standards with oversight by regulatory agencies. After these initial formative evaluations are performed, pacemakers are subjected to rigorous summative evaluations of safety and efficacy (also under regulatory guidance) to determine whether persons really are better when these devices are used. Often, they are followed by health technology assessments that evaluate the devices in usual care settings and include economic analyses (tests of effectiveness and efficiency). Because biomedical informatics systems typically do not receive the level of regulatory scrutiny given to other medical technologies, users (or their representatives) of necessity will have to play a larger role in both the formative and summative evaluation of these systems.

Table 1: Formative vs. Summative Evaluation

	Formative Evaluation	**Summative Evaluation**
Objective	Perfect the information intervention	Measure the information intervention's benefits and harms (changes in care processes, clinical, and economic outcomes)
Focus	Persons interacting with an information resource	Persons potentially benefiting from the information resource (system users, health care providers, and patients)
Methods	Management and systems engineering	Health technology assessment
Examples	Usability, workflow, and implementation fidelity analyses	Safety, health outcomes, and health economic studies

3. Evaluation Mechanisms

Biomedical informatics systems can be conceived of as a series of interconnected mechanisms (interventions) that collectively seek to create value for society (increase health benefits or reduce medical costs). Some of these mechanisms are contained within the socio-technical systems (person + information resource) that produce information interventions; whereas, other mechanisms are parts of the wider health care environment. The distinction between formative and summative evaluations presented in the previous section can be useful when determining which mechanisms will be the subject of a specific evaluation study (Figure 2).

Biomedical Informatics Value Chain

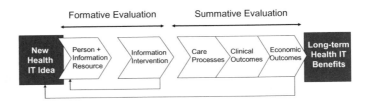

Figure 2. Biomedical Informatics Value Chain Mechanisms

Formative evaluation is concerned with those mechanisms that begin with a new health information technology idea and end with the creation of specific information interventions; whereas, summative evaluation begins with the health care processes that are impacted by the information interventions and ends with potential improvements in society's long-term health benefits. Both types of evaluation provide feedback to improve the person + information resource that creates the information intervention.

While the formative vs. summative distinction is a useful starting point in identifying mechanisms for evaluation, it is not sufficient to identify the specific mechanisms that are thought to provide value and which would be the most important to evaluate. In this regard, the Stead-Lin typology of health information technology domains becomes an important component in our evaluation framework as it provides a means for classifying biomedical informatics systems according to their primary functions (Table 2) [4]. Although the discussion below focuses on the use of the Stead-Lin typology in summative evaluation, we believe that is has similar utility in formative evaluations.

Table 2. Health Information Technology Domains

Domain Name	Domain Description	Example Applications
Automation	Performs tasks with little modification	Administration, lab results, invoicing
Connectivity	Connects systems to each other	Wide are networks, wireless infrastructure
Decision Support	Facilitates or improves decisions	Rule-based alerts, statistical / heuristic support
Data-Mining Capabilities	Recognizes relationships	Provides inputs for evidence-based medicine

Each biomedical informatics system will have one or more information technology functions that are presumed to drive value. When relationships are specified between these information technology mechanisms and resultant changes in health care mechanisms (care process, clinical outcomes and medical costs), they form a value proposition. Typically, this proposition will suggest that medical costs will be reduced or health benefits will be increased through the use of the information mechanism.

When we formulate a value proposition, we begin with the intervention, envision how the intervention's mechanisms will drive benefits and then formally state those benefits. The Stead-Lin typology can be useful in this process as it suggests four ways in which a specific information mechanism may create value for society. Specifically, information mechanisms may automate existing process and lead to more consistent and efficient health care processes; they may connect systems together and provide health care personnel with greater access to information; they may facilitate decision making and improve health care quality; or they may recognize new relationships in data that will support changes in health care systems. By using the Stead-Lin typology as a guide, we can focus our evaluation efforts on those mechanisms that presumably will be the source of the greatest overall benefit.

4. Evaluation Timing

The amounts and types of information available for evaluators changes throughout a biomedical informatics system's lifecycle. When the new health information technology is conceived, there is no direct information for use in evaluation. This means that early phase evaluations must be performed using models and simulations that are based upon information derived from other sources. As a technology is developed, some aspects of evaluation can be performed using the new technology as a source for evaluation information; whereas, other aspects can only be performed using models or simulations. It is only after the technology has been implemented and in use for a while that evaluations can be performed using historical data.

The location of a biomedical informatics technology along the System Development Life Cycle (SDLC) provides a useful perspective when considering the dimension of timing. This cycle describes a continuum of phases starting with project planning, requirements analysis, design, implementation and finally reaching the support phase during post-implementation [5,6]. SDLC phase will have a strong impact on not only the type of applicable evaluation methods but also the setting and overall nature of the evaluation as well as the extent of opportunity for iterative feedback.

A formal recognition of the role information availability plays in evaluations can be shown using a pre- vs. post-implementation comparison (Table 3). At the pre-implementation stage, formative and summative evaluations can be performed. However, they will be conducted in the form of models or simulations that rely upon sources other than the new information technology for their inputs. The major limitation to these pre-implementation models and simulations is that they rely upon assumptions that may not be correct in post-implementation reality. Nonetheless, the results of pre-implementation models and simulations can be useful in assessing in a general manner whether the proposed information technology is likely to produce value for society and in suggesting ways in which it can be modified to optimize the tradeoff between increased costs and increased health care benefits. To the extent that these evaluations can be made with some degree of accuracy, they will improve the development process.

Table 3. Pre- vs. Post-Implementation Evaluation

Attribute	Pre-Implementation	Post-Implementation
Focus	Future	Past and current
Study Data	Other sources	Historical, real data
Study Analyses	Models / projections	Descriptions / observational / empirical
Limitations	Assumptions	Context / generalizability
Accuracy	Variable	More precise
Utility	Good idea?	How did it work?

After implementation, the evaluation question changes from one of what might happen to one of what did happen. This is the time that the presumed relationships identified in pre-implementation evaluation are tested. The objective is to determine whether the information intervention changed elements of the health care environment (care structure, care processes, clinical outcomes, population health and medical costs) in ways that were expected so as to create value for society. If the presumed benefits are not achieved, the evaluator must determine the extent and reasons for these discrepancies and provide this information to system developers.

5. Conclusion

In this paper, we have described a framework for biomedical informatics system evaluation. The three elements of this framework (domain, mechanism, and timing) identify generic evaluation types that frame how a particular evaluation study will be designed and conducted. When these types are combined with details of the evaluation context such as those found in the STEEPLE model, they define unique biomedical informatics evaluation problems [7].

References

[1] C.P. Friedman, A "fundamental theorem" of biomedical informatics, *J Am Med Inform Assoc.* **16** (2009), 169-170.

[2] M.S. Scriven, *The methodology of evaluation, in perspectives of curriculum evaluation, AERA Monograph Series on Curriculum Evaluation,* Rand McNally, Chicago, 1967.

[3] M.S. Scriven, Beyond formative and summative evaluation, in evaluation and education: At quarter century, in: M.W. McLaughlin, D.D. Phillips, editors, *Nineteenth Yearbook of the National Society for the Study of Education,* University of Chicago Press, Chicago, 1991.

[4] W.W. Stead, H.S. Lin, *Computational Technology for Effective Healthcare: Immediate Steps and Strategic Directions,* The National Academic Press, Washington, D.C., 2009.

[5] A. Kushniruk, Evaluation in the design of health information systems: application of approaches emerging from usability engineering, *Comput Biol Med* **32** (2002), 141-149.

[6] S. McConnell, *Rapid Development: Taming Wild Software Schedules,* Microsoft Press, Redmond, Washington, 1996.

[7] J.D. Brehaut, D. Juzwishin, *Bridging the gap: the use of research evidence in policy development,* Health Technology Assessment Unit HTA Initiative #18, Alberta Heritage Foundation for Medical Research, 2005.

Health Records

International Perspectives in Health Informatics
E.M. Borycki et al. (Eds.)
IOS Press, 2011
doi:10.3233/978-1-60750-709-3-103

Use of Ontologies for Monitoring Electronic Health Records for Compliance with Clinical Practice Guidelines

Pam WHITE[a,1], Abdul ROUDSARI[a,b]

a Centre for Health Informatics, School of Informatics, City University, London, UK
b School of Health Information Science, University of Victoria, BC, Canada

Abstract: Ontologies can assist with translating information from an electronic health record to a clinical practice guideline and reformatting it into a compliance report. A 2009 literature search reviews publications on the use of ontologies to support automated reporting of compliance with clinical practice guidelines via electronic health records. Research stage, data-pulling capabilities, ontologies used, and issues raised are some of the comparative data pulled from 13 articles from the literature review results. Suggestions for further research are given.

Keywords: clinical practice guidelines, electronic health records, ontologies, compliance

Introduction

Use of computer-interpretable guideline (CIG) systems has been shown to improve quality of health care [1]. While literature reviews have been published regarding the development of CIG systems, the focus has largely been on guideline structure, execution, and effectiveness [1,2,3,4,5]. Discussions of ontologies in these reviews mostly emphasise supporting guideline access, rather than monitoring for compliance.

Relatively new to the field of health informatics, ontologies are the "specifications of the entities, their attributes and relationships among the entities in a domain of discourse" [6]. Use of terminologies and classifications, facilitation of data exchange among applications, and natural language processing are some functions of ontologies that may facilitate monitoring compliance with clinical practice guidelines (CPGs). A literature review on the use of ontologies for monitoring compliance with CPGs via electronic health records (EHRs) was conducted in 2009.

---

[1] Corresponding Author: Pam White, MLS, Centre for Health Informatics, City University, Northampton Square, London, EC1V 0HB, UK   Email: Pamela.white.1@soi.city.ac.uk

1. Method

Database searches in PubMed MEDLINE, CINAHL, Cochrane, and Web of Science were conducted to identify relevant literature from 2000-2009. Database searches were supplemented by hand-searches of reference lists of the selected articles. The Related Articles search link was used in PubMed for relevant articles. Authors of relevant articles were also searched under a 'Cited Articles' search in Web of Science and/or Google Scholar for follow-up articles by the original first author.

Search statements were based on the following concepts: Clinical Practice Guidelines, Electronic Health Records, Compliance, Ontologies. The PubMed search was stored in NCBI's database and set to send updates.

1.1 Inclusion/exclusion criteria

Titles and abstracts of results were reviewed to determine whether the article was about using ontologies to audit EHRs for compliance with clinical practice guidelines. Articles published in languages other than English were excluded. Articles about single reminder systems were excluded, as clinical practice guidelines tend to be multi-faceted. When an author or group of authors had published more than one article on substantially the same topic, the most recent article was selected. Primary literature was reviewed as a priority, with grey literature included if it met all other criteria. Review articles and commentary were marked for background reading.

1.2 Data Extracted for Comparison

Articles with all 4 concepts were screened for nine comparative pieces of information:
1) Stage of study (proposal, in progress, complete)
2) Whether data was retrieved from an electronic health record
3) If data was retrieved from an electronic health record, could it be retrieved from more than one type of electronic health record model?
4) Ontologies or vocabularies used
5) Whether testing was done in a condition-specific trial
6) Which modelling tools, if any, were used for guidelines?
7) Location of study/authors
8) Length of study
9) Issues raised

2. Results and Discussion

This discussion will synthesise the results from the thirteen studies that met the inclusion/exclusion criteria [7-19]. Issues for monitoring compliance with CPGs via EHRs, drawn from the articles that met the criteria for inclusion, will be described. Issues raised include: scalability and framework, vocabulary and text, coding errors, stage and level of EHR implementation, and CPG content and interpretation.

Table 1 shows the study stage, length and EHR flexibility of the studies analyzed in this review. Eight [9,12,13,14,15,16,17,18] studies have been completed, including those with follow-up articles. Eight studies involved retrieving data from an EHR

[9,10, 13,14,15,16,17,19] though two of these [10,19] were still a work in progress at the time of the submission of this review. Two researchers who had completed their studies were able to retrieve data from more than one type of EHR [14,16].

The longest of the thirteen studies was a four-year retrospective study [15], which has been completed and able to pull data from a single type of EHR. Two studies were in the proposal phase and a third, though in progress, did not state a study length.

Natural language processing or text mining featured in three of the studies [8,13,14]. Techniques for this differed from study to study.

Table 2 shows the number of studies covering a particular condition and assigns codes to the conditions. Table 3 shows which ontologies were used in studies for particular conditions. Although hypertension and diabetes were the most popular conditions involved in the studies, no terminology was exclusively linked to either condition. Six different ontologies were used with hypertension [13,15,16,17,18,19]. International Classification of Diseases (ICD) and Current Procedural Terminology (CPT) were the only two ontologies used by different studies for some of the same conditions [9,11,15,16]. Study location may have been an influential factor in choice of terminologies or ontologies. The majority of the studies have taken place in the United States, with some international author partnerships. One study took place in six European countries [14] and included language translation capabilities.

Table 1: Study Stage, Length, and EHR Flexibility

	Articles about the use of ontologies to measure compliance with CPGs via EHRs
Proposed study	2 [7, 8]
Work in progress	[9] [10], [11], [14] , [12], [13], [18], [19]
Complete	[15], [16], [17]
Able to pull data from EHR,	8 [15], 9, [10], [14], 13, 15, 16,[19]
More than one type?	2 [14], 16)
Updated, including updates by different authors	[8] updated 2007 Not known whether complete [14] updated 2002, now complete [17] updated 2009, built upon completed study [9]) updated 2009, now complete [12] updated 2007, now complete [18] updated 2004, now complete [13] updated 2008, now complete

Table 2: Condition/Procedure Codes (number of studies*)

Condition/Procedure	Code	Number of Studies
Diabetes	Di	5
Cancer waiting times	CW	1
Cardiovascular disease	CD	3
Cholesterol	Ch	3
Preventive services	PS	2
Hypertension	Hy	6
Maternal-Child Health	MCH	1
Endoscopy	En	1

*Some studies covered more than one condition.

Table 3: Ontologies and Conditions

Ontology	# of Studies	Condition/Procedure Code
Systematized Nomenclature of Medicine Clinical Terms	3	Di, CW [7], En [14], PS [12]
Unified Medical Language System	1	CD [11]
International Classification of Diseases	2	Di, Ch, CD [15], Di, MCH [9]
Current Procedural Terminology	3	Di, Ch, CD [15], Di, CD, Ch, Hy [16], CD [11]
National Drug Code	1	Di, Ch, CD (Stanek)
Not specified and local (proposed)	2	Hy [8], CD [11]
Omaha Nursing	1	Di, MCH [9]
International Classification of Primary Care	1	Ch [10]
World Health Organisation Anatomical Therapeutic Chemical classification system	1	Ch [10]), Di, Hy [17]
Minimal Standard Terminology for gastrointestinal endoscopy	1	En (14)
Logical Observation Identifiers Names and Codes	1	PS [12]
Operational Conceptual Modelling Language	1	Hy (13)
Quality Indicator Language	1	Hy [18]
Advisory Adherence Evaluator	1	Hy [19]
Guideline Interchange Format 3, Guideline Execution Engine, and Guideline Expression Language	1	PS [12]
LISP-Miner	1	Hy [13]
MedCritic, EON, Asgaard architectures (author-developed)	1	Hy [18]
EBM Connect (commercial software)	1	Di, CD, Ch, Hy [16]
Knowledge-Based Temporal Abstraction	1	Di, Hy [17])
Assessment and Treatment of Hypertension: Evidence-Based Automation (locally developed)	1	Hy [19]

2.1 Issues Raised

Issues raised include: scalability and framework, vocabulary and text, coding errors, stage and level of EHR implementation, and CPG content and interpretation. While other issues may have been discussed in the articles, these were most prominent and most relevant to the use of ontologies for monitoring compliance with CPGs via EHRs. Each of these issues has a direct bearing on or is an example of an entity, attribute, or relationship, which shows a connection with the realm of ontologies.

2.1.1 Scalability and Framework

Warren [17] and Advani [18] note that scalability can be an issue when building upon trials of EHR monitoring for compliance with CPGs. Advani explains one reason is that successful systems may focus on just one element or stage of guideline audit. Stanek [15] cautions that researchers must avoid patient selection bias and watch for other misleading variables, such as missing data and temporal issues. Advani indicates the need for a method for determining full versus partial compliance.

2.1.2 Vocabulary and Text

There are vocabulary and text issues from both guideline and EHR sides for compliance monitoring. Hung [11] and Monsen [9] warn that the limited granularity of controlled vocabularies used to code guidelines may cloud audit processes. Svatek [13] and Delvaux [14] state that there are difficulties in processing text in patient records. Free text tends to be used for technical issues. The ability to assign attributes within controlled vocabularies is a possible solution to mapping technical components of EHRs. Delvaux explains a method to partially automate identification of frequently associated findings, thus reducing the need for multiple initial terms.

2.1.3 Coding Errors

Most of the studies covered in this analysis have emphasised audit via clinical coding. The software used in Welch's research, EBM Connect, relies on clinical coding to audit EHRs for compliance with CPGs [20]. Stanek [15] and van Wyk [10] warn that audit of EHRs can be challenged by miscoding. For example, miscoding a drug for the wrong condition may falsely skew audit statistics for incidence and prevalence.

2.1.4 Stage and Level of EHR Implementation

Welch [16] noted that stage and level of EHR implementation has an impact on the cost effectiveness of EHR use, including the cost-effectiveness of the use CIGs. Measuring the cost-effectiveness of CIGs requires the monitoring of compliance with the CIGs.

2.1.5 CPG Content and Interpretation

The content of CPGs may interfere with compliance, sometimes in ways that are not undesirable. Treatment decisions for some patients may not be covered by a guideline [8,13,18]. Guidelines may be outdated or have errors in the text [13]. They may be inadequate with respect to data chosen for analysis or their formalisation may have been erroneous [12,13,18]. Interpretation of guidelines may differ amongst clinicians [12]. Patient compliance may also be a factor [10].

2.2 Limitations

There were several limitations to this review. Some articles mentioned pulling data from EHRs, but did not specify the methodology or note any ontology used and could not be used in this review. Some articles that were determined to include all four concepts did not actually test their software against an EHR. These articles focussed on methodologies for improving technologies for auditing EHRs, rather than the actual testing of those technologies on an EHR. These articles were included in the review.

Because 'ontology' is such a broad concept, with little agreement on specific terms to describe its functions [21,22], it was near impossible to include all possible relevant terms in the literature search statements.

This review did not determine which studies covered audit mechanisms that were part of a larger guideline implementation system.

3. Conclusions

Many studies on computer-interpretable guidelines emphasise guideline modelling and accessibility via EHRs. Some decision support systems have the potential to integrate monitoring for guideline compliance into the workflow [5]. There are relatively few published studies on using ontologies to audit EHRs for compliance with CPGs without necessarily incorporating guideline modelling and/or access. A modular, rather than standalone system may be better due to the flexibility offered by a modular approach.

This paper has explored the use of ontologies to audit electronic health records for compliance with clinical practice guidelines. Suggested areas for further research include: scalability of and framework for CPG audit systems, mapping vocabularies and text, controlling coding errors, and determining appropriate stage and level of EHR implementation for suitability of introducing a CPG audit system.

References

[1]   G. Damiani, L. Pinnarelli, S. C. Colosimo, et al. The effectiveness of computerized clinical guidelines in the process of care: a systematic review. *BMC Health Serv Res.* **10** (2010), 2.
[2]   F. A. Sonnenberg, C. G. Hagerty. Computer-interpretable clinical practice guidelines. Where are we and where are we going? *Yearb Med Inform.* (2006) 145-58.
[3]   T. Y. Leong, K. Kaiser, S Miksch. Free and open source enabling technologies for patient-centric, guideline-based clinical decision support: a survey. *Yearb Med Inform.* (2007) 74-86. Erratum in: Yearb Med Inform. (2008) 19.
[4]   M. Peleg M, Tu S, Bury J, et al. Comparing computer-interpretable guideline models: a case-study approach. J Am Med Inform Assoc. **10** (2003), (1):52-68.
[5]   Isern, D; Moreno A. Computer-based execution of clinical guidelines: A review. International journal of medical informatics **77** (2008), 787–808.
[6]   Rubin DL, Shah NH and Noy NF. Biomedical Ontologies: a functional perspective. Briefings in Bioinformatics **9** (2008), (1):75-90.
[7]   Bernstein K, Andersen U. Managing care pathways combining SNOMED CT, archetypes and an electronic guideline system. Stud Health Technol Inform. **136** (2008), 353-8.
[8]   Steichen O, Daniel-Lebozec C, Charlet J, et al. Use of electronic health records to evaluate practice individualization. AMIA Annu Symp Proc. (2006), 1110.
[9]   Monsen KA, Fitzsimmons LL, Lescenski BA, et al. A public health nursing informatics data-and-practice quality project. Comput Inform Nurs. **24** (2006), (3):152-8.
[10]   Van Wyk JT, Van Wijk MA. Assessment of the possibility to classify patients according to cholesterol guideline screening criteria using routinely recorded electronic patient record data. Stud Health Technol Inform. **93** (2002), 39-46.
[11]   Hung PW, Stetson PD. Development of a quality measurement ontology in OWL. AMIA Annu Symp Proc. (2007) 984.
[12]   Wang, DW; Peleg, M; Tu, SW; et al.. Design and implementation of the GLIF3 guideline execution engine. *Journal of Biomedical Informatics* **37** (2004), (5):305-318.
[13]   Svátek V, Ríha A, Peleska J, et al. Analysis of guideline compliance--a data mining approach. Stud Health Technol Inform. **101** (2004), 157-61.
[14]   Delvaux M, Crespi M, Armengol-Miro JR, et al. Minimal standard terminology for digestive endoscopy: results of prospective testing and validation in the GASTER project. Endoscopy. **32** (2000), (4):345-55.
[15]   Stanek EJ, Sarawate C, Willey VJ, et al. Risk of cardiovascular events in patients at optimal values for combined lipid parameters. Curr Med Res Opin. ;**23** (2007), (3):553-63.
[16]   Welch WP, Bazarko D, Ritten K, et al. Electronic health records in four community physician practices: impact on quality and cost of care. J Am Med Inform Assoc. **14** (2007), (3):320-8.
[17]   Warren J, Gadzhanova S, Stanek J, etal. Understanding caseload and practice through analysis of therapeutic state transitions. AMIA Annu Symp Proc. (2005), 784-8.
[18]   Advani A, Shahar Y, and Musen MA, Medical Quality Assessment by Scoring Adherence to Guideline Intentions, Proc AMIA Symp. (2001), 2-6.

[19] Chan AS, Coleman RW, Martins SB, et al. Evaluating provider adherence in a trial of a guideline-based decision support system for hypertension. Stud Health Technol Inform. 107 (2004), (1):125-9.
[20] Ingenix. Symmetry EBM Connect Product Sheet. Accessed online, 24/06/10 at: http://www.ingenix.com/content/attachments/SymmetryEBMConnectproductsheet.pdf
[21] Bodenreider O. Biomedical Ontologies in Action: Role in Knowledge Management, Data Integration and Decision Support. Methods Inf Med 47 (2008), Suppl 1;:67-79.
[22] Rubin DL, Shah NH and Noy NF. Biomedical Ontologies: a functional perspective. Briefings in Bioinformatics 9 (2008), (1):75-90.

International Perspectives in Health Informatics
E.M. Borycki et al. (Eds.)
IOS Press, 2011
doi:10.3233/978-1-60750-709-3-110

The Use of Biometrics in the Personal Health Record (PHR)

Wilfred BONNEY[1]

School of Business and Technology, Capella University, USA

Abstract. The emergence of the Personal Health Record (PHR) has made individual health information more readily accessible to a wide range of users including patients, consumers, practitioners, and healthcare providers. However, increased accessibility of PHR threatens the confidentiality, privacy, and security of personalized health information. Therefore, a need for robust and reliable forms of authentication is of prime concern. The concept of biometric authentication is now highly visible to healthcare providers as a technology to prevent unauthorized access to individual health information. Implementing biometric authentication mechanisms to protect PHR facilitates access control and secure exchange of health information. In this paper, a literature review is used to explore the key benefits, technical barriers, challenges, and ethical implications for using biometric authentication in PHR.

Keywords. biometrics, personal health record, confidentiality, privacy, security

Introduction

The emergence of electronically stored medical records has made medical information more readily accessible to a wide range of users, including patients, consumers, practitioners, and healthcare providers [1]. Popular amongst these stored medical records is the Personal Health Record (PHR). PHR is a consumer-centric "tool to use in sharing health information, increasing health understanding, and helping transform patients into better-educated consumers of health" [2]. However, increased accessibility of PHR threatens the confidentiality, privacy, and security of personalized health information [3,4]. Therefore, a need for robust and reliable forms of authentication is of prime concern [4].

The need for secure Healthcare Information Systems has become critical as a result of the security requirements of Health Insurance Portability and Accountability Act (HIPAA); and Personal Information Protection and Electronic Document Act (PIPEDA) [4-6]. As patients continue to access and use PHR to document their personal health information such as medical history, medical and emergency contacts, outpatient and hospital visits, immunization tracking, insurance records, and health-related alerts; there is an increasing necessity to have a reliable forms of authentication in place to verify their individual identities [5,7]. Any secure authentication mechanism

---

[1] Corresponding Author: Wilfred Bonney, School of Business and Technology, Capella University; E-mail: bonney@cs.dal.ca

developed must be based on a solid understanding of the intended uses and business requirements of the PHR.

Inadequate security of Healthcare Information Systems such as Electronic Health Record (EHR) and PHR poses a potential liability to the organization associated not only with HIPAA and PIPEDA requirements but also with loss of confidential information, denial of service, and compromised data integrity [5,6,8,9]. Biometric authentication is often considered as a technology that would help protect the integrity, confidentiality, privacy, and security of sensitive electronic health data contained in the PHR [5,6,10]. The objective of this paper is to explore the key benefits, technical barriers, challenges, and ethical implications for using biometric authentication in PHR. The first part of the paper gives an overview of biometrics and PHR. In the second part, the focus is on the key benefits, challenges, and technical barriers for implementing biometric authentication in PHR. The third part focuses on ethical implications for integrating biometric authentication with PHR.

1. Introduction to Biometrics

According to Pocovnicu [11], the "etymology of the word biometrics comes from the ancient Greek words: 'bios' - life and 'metros' – measure" (pg. 1). Biometrics, in its purest form, is a science that focuses on the statistical analysis of biological phenomena and measures to determine individual identity [5,6,8,12]. Biometrics is a rapidly advancing field and is gaining popularity in the IT industry because of its ability to provide a methodology for determining authorized persons for access to facilities and services based on their physiological or behavioral characteristics [8,12-15].

The biometric technology enables an automatic authentication and/or identification of individuals based on some physiologically and behavioural characteristics such as fingerprints, iris, retina, voice, gait, odour, or facial features [8,12,16-18]. In distinguishing the differences between biometric authentication and identification, Zorkadis and Donos [18], asserted that biometric authentication answers the question: "Am I who I claim to be?" and the biometric identification answers the question: "Who am I?". Whereas the authentication mechanism "verifies the identity of the person by processing biometric data, which refers to the person who asks and takes a yes/no decision (1:1 comparison)" [18], the identification mechanism recognizes the "individual who asks by distinguishing him from other persons whose biometric data is also stored in the database and takes 1-of-n decision" [18]. Compared to other non-biometric identifiers, biometric authentication provides some inherent usability advantages that correspond to a direct evidence of the personal identity versus possession of secrets which can be potentially stolen [8,14,16].

When it comes to securing Healthcare Information Systems hosted in an online environment, a reliable user authentication method is very crucial and any attempt to maximize security vulnerabilities is of great essence. This is because the security of personalized health data is one of the most important parts of privacy protection legislation [18] and the "consequences of an insecure authentication system in a corporate or enterprise environment can be catastrophic, and may include loss of confidential information, denial of service, and compromised data integrity" [13]. Fortunately, the availability of automated biometrics authentication methods such as fingerprint, face, iris, and speech recognition can provide a much more accurate and reliable user authentication method [12,13,18,19].

In the context of Health Information Exchange, biometrics technologies are increasingly being viewed as a means of managing access to information systems, facilitating easier access to medical information, protecting health records, preventing the unauthorized use of system resources, developing new measures for combating bio-terrorism, defending health care consumers against fraud, and ensuring the security of financial and patient records [5,17,20]. These properties of biometrics make the technology more attractive and popular in many healthcare organizations worldwide.

2. Introduction to PHR

PHR is a modern healthcare information system or software application that can strengthen patients' ability to actively manage their own health and healthcare [1,7]. The key features of the PHR are that "it is under the control of the subject of care and that the information it contains is at least partly entered by the subject (i.e. consumer, patient)" [21].

Healthcare providers benefit enormously from the increasing use of PHR by patients and/or consumers. PHR "offer the promise of reducing medical errors, improving disease management, and reducing the overall costs of healthcare delivery by empowering patients as active participants in their own health care" [1]. PHR is also considered as an innovative and transformative health technology that fundamentally change self-care and healthcare delivery in ways that add substantial value to individuals and society [7].

PHR has many functionalities and capabilities in supporting and improving healthcare delivery. Some of the capabilities includes the ability to (a) improve the availability of patient information at the point of care; (b) enable electronic connectivity between clinical care managers and patients or their caregivers; (c) enable a shift in the health care locus of control to consumers by moving the control of health information from providers to patients or to a more shared control; and (d) reduce costs and improve healthcare delivery by facilitating the sharing of patient and administrative information among health care systems, thereby, reducing redundant transactions and tests [7].

These capabilities of the PHR require that information stored in the PHR is transmitted securely and accessed only by the authorized users. The security of health data is, therefore, of great concern when it comes to the adoption and implementation of PHR. Many patients entrust healthcare providers with their primary care data with the expectation that their privacy and confidentiality will not be violated. However, in many cases, the security vulnerabilities of Healthcare Information Systems lead to unauthorized access of personalized health information. The use of biometric authentication in PHR has the potential to maximize the secure exchange of health information and limit access only to authorized users [17,20].

3. Key Benefits of Integrating Biometrics with PHR

There are tremendous opportunities, by researchers, to integrate biometric authentication with PHR in the healthcare domain. With an increasing adoption of EHR and PHR, the biometric authentication technology is slowly gaining traction in the healthcare domain. Security and privacy are the main driving force for the utilization of biometrics in PHR. The ultimate goal of using PHR is to ensure that personalized health information is transmitted securely and is accessible only by the authorized users in a secure environment. The use of biometrics will not only enable much tighter control over patients and/or consumers access to the PHR but also provide tighter audit trails for tracking patients' activities and encounters in the continuum of integrated Healthcare Information Systems [7].

In the context of healthcare interoperability, the most significant feature of the PHR is its ability to share information between different authorized users in a secure environment [21]. There is an expectation that the adoption rates of PHR will increase with increasing security and protection of personal health information. Increase in the adoption of PHR is a "necessary means to improving patient safety, quality, and evidence-based practice" [22]. Healthcare providers who adopt PHR will require that clinical information be protected and private at all time; and that storage and secondary uses of the primary care data be approved by patients [2,23].

4. Technical Barriers

There is a widespread misapprehension in the healthcare IT community as to what constitutes PHR. This misapprehensions emanates from the fact that the PHR is considered to be a completely different entity from the EHR if it is to meet the requirements of patients/consumers to create, enter, maintain, and retrieve data in a form meaningful to them and to control their own health record [21]. Depending on whether the PHR should use different architecture than the EHR presents different security architecture, challenges, and protocols that might not necessarily satisfy the requirements of participating healthcare providers. This might lead to different levels of security that could complicate the implementation of a biometric authentication in integrated Healthcare Information Systems.

There is also an issue of who owns the clinical information contained in the PHR. There is no clear consensus among healthcare providers as to whether the clinical data stored in the PHR is owned by patients/consumers, healthcare providers, or third party organizations such as a Web service provider [15]. This also presents security challenges in implementing the biometric technology. Knowing the data ownership is important in defining access control to various files stored in the repository of the PHR.

5. Key Challenges

The biometric technology has challenges on its own. The drawback of using biometrics in PHR is that of privacy and security concerns associated with handling health data. The storage of "biometric information in repositories along with other personally identifiable information raises several security and privacy risks" [16]. This is because the databases storing the biometric data are vulnerable to attacks by insiders or external adversaries and may be searched or used outside of their intended purposes [14,16].

Biometrics uses matching algorithms that are probabilistic in nature, meaning that two samples of the same individual are never exactly the same [16]. The fact that the biometric systems cannot rely on the same process for authenticating individuals makes it very hard to revoke and change biometrics in case biometric data are compromised [14,16]. Hence in a situation whereby the security is compromised, fixing the problem will take some time compared to problems related to changing passwords of non-biometric systems.

Moreover, the extent to which authorized users of a biometric system have to go through in order to access clinical information is often time-consuming and challenging. It brings out the question of how much security protocols are needed in order to access a single patient record. The biometric technology is seen, by many people, as "being intrusive, a potential tool for demographic profiling, and a means of eroding individual privacy" [20]. This viewpoint of the public has often affected its implementation efforts worldwide. Other challenges facing the implementation of the biometric technology include physical traits of individuals; and system, business, operational and legal issues [14,18,20].

6. Ethical Implications

The ethical implications on the use of biometric authentications in PHR often stem from the fact that PHR contains digitized personal health information and is complicated with the ethical considerations associated with the use of electronic health data. According to Myers et al [3], confidentiality and privacy concerns are even more sensitive in the digital age and high-profile "breaches of individuals' health information have heightened anxiety about privacy, as have plans to create interconnected electronic health information networks".

Electronic health data formats can improve performance of healthcare delivery and core public health functions, but potentially threaten confidentiality and privacy because they can be easily duplicated and transmitted to unauthorized people [3]. Although such security breaches is common and do occur, electronic health data can be better secured than paper charts, "because authentication, authorization, auditing, and accountability can be facilitated" [3].

These characteristics of electronic health data call for the development of a strict governance policy for managing the accessibility of PHR. The policy process for PHR can be improved by having a minimum PHR governance structure. The governance structure should accurately reflect and serve a broad purpose for PHR, thereby, facilitating the communication between clinicians and patients [1]. Reti et al [1] proposed a governance structure that recognizes clinicians and patients as key stakeholders of PHR and include them as members.

7. Conclusion

There is no doubt that the biometric technology seemingly has tremendous potential in facilitating cost reductions, enhanced information security, increased quality of care, improved accessibility, and even greater geographic equity of healthcare delivery [20]. Secure authentication of personal health information is a critical component of the consumer-driven healthcare applications such as EHR and PHR [4]. These requirements can be effectively handled using biometric authentication technology to maximize the confidentiality, integrity, privacy and security of personalized health information. Kahn et al [2] claimed that the adoption of the PHR is not possible until all issues relating to technical barriers, policy barriers, and consumer satisfactions are resolved by dedicated national bodies.

It is therefore recommended that the biometric technology is implemented in a phased approach to ensure that all security loopholes are addressed during the deployment phase. Although the use of biometrics in PHR has enormous benefits, the cost of implementation cannot be ignored [6,8,14]. Many healthcare providers are not willing to implement a biometric-based technology that is very costly only to find out that the security of the health data is still vulnerable to some phishing and spoofing attacks [13,16]. Future research should focus on combining biometric authentication with other cryptographic techniques to ensure that electronic health data is highly protected and secured.

References

[1]   S.R. Reti, H.J. Feldman, C. Safran, Governance for personal health records. *JAMIA.* **16(1)** (2009),14-17.
[2]   J. Kahn, V. Aulakh, A. Bosworth, What it takes: Characteristics of the ideal personal health record. *Health Aff.* **Mar/Apr;28(2)** (2009), 369-376.
[3]   J. Myers, T.R. Frieden, K.M. Bherwani, K.J. Henning, Privacy and public health at risk: Public health confidentiality in the digital age. *Am. J. Public Health* **May 98(5)** (2008), 793-801.
[4]   U. Sax, I. Kohane, K.D. Mandl, Wireless technology infrastructures for authentication of patients: PKI that rings. *J Am Med. Inform Assoc.* **May/Jun;12(3)** (2005), 263-268.
[5]   R.A. Perrin, Biometrics technology adds innovation to healthcare organization security systems. *Healthc. Financ. Manage* **Mar;56(3)** (2002), 86-88.
[6]   R.L. Simpson, Eyeing IT trends and challenges. *Nurs. Manage.* **Dec;33(12)** (2002), 46-47.
[7]   D. Detmer, M. Bloomrosen, B. Raymond, P. Tang, Integrated personal health records: Transformative tools for consumer-centric care. *BMC Med. Inform. Decis. Making* **8(1)** (2008), 45-58.
[8]   C.L. Smith, The science of biometric identification. *Aust. Science Teachers J.* **Sep;49(3)** (2003), 34-39.
[9]   L.A. Gordon, M.P. Loeb, The economics of information security investment. *ACM Trans. on Inf. and Syst. Secur.* **5(4)** (2002), 438-457.
[10] P. Starr, Health and the right to privacy. *Am J. of Law and Medicine* **25(2/3)** (1999), 193-201.
[11] A. Pocovnicu, Biometric Security for Cell Phones. *Informatica Economica* **13(1)** (2009), 57-63.
[12] P.M. Corby, T. Schleyer, H. Spallek, T.C. Hart, Using biometrics for participant identification in a research study: A case report. *J Am Med. Inform Assoc.* **Mar/Apr;13(2)** (2006), 233-235.
[13] N.K. Ratha, J.H. Connell, R.M. Bolle, Enhancing security and privacy in biometrics-based authentication systems. *IBM Syst. J.* **40(3)** (2001), 614-634.
[14] J. Langenderfer, S. Linnhoff, The emergence of biometrics and its effect on consumers. *J. Consum. Aff.* **Winter;39(2)** (2005), 314-338.
[15] S. Venkatraman, I. Delpachitra,. Biometrics in banking security: A case study. *Inf. Manage. Comput. Secur.* **16(4)** (2008), 415-430.
[16] A. Bhargav-Spantzel, A.C. Squicciarini, S. Modi, M.Young, E. Bertino, S.J. Elliott,. Privacy preserving multi-factor authentication with biometrics. *J. Comput. Secur.* **10;15(5)** (2007), 529-560.
[17] A.E. Flores Zuniga, K.T. Win, W. Susilo, Biometrics for electronic health records. *J. Med. Syst.* **34(5)** (2010), 975-983.
[18] V. Zorkadis, P. Donos, On biometrics-based authentication and identification from a privacy-protection perspective: Deriving privacy-enhancing requirements. *Inf. Manage. Comput. Secur.* **12(1)** (2004), 125-137.
[19] O.T., Song, A.T.B. Jin, T. Connie, Personalized biometric key using fingerprint biometrics. *Inf. Manage. Comput. Secur.* **15(4)** (2007), 313-328.

[20] A. Chandra, R. Durand, S. Weaver, The uses and potential of biometrics in health care. *Int. J. Pharm. and Healthc. Mark.* **2(1)** (2008), 22-34.

[21] International Organization for Standardization (ISO/TC 215). Health informatics — Electronic health record — Definition, scope, and context. (2005), 1-27.

[22] T.J. Watkins, R.E. Haskell, C.B. Lundberg, J.M. Brokel, M.L. Wilson, N. Hardiker, Terminology use in electronic health records: basic principles. *Urol. Nurs.* **29(5)** (2009), 321-327.

[23] J. Adler-Milstein, D.W. Bates, Paperless healthcare: Progress and challenges of an IT-enabled healthcare system. *Bus. Horiz.* **4;53(2)** (2010), 119-130.

International Perspectives in Health Informatics
E.M. Borycki et al. (Eds.)
IOS Press, 2011
doi:10.3233/978-1-60750-709-3-117

Longitudinal Analysis on Utilization of Medical Document Management System in a Hospital with EPR Implementation

Shigeki KUWATA[a,1], Hitomi YAMADA[b], Keunsik Park[b]

[a]*Division of Medical Informatics, Tottori University Hospital, Yonago, Tottori, Japan*
[b]*Department of Medical Informatics, Osaka City University Hospital, Abeno, Osaka, Japan*

Abstract. Document management systems (DMS) have widespread in major hospitals in Japan as a platform to digitize the paper-based records being out of coverage by EPR. This study aimed to examine longitudinal trends of actual use of DMS in a hospital in which EPR had been in operation, which would be conducive to planning the further information management system in the hospital. Degrees of utilization of electronic documents and templates with DMS were analyzed based on data extracted from a university-affiliated hospital with EPR. As a result, it was found that the number of electronic documents as well as scanned documents circulating at the hospital tended to increase. The result indicated that replacement of paper-based documents with electronic documents did not occur. Therefore it was anticipated that the need for DMS would continue to increase in the hospital. The methods used this study to analyze the trend of DMS utilization would be applicable to other hospitals with with a variety of DMS implementation, such as electronic storage by scanning documents or paper preservation that is compatible with EPR.

Keywords. document management system, electronic document, electronic patient record, scanned document, template

Introduction

A trend of information technology concerning medical records has drastically turned from the former paper-based storage into the EPR system. Some of paper-based documents, however, still tend to remain unchanged as flexible media even after the introduction of EPR. With a variety of the documents, it is highly effective to store the document information into the electronic database to organize and utilize the contents of the documents as beneficial resources in hospitals. In Japan, document management systems (DMS) have widespread in major hospitals in response to such need as a platform to digitize the paper-based records being out of coverage by EPR [1].

This study aimed to examine longitudinal trends of actual use of DMS in a hospital in which EPR had been in operation, which would contribute to planning the further information management system in the hospital.

---

[1] Corresponding Author: Dr. Shigeki Kuwata; shig@med.tottori-u.ac.jp

1. Methods

1.1. Target Facility in This Study

The target medical facility in this study was a university-affiliated hospital with 35 clinics and 1,005 beds at an urban area in Japan. The hospital had 2,100 outpatients visits per day and 1,300 discharged patients per month in average as of 2009. Accompanied with the adoption of EPR, HOPE/EGMAIN-EX [2], to the hospital in 2007, a medical document management system (DMS), Yahgee [3], was also introduced to replace large part of conventional paper-based medical documents with electronic documents. The system had characteristics as follows: 1) it was able to preserve the original format of pre-existing paper documents as electronic templates, 2) it enabled end users to create and customize the templates, and 3) all data input by users in documents were stored into its database that would be useful for secondary use of clinical data.

Documents within coverage of the system were linked to EPR that possessed indexes for the documents. Accordingly users were able to access the documents through interfaces of EPR. On the other hand, paper documents being out of coverage by DMS were scanned and registered into EPR.

1.2. Data Extraction

Logged data for created documents and templates from May 2007 to November 2009 (31 months) were extracted from DMS. In addition, logged data for documents scanned and registered to EPR in November from 2007 to 2009 were also collected from a data warehouse system equipped with EPR.

1.3. Trends of Document Creation and Template Utilization

Frequencies of newly created electronic documents with DMS were compared with the total number of patients, calculated as the amount of inpatients and outpatients, at the hospital. Subsequently frequencies of (1) newly registered electronic templates, (2) "active" templates, defined as templates that actually circulated in past six months, and (3) templates in use with DMS were counted and analyzed to examine if the templates "actively" circulated in the hospital. All data were added up for each month during the target period.

2. Results and discussion

Figure 1 shows the longitudinal course of document creation with DMS. The number of documents and also the number per capita (patient) tended to increase. As seen in 6-month moving average plots, a remarkable rise of the number of documents was found. In addition, the increase was accompanied with that of the total number of patients, as well as a with the increase of documents per capita (Figure 2). It was likely that both paper-based and electronic documents circulating in the hospital increased, since scanned documents, being out of coverage by DMS, also increased with the same trend as shown in Figure 3.

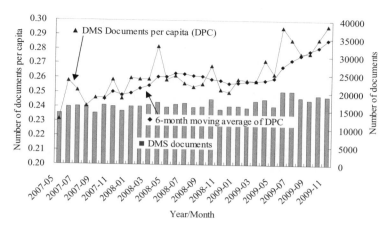

Figure 1. Longitudinal course of the relationship between the number of newly created documents and the number of newly created documents per capita (patient) in the document management system (DMS).

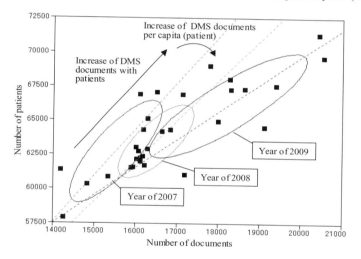

Figure 2. Longitudinal course of the relationship between numbers of patients and newly created documents in the document management system (DMS). Each plot corresponds to data for each month of the year. Circle represents bivariate normal ellipse by orthogonal regression (P=0.5).

Figure 4 represents the longitudinal course of registered templates, "active" templates and templates in use. The accumulated number of templates registered in DMS increased almost constantly reaching to approximately 1,000 entries at the end of the period, while active templates remained almost constant until May 2009 followed by substantial increase of active templates. The increase was also found at the number of templates in use, but it reduced to the previous level at the end. It was noted that a similar rise occurred at the same period in the number of newly created documents, as found at 6-month moving average plots in Figure 1. From those findings it was concluded that considerable amount of templates that frequently circulated was registered in May 2009, which caused the increase of documents and active templates. The occasional rise, however, did not greatly affect the number of templates in use.

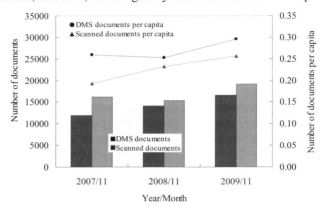

Figure 3. Longitudinal course of number of documents in the document management system (DMS) and scanned documents (out of coverage by DMS).

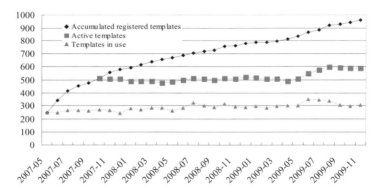

Figure 4. Longitudinal course of number of registered templates and their utilization in the document management system.

Of 766 templates registered at the beginning of the period (May 2007), 265 (35%) were constantly circulated throughout the period (26 months as active templates), whereas 128 (17%) were never used as active documents (Figure 5).

Figure 6 shows the distribution of the number of newly created documents per month against frequency of active template utilization with DMS. For the templates being active for 26 months, approximately 40% of them circulated with more than 100 documents that were monthly created with DMS. On the contrary, 90% of other templates circulated with only less than 10 documents per month. It was likely that documents that kept longer active status generally tended to originate from templates that frequently circulated in the hospital.

It should be noted that the findings from this study would not be applied to other hospitals without considering differences between facilities on several conditions, *e.g.*, coverage by DMS, EPR and other systems, business workflow of medical professionals, and so on. The analysis methods of the study, however, would be useful to other facilities regardless of those conditions.

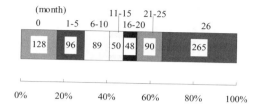

Figure 5. Active utilization of templates in the document management system (unit in month).

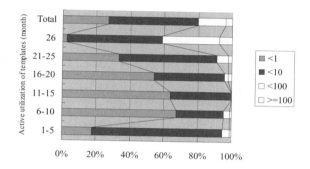

Figure 6. Distribution of number of newly created documents per month against frequency of active utilization of templates in the document management system.

3. Conclusion

The number of electronic documents in DMS increased even in the hospital in which EPR had been in operation. The cause attributed to the increase of both patients and circulated documents per capita. The results of the study also indicated replacement of paper-based documents with electronic documents did not occur, since scanned documents also increased with electronic documents. Therefore it was anticipated that the need for DMS would continue to increase in the hospital. The methods used this study to analyze the trend of DMS utilization would be applicable to other hospitals with a variety of DMS implementation, such as electronic storage by scanning documents or paper preservation that is compatible with EPR.

References

[1] K. Kunimoto, Document Management with EPR, *Japan J Med Inf* **29**(suppl.) (2009), 48–49.
[2] HOPE/EGMAIN-EX, Fujitsu Limited. http://segroup.fujitsu.com/medical/products/egmainex [accessed: May 31, 2010] (in Japanese)
[3] Yahgee Co.,Ltd. http://www.yahgee.jp/ [accessed: June 16, 2010] (in Japanese)

International Perspectives in Health Informatics
E.M. Borycki et al. (Eds.)
IOS Press, 2011
© *2011 ITCH 2011 Steering Committee and IOS Press. All rights reserved.*
doi:10.3233/978-1-60750-709-3-122

Early Development of an Enterprise Health Data Warehouse

Mowafa Said HOUSEH[a,1], Majid AL-TUWAIJRI[a]

[a] *College of Public Health and Health Informatics, King Saud Bin Abdul Aziz University for Health Science, Riyadh, Kingdom of Saudi Arabia*

Abstract. The purpose of this study is to describe early development challenges of an enterprise data warehouse within a Saudi Arabian academic healthcare facility. An action case research method was selected for this paper. The study took place between December 2009 and February 2010. Data collection included interviews, meeting observations, and meeting minutes. Early development challenges centered on the development of clear contracts with vendors; development of a clear project plan; a need to fast-track bureaucracy; and educate clinicians and staff about the project; and lack of data standardization

Keywords. electronic data warehouse, Saudi Arabia, healthcare, challenges

Introduction

A challenge healthcare organizations face today is the ability to link various databases with each other to create reports that are useful for decision-makers. Part of the problem can be attributed to the vertical organizational design that has led to the creation of information silos. These legacy organizational designs do persist and contribute to the problem of information processing within healthcare organizations.

Tomorrow's successful healthcare organizations will be designed around the building blocks of information technology. The success of these organizations will be a result of their ability to use information as a main driver for clinical and administrative decision-making. In this type of organization, decisions will be informed through data. Clinicians and administrative staff will be more informed and able to make more informed decisions for quality improvement.

Along the way towards this type of organization, there will be mistakes made and lessons to be learned. In this paper, we explore early development challenges of an Enterprise Data Warehouse (EDW) project within a large healthcare institution in the Kingdom of Saudi Arabia. Lessons learned from the early development challenges are discussed.

---

[1] Dr. Mowafa Househ, King Saud Bin Abdul Aziz University for Health Sciences, College of Public Health and Health Informatics, Riyadh, Kingdom of Saudi Arabia; Email: househmo@ngha.med.sa

1. Background

The study was conducted within National Guard Health Affairs (NGHA), King Abdul Aziz Medical city, located in Riyadh, the Kingdom of Saudi Arabia. NGHA is a leading public healthcare institution within Saudi Arabia. In December 2009, NGHA received the Joint Commission International Accreditation Gold seal of approval. In February of 2010, NGHA won a regional award for their successful implementation of electronic health records.

NGHA facilities are located in the eastern, western, and the largest, is located in the central region of the country. NGHA covers the health of all National Guard employees as well as their families. There are approximately 106,000 inpatient visits, 1,000,000 outpatient visits (exc. Dental), 26,000 surgical operations and 22,000,000 laboratory investigations. Most of the clinical and administrative activities take place in the central region of the country at the King Abdul Aziz Medical City, which houses a tertiary academic hospital facility.

NGHA has been dedicated to improving the state of health informatics within the region. For example, in 2005, NGHA created the college of Health Informatics at King Saud bin Abdulaziz University for Health Science. It is a graduate level program focused on training leaders in health informatics within the Gulf region. NGHA also works in collaboration with the Saudi Association of Health Informatics which has spurred investments electronic health records within NGHA facilities.

In August of 2009, NGHA created a plan to create an enterprise health data warehouse that would aggregate information from clinical and administrative databases within all three NGHA regions. The impetus behind the project was from a growing need to create an accountability and performance structure within the organization and the frequent requests by clinical and administrative staff for various types of reports spanning from several different systems. Figure 1, shows the various inputs that will be housed in the EDW. The information sources span both clinical and non-clinical systems.

There have been various stages identified for project implementation. Thus far the project management group created a workshop and presentation for information technology personnel around the project; completed preliminary data capturing reports; have completed a project scope document. The project management group is currently working towards creating an implementation plan for the project.

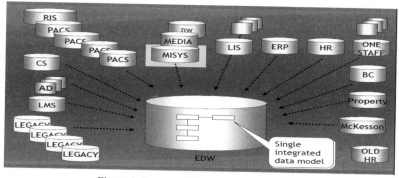

Figure 1. Sources of Information for EDW

2. Methodology

For this research, an action case study approach was selected as an appropriate method. An action case study examines a phenomenon within its natural setting with the researcher acting as a participatory agent within the research project [1]. Action Case uses similar data collection methods (e.g., observations or interviews) found in qualitative case studies. The major difference between action case and case studies is the researcher's role as an active participant within the group. This research method has been primarily used in information system research and rarely has it been used in health informatics research.

The study took place over a three month period, between December of 2009 and February of 2010. The researcher was a participant in the project management group. The researcher's role was to participate in helping manage the project and fulfill its implementation by the end of 2010. The project is seen as important objective for NGHA senior management.

The project management group met on a weekly basis. The project management group involved technical staff, I.T. consultants, and a project manager. A steering committee was also formed in 2009 that included various technical and user groups. The purpose of the steering committee was to guide the project team towards fulfilling the enterprise data warehouse (EDW) mandate.

Data collection methods included research observation notes, semi-structured interviews with participants, and meeting minutes. Observation notes were collected between December of 2009 and February of 2010 by the researcher. Meeting minutes from August 2009 to February 2010 were obtained from the project manager of the group. Seven different stakeholders were interviewed using a semi-structured interview that focused on understanding the development challenges as a result of EDW development within NGHA. Four individual interviews with members from the steering committee were carried out, as well as two individual interviews with the project management team. One group interview with EDW technical consultants consisting of five individuals was also carried out. On average, each semi-structured interview lasted between 40 and 60 minutes. Two interviews lasted for only 15 minutes. The interviews were not recorded. Rather, detailed notes on each conversation were captured.

Content analysis was utilized to analyze the data. In general, content analysis is a data analysis approach that can be used to analyze qualitative data; it is a systematic process of analyzing communication messages and making inferences based on the analysis [2], [3]. Content analysis involves the interpretation of textual data that has been categorized into concepts. Once the identification of concepts or categories has taken place, they are categorized into themes based on their relationships with each other [4]. An open source qualitative analysis program was used in the analysis of the data.

3. Results

Several key findings were identified relating to issues the group had with the development. The statements made by the participants are paraphrased.

Finding 1: Clear Contracts with Vendors Needed: A major stumbling block reported by most users was around vague roles around two vendors involved within the project. One vendor whom implemented the electronic health record system within NGHA used the Massachusetts General Hospital Utility Multi-Programming System (MUMPS), which is a programming language created in the late 1960's used in the programming of clinical applications. There were many data reliability and validity issues with regards to the data extraction tool provided by the vendor. Another vendor approached NGHA with a data extraction tool that would solve the problem. NGHA agreed to allow the vendor to extract the data, but the EHR vendor refused to provide them access to their EHR. This caused unnecessary delay within the project. Most stakeholders noted that a clearer contract should have been conducted with both vendors, which could have avoided such an unnecessary delay.

Finding 2: Clear Project Direction Needed: Most stakeholders noted the importance of project clarity. A few stakeholders were confused about the scope of the project and the purpose of the EDW. For example, because much of the focus had been on data extraction from clinical systems, one stakeholder was confused about the scope of the project. They noted: "I'm not sure if this is a clinical data warehouse project or an enterprise health data warehouse project." Other confusions were around reporting requirements related to key performance indicators (i.e., measurement performance indicators). One member noted:

> *Which KPI's are we going to use? What is the selection process going to be? When are they going to be delivered? How many reports are we supposed to produce? What is the number of KPI's we are selecting? These are all questions that are unclear to me.*

Finding 3: Fast-Track Bureaucracy: In a large organization where there is a high level of bureaucracy, many stakeholders felt that to move the project forward, bureaucracy needed to be fast-tracked within the organization. One stakeholder noted that it took nearly six months to hire an individual, and a similar time period to sign and approve a contract. Payment of contractors was also delayed. Stakeholders recognized bureaucracy as an obstacle to move things forward in an appropriate manner. As one stakeholder noted, "to get something done you need authorization from management, send several communiqués, and must talk to several departments to get things approved."

Finding 4: Staff Education and Awareness: Several stakeholders noted that many people, especially in the eastern and western regions, were not aware of the EDW project and its purpose. The stakeholders noted that it was important to involve users in the development process. One stakeholder noted: "the success of the project relies heavily on good project management that involves the users from day one".

Finding 5: Lack of Data Standards: Several stakeholders identified that a lack of standardization in data entry through the clinical system compromised the data quality and reliability of the electronic data warehouse. For example, in the western region the "fasting blood sugar" was used as a field for measuring glucose levels. In the central region, "fasting glucose" was used. The stakeholders have started to indentify a need to begin standardizing terms within the clinical system. Discussion is taking place on how to address this issue.

4. Discussion and Conclusion

This paper discussed some of the early development challenges faced by the NGHA EDW project. The project team is currently trying to find ways to learn from this new experience. They are discussing new ways to create clearer contracts, a detailed project charter with clearer roles, responsibilities, timelines, milestones, ways to involve users, and attempt to fast-track bureaucracy. Discussions are taking place on how to standardize data entry. These changes are anticipated to move the project forward and lead towards a successful development and future implementation of an EDW project. Sanders and Protti (2007), discuss the risks to success of an EDW within a healthcare institution. They list ten risks that can cause an EDW project to fail. These risks include [5]:

- Lack of standards
- Inadequate metadata
- Insufficient resources
- Lack of support
- Scalability in meeting future demand
- User not provided with correct training
- Limited co-operation from departments
- Data quality and reliability issues
- Lacking of one person with expertise of all EDW life cycle phases
- Lack of adequate source information systems

Some of these risks identified by Sanders and Protti have been identified in the project and are being addressed. Other risks to success factors described by the authors are under consideration and have been flagged as potential problems. The project management team will address them as the project moves on. The current challenges represent early attempts in the planning of an enterprise health data warehouse project. Future studies around this project will focus on issues relating to those described by Sanders and Protti (2007) and how they were resolved.

References

[1]   K. Braa, R. Vidgen, Interpretation, Intervention, and Reduction in the Organizational Laboratory: a Framework for In-Context Information Systems Research, *Acc Manage Inf Tech* **1** (1999), 25-47.

[2]   B. Berg. *Qualitative Research Methodology*. 3rd ed. Allyn & Bacon, Boston, 1989.

[3]   N. Kondracki, N. Wellman, and D. Amundson, Content Analysis: Review of Methods and their Applications in Nutrition Education, *J Nut Educ Behav* **34(4)** (2002), 224-230.

[4]   F. Lau, R. Hayward, Building a Virtual Network in a Community Health Research Training Program. *JAMIA*, **7** (2000), 361-377.

[5]   Sanders, D. Protti, Data Warehouses in Healthcare: Fundamental Principles, *Healthcare Quart*, **11** (2007), 1-16.

International Perspectives in Health Informatics
E.M. Borycki et al. (Eds.)
IOS Press, 2011

doi:10.3233/978-1-60750-709-3-127

Informed Use of Patients' Records on Trusted Health Care Services

Tony SAHAMA[a,1] , Evonne MILLER[b]

[a]*Faculty of Science and Technology (QUT), Brisbane, Australia*
[b]*Faculty of Built Environment and Engineering (QUT), Brisbane, Australia*

Abstract. Health care is an information-intensive business. Sharing information in health care processes is a smart use of data enabling informed decision-making whilst ensuring. the privacy and security of patient information.. To achieve this, we propose data encryption techniques embedded Information Accountability Framework (IAF) that establishes transitions of the technological concept, thus enabling understanding of shared responsibility, accessibility, and efficient cost effective informed decisions between health care professionals and patients. The IAF results reveal possibilities of efficient informed medical decision making and minimisation of medical errors. Of achieving this will require significant cultural changes and research synergies to ensure the sustainability, acceptability and durability of the IAF.

Keywords. informed decision, information accountability, security, privacy, data encryption, sharing information, electronic health information

Introduction

Health care is an information-intensive business. E-health, the combination of electronic health information and communications technology (HICT) which supports decision making processes is central to facilitating knowledge sharing, safety and quality in a contemporary patient-centered health care system. In Australia, the implementation of HICT is a public policy priority, with the government advocating a vision for all patients to have, hold and control their personal e-health record by 2012 [1]. Achieving this target is a challenging undertaking that requires addressing issues of technological viability, social acceptance and multiple internal organisational barriers (e.g., data computability, privacy, culture of information sharing among patients and health professionals [10]).

Establishing a free flow of health information and communications between health professionals and patients involves more than just the technological development of an interface, as the perceived risks, barriers to social acceptance and the health care delivery mechanism that must be understood. Whilst there are significant pockets of investment in e-health data and information exchange across Australia to date, attempts to develop HICT and linked e-health infrastructure have been fragmented and fraught with difficulty[2].

Dr. Tony Sahama, Computer Science Discipline, Faculty of Science and Technology (FaST), Queensland University of Technology (QUT), PO Box 2434 Gardens Point, Brisbane, QLD 4001, Australia. t.sahama@qut.edu.au

1. The Approach

This paper explores an effective and efficient data integration technique using data encryption protocol and the use of Information Accountability Framework (IAF) in health care decision making when sharing sensitive information. The first approach allows the computer to communicate with another computer, keeping only the accountable human in the communication loop. This can be achieved via data encryption techniques (thus protecting sensitive data [15]) and will enhance faster data accessibility and establish trust; however, once encrypted, data can no longer be easily queried and sharing will be difficult for humans. Database performance depends on how sensitive data is encrypted. Thus, we review the conventional encryption method (which can be partially queried) and propose an encryption method for numerical data, which can be effectively queried in the human readable version. The proposed system includes the design of the service scenario, a metadata model to enhance data accessibility, facilitate speedy indexing and querying, and allow auditing of healthcare record data, while keeping patient's private data securely encrypted. The second approach, which requires public and professional trust, is a policy driven approach letting both computers and humans interact at any time with a set of constraints imposed by the proposed IAF framework.

1.1. Significance of the Concept

The first necessary step in patient-controlled e-health record is to investigate how and when clinical information is revealed (or shared) to proper stakeholders – e.g., doctors, nurses, patients, researchers, and all health care decision making organisations. To keep conversations private but accessible, there must be a special mechanism that preserves and manages sensitive patient information. One approach to build synergistic capabilities is to use both the capabilities of the Machine power (e.g., Computer power: of Speed, Accuracy and Attention-to-details) and human power (e.g., Intuition, Creativity and Judgment). This is an achievable goal, as the Computer power is readily available, but it is a challenging task. Figure 1 illustrates how we propose to utilise machine and human power in the IAF to tackle such cognitive barriers.

1.2. Information Accountability Framework (IAF)

The IAF requires information accountability and transparency, monitoring whether a particular use is appropriate under a given set of rules via a system that holds both individuals and institutions accountable for misuse [3] via accountability protocols, which provides lasting evidence - through digital signatures - of actions by users IAF Audit Trail and Workflow.

The second stage of the IAF involves connecting requests from the public space to the professional space. A solid integration between Operating System-based security and Operating System-based communication protocols, embedded data access and the retrieval architecture is the ideal framework with strict protocols for information accountability and auditing processes. Figure 1 depicts a possible architecture for IAF patient care systems, with each different layer embedded with its architecture to accommodate necessary functionalities (including the Operating System-based security [4] model and Health Information Access Control (HIAC) model[5]).

1.3. Implications of the Concept and Our Approach

Figure 2 and Table 1 illustrate an experiment utilising secured database service scenario with simulated data on general medical data flow within Australian Health Care Workflow context that accommodates all stakeholders in the decision making process: Administrator for Systems perspective (AD), Patient (PT), General Practitioners (GP), Specialists (SP) and other allied entities [e.g., Nurses (NS); Analyst (AT)]. Figure 2 illustrates an simple health care workflow experiment using Bucket Index (an Index mechanism on character data, which has close relationship with all of its characters) and data encryption; we hypothesized that the Bucket Index encryption techniques would be efficient protocols when computer power is utilized,

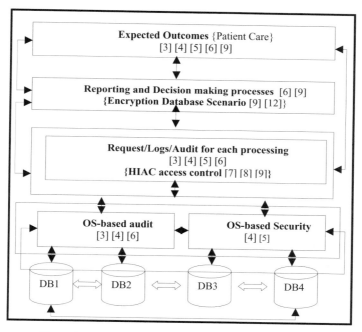

Figure 1: Proposed IAF Audit and Log Trail Workflow [6]

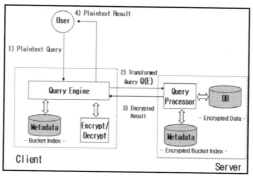

Figure 2: The Encrypted Database (DB) Service Scenario [9]

Table 1: Data Access Permission by User's and Roles
(Legend:- R = Read; W=Write; R/W= Read and Write)

User Role / Table Name	AD	GP	NS	SP	AT	PT
Patient_Base	R/W					R
Patient_Identity		R/W	R/W	R/W	R	
Patient_Record		R/W	R	R/W	R	
Patient_Chart		R/W	R	R/W	R	
Disease		R	R	R	R	R*
AD	R/W					
GP		R/W				
NS			R/W			
SP				R/W		
AT					R/W	
PT						R

1. User (human entity) requests queries to the system
2. Client (front end) transforms queries posed by user(s) into equivalent queries operating on the encrypted data stored on the server
3. Server (Database) stores the encrypted data from one or more data owners and makes them available for distribution to clients
4. Query Processor in client module transforms original plaintext query to the transformed query according to cryptographic algorithm
5. The Query Executor in server processes the transformed query and returns the encrypted query result to clients

2. Results and Discussion

The results are based on a general scenario e.g., Health Clinic visit (Table 1). To ensure accuracy, the specialist (SP) can read/write only when General Practitioner (GP) permits him/her to be involved in the patient's treatment; whilst analyst (AT) can only read the old patient's records after GP or SP finalise the case. Initially Admin (AD) records the first information of the patient and assigned GP to the patient.

3. Conclusion and Future Work

These results are the first step toward constructing the secured health database embedded information accountability scenario, with both approaches practicable when information sharing is accepted by the user (e.g., patients). As the information sharing culture is in its infancy, high performance accountability and privacy protocols [11] are required to develop a more effective algorithm that can directly be executed over the encrypted data [10,12] and with effective homomorphism properties [13]. This approach requires access control, ID based or attribute based encryption algorithm, health-care professionals support and the candidate (e.g., Patients') active participation, where all of which requires time and synergies. We presented, outcomes of the proposed IAF concept include enabling understanding of the power, importance and protocols of sharing electronic-data between health care professionals and patients, as well as improving the health system [14].

References

[1]   National Health and Hospitals Reform Commission (NHHRC), http://www.nhhrc.org.au/ Accessed on 10 October 2009.

[2]   "Towards Q2: Tomorrow's Queensland -http://www.towardq2.qld.gov.au/tomorrow/index.aspx. Accessed on 05 October 2009.

[3]   D. J. Weitzner, H. Abelson, T. Berners-Lee, J. Feigenbaum, J. Hendler, G. J. Sussman. Information Accountability. *Comm of the ACM* **51**(6) (2008),82-87.

[4]   L. Franco, T. Sahama, P. Croll P. Security Enhanced Linux to Enforce Mandatory Access Control in Health Information Systems. In Australasian Workshop on Health Data and Knowledge Management, the Australian Computer Science Week. *Conference in Research and Practice in Information Technology Series* **327**(2008), 27-33.

[5]   V. Liu, W. Caelli, L. May, P. Croll. Open and Trusted Health Informatics Structure, In Australasian Workshop on Health Data and Knowledge Management, the Australian Computer Science Week. *Conference in Research and Practice in Information Technology Series* **327** (2008) 35-43.

[6]   T. Sahama, J. Kim, "Role of Ubiquitous Sensor Network in Patient Care".2009 *International Conference of Korea Institude of Maritime Information & Communicaiotn Sciences (ICKIMICS2009)* (2009).

[7]   G. Schadow, S. J. Grannis, C. J. McDonald. Discussion Paper: Privacy-Preserving Distributed Queries for a Clinical Case Research Network. *IEEE International Conference on Data Mining Workshop on Privacy, Security, and Data Mining*, Maebashi City, Japan. *Conference in Research and Practice in Information Technology*, **14** (2002).

[8]   Y, Yang, R. H. Deng, F. Bao, Fortifying Password Authentication in Integrated Healthcare Delivery Sustems, *ACM ASIACCS'06*, March 21—24, 2006, Taipei, Taiwan: (2006) 255—265.

[9]   J. Kim, T. Sahama, A Study on the Encryption Model for Numerical Data. *Int J KIMICS*, **7**(4) (2009) 30-34

[10] J. Grimson, W. Grimson, W. Hasselbring. The SI Challenge in Health Care. *Comm ACM* **43**(6) (2009) 49-55.

[11] S. H. Cannoy, A. F. Salam. A Framework for Health Care Information Assurance Policy and Compliance. *Comm of ACM*, **53**(3) (2010) 26—130.

[12] R. J. Rincon, M. Paselli, J. Recas, Q. Zhao, M. Sanchez-Elez, D. Atienza, J. Penders, G. De Micheli. OS-Based Sensor Node Platform and Energy Estimation Model for Health-Care Wireless Sensor Networks. Design, Automation and Test in Europe 2008: 10-14 March (2008), 1027-1032.

[13] J. Lee. Health Care Reform in South Korea: Success of Failure? *Amer J Pub Health*, **93**(1) (2003) 48—51.

[14] L. Liu, J. Gai, A Method of Query over Encrypted Data in Database IEEE 2009 International *Conference on Computer Engineering and Technology*, (2009) 23—27.

[15] W. C. *Barker Recommendation for the Triple Data Encryption Algorithm (TDEA) Block Cipher: Information Security*, NIST Special Publication 800-67 Ver 1.1, Natl.Inst.Stand.Technol.Spec.Publ.800-67, May (2004).

[16] D. Shin, T. Sahama, J. T. Kim, H. H. Kim. Data Encryptions Techniques for Electronic Health Record Exchange: to appeared in Conference for *Information Technology and Communications in Health (ITCH)* to be held in Victoria, British Columbia from February 24 through February 27, 2011.

International Perspectives in Health Informatics
E.M. Borycki et al. (Eds.)
IOS Press, 2011
© 2011 ITCH 2011 Steering Committee and IOS Press. All rights reserved.
doi:10.3233/978-1-60750-709-3-132

Scenario-based Stress Testing of an Electronic Patient Record System in a Thin-client Computing Implementation

Kei TERAMOTO [a,1], Shigeki KUWATA [a], Andre W. KUSHNIRUK [b],
Elizabeth M. BORYCKI [b], Masaki MOCHIDA [c], Katsuhiro FUJII [c],
Kenta KURANAKA [c], Hiroshi KONDOH [a]

[a] *Division of Medical Informatics, Tottori University Hospital, Yonago, Tottori, Japan*
[b] *School of Health Information Science, University of Victoria, Victoria, British Columbia, Canada*
[c] *Division of System Design, SECOM.SANIN Co., Ltd, Matsue, Shimane, Japan*

Abstract. Implementation of thin-client computing (TCC) generally requires an elaborate process of determining appropriate specifications of the centralized servers (server sizing). This study aimed to assess the usefulness of the server sizing methods with eight scenarios based on practical usage of an electronic patient record. Actual data obtained from a hospital, where TCC was introduced based on the methods of the study, showed that the stress testing of one of server sizing methods contributed to steady operation of the system, while the scenarios should be improved to reflect more practical workflow in real settings to achieve more precise estimation of the centralized server performance in TCC.

Keywords. electronic patient record, scenario-based testing, server sizing, thin-client computing, usability

Introduction and Objectives

In recent years thin-client computing (TCC), comprising centralized servers and low-cost thin-clients (Figure 1) for security strategy, has aroused widespread attention [1-4]. Prior to implementation, this architecture generally requires an elaborate process of server sizing, *i.e.*, determining appropriate specifications of the centralized servers. Only a few attempts, however, have so far been made at the evaluation of server sizing for Electronic Patient Record (EPR) systems in large medical facilities [5, 6]. This study aimed to assess the usefulness of the server sizing methods the authors employed in introducing TCC to EPR systems developed on the conventional server-client model, with eight scenarios based on practical EPR usage.

---

[1] Corresponding Author: Kei Teramoto, Division of Medical Informatics, Tottori University Hospital, 36-1 Nishi-cho, Yonago, Tottori, 683-8504, Japan; E-mail: kei-tera@umin.net

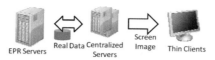

Figure 1. A typical system configuration and data transfer method of thin-client computing

1. Methods

1.1. Experimental Environments

Figure 2 and Table 1 show experimental environments and devices used in the testing for server sizing. EPR applications were installed in the centralized server that performed the role of the PC client in which they would be installed in the server-client model. The package products of the applications, Clinical Information System developed by IBM Japan, Ltd., included full functioned physician's order entry, patient records and some departmental systems [7]. Windows Server 2003 Enterprise Edition was installed in the centralized server to avoid physical memory limitations (up to 4Gbytes for the Standard Edition). Only virtualization software was installed in the client PCs for connecting the centralized server.

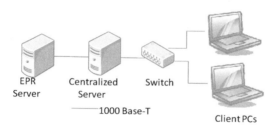

Figure 2. Experimental system configuration for server sizing.

Table 1. Specifications of experimental devices for server sizing.

Role/Model	Hardware/OS	Software
EPR Server	• Proliant BL460c Server Blade/ Dual Core Intel Xeon processor 5160 (3GHz, 1333MHz FSB)/ 6Gbytes memory, Hewlett-Packard	• Clinical Information System (Server), IBM Japan
Centralized Server	• Windows 2003 Server Enterprise Edition, Microsoft	• Clinical Information System (Client), IBM Japan • GO-Global 3.2.1 (Server), GraphOn
Switch	• Catalyst 2960S-48TS-S, Cisco	–
Client PC	• Probook 4710c, Hewlett-Packard • Windows XP Professional, Microsoft	• GO-Global Native Client 3.2, GraphOn

1.2. Stress Testing for Server Sizing

The stress testing was executed to determine the maximum number of clients, being identical to that of users that were able to simultaneously connect to the server with the specifications described in Table 1. Load status of the centralized server was measured during the testing including eight scenarios (Table 2) based on practical EPR usage. Testers had over five-years of experience in PC operations and received practical training of the EPR application before the testing. To observe how the server load and the usability vary with the stress, the testing was repeated four times starting with five testers, subsequently with 10, 15 and 20 testers.

All the testers reported problems occurred during the testing in a free-style format. The reports by the testers were categorized into two groups composed of response delays and abnormal halts of the application. Microsoft Management Monitor Console (MMC) was used to monitor CPU and memory usage in a centralized server. Load data obtained by MMC were recorded and compared with those obtained from a TCC-featured EPR system, which was actually introduced after the stress testing of this study and had been in operation in a university-affiliated hospital with daily 1,200 outpatients and 697 beds located in a rural area of Japan.

2. Results

2.1. Load Data in the Centralized Server

Figure 3 represents the results of the centralized server performance with stress testing. The left chart indicates the ratio of CPU usage and the right chart does memory available in the server. Horizontal axes represent the number of testers who logged in the server. The average of CPU usage increased almost linearly with the number of users, while the maximum usage reached to 100% for more than 10 users. The average of available memory also linearly decreased, but the minimum availability still exceeded 2.5Gbytes for 20 users, which indicated that the memory of the server specified in Table 1 was enough to allow 20 users to login.

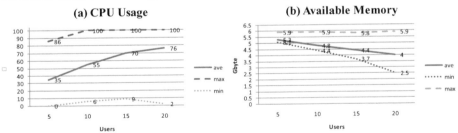

Figure 3. Results of CPU usage and memory available on the centralized server with stress testing.

Table 2. Scenarios and corresponding reported problems with CPU usage during the testing for 20 testers.

No.	Scenario Title	Response delays (Reported Testers)	Abnormal Halts (Reported Testers)	CPU Usage (%)
1	Terminate the EPR application	0	0	19
2	Switch items for the blood test order	2	4	21
3	Switch schema images	14	2	86
4	Scroll order windows	6	7	64
5	Expand and shrink folders	5	0	24
6	Switch windows of bed maps	3	4	61
7	Search disease names by keywords	6	4	71
8	Boot the multiple EPR applications	2	3	81

2.2. The Relationship Between CPU Load and System Problems

Table 2 represents the scenarios used, corresponding reported problems and CPU usage (two minutes average) during the stress test. Values at the problems represent the number of testers who reported those abnormalities. Though no obvious correlation between the problem frequencies and CPU usage was observed, an extremely high frequency of abnormalities, as found in scenario #3 and #4, should be avoided for practical use of the system. Accordingly, it was recommended in the stress testing that the heavily loaded centralized server, *e.g.* approximately more than 60-70% of CPU usage, would cause serious usability problems.

2.3. Comparison with the Data Obtained from the Actual EPR System in Operation

Figure 4 shows the data obtained from the university-affiliated hospital in which the EPR system has been in operation. The server configuration was determined according to the results of server sizing as stated to allow 1,050 simultaneous connections from thin-clients, resulting in 70 centralized servers with maximum 15 connections for each server. The figure includes: (a) the number of users calculated as that of client PCs connected to one centralized server, (b) CPU usage and (c) memory usage. All the values were the averages for five-minute periods. Horizontal axes indicate a time course of 36 hours starting with 0 a.m. on the day of the observation that was chosen randomly from weekdays with typical business activities at the hospital.

The number of client PCs increased from 8 a.m. and marked the highest value as 13 users at around 5 p.m. CPU usage correlated much less with the number of users than available memory did, contrary to the results from the stress testing showing a linear correlation with the number of login users. Peak values of CPU usage did not exceed 50% being lower than the "heavily loaded" situation stated above, indicating that the server was working in a stable situation.

On the other hand, consumed memory tended to be underestimated in the stress testing, for instance, applications for 13 users occupied 49% of memory (corresponding to approximately 3Gbytes) at the peak in the actual settings, while applications for 20 users occupied only 2Gbytes of memory in the testing. To compare more accurately, the relationship between the number of EPR users and memory consumption in the EPR system was measured with the Windows Task Manager, generally installed with Windows OS, which can provide the information on how much memory is currently consumed for running individual application processes. The results presented that 10 out of 13 users actually operated the EPR system (3 users operated other applications) and that memory consumption reached approximately 2.5 Gbytes for 10 users. In the case of 5 EPR users, memory consumption reached approximately 1.2 Gbytes. Since the values of consumed memory for 5 and 10 users in the stress-testing were 0.7 and 1.2 Gbytes respectively, the data for real settings ranged 1.7-2.1 times higher than those for the stress-testing.

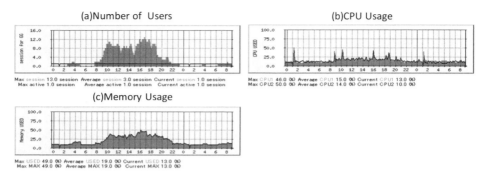

Figure 4. Diagram showing performance of the centralized server in actual settings after the testing.

3. Discussion

3.1. Evaluation of the Stress Testing

Discrepancies were found between the results of the stress testing and the actual data, although the testing contributed to steady operation of the system. It was likely that the higher intensity of the user's activity, *i.e.*, frequency of user's keyboard and mouse operation, than in the actual settings of the EPR system, led to the overestimate of CPU usage. The testers constantly operated the EPR during the time designated in the scenarios, which does not follow in the actual hospital settings. More detailed scenarios would be required to reflect the actual usage of the system, as the intensity may vary with the user's workflow. On the other hand, the underestimate of memory consumption would stem from the exclusion of various departmental applications in the testing that were used in the actual settings.

It is noted that the performance of the centralized server depends on EPR and virtualization applications selected in the testing. Parameter setting for the applications also affects the performance.

3.2. Relevant Issues on Virtualization of the EPR System

The client-side application of the EPR system developed based on the server-client model often assumes that a single user executes it on a client PC, therefore its functions, *e.g.* user's profile, registry and file system location, are not usually designed to allow simultaneous multiple users' processing (MUP) on the client. MUP, however, is the first requisite of the virtualization for the applications on the centralized server: To give virtual environments to users who login the server, programs of the applications should be coded to allow multiple users to share the system resources such as memory, CPU and master files. Otherwise some serious usability problems of the applications, *e.g.* response delays and partial omission of screen information, would occur, being distinctive particularly when the server is heavily loaded. The most authentic but infeasible way of adapting the programs to MUP is to review and rewrite all the program codes. Instead, the stress testing by multiple human testers could be adopted to locate the problems about MUP within the EPR application. As partly illustrated in Table 2, some abnormalities deriving from EPR application problems were detected, which would also be useful to improve the quality and usability of the system. Further studies of the authors will be focused on the analyses of these issues.

4. Limitation

4.1. Difference Between the Real EPR Operation by Medical Professionals and the Scenario-based Stress Testing by Testers

Though the testers who participated in this experiment had adequate skills for the EPR operations of the scenario-based stress testing, the results of server-sizing were different from with the actual data obtained from the target hospital: The higher intensity of the EPR operation by the testers than actual medical professionals led to the overestimate of CPU usage and the underestimate of memory consumption. To obtain the high accuracy of server-sizing, the scenarios should include more practical EPR operations in frequency and timing of user-interface usage by medical professionals, as well as in multiple applications running simultaneously on the centralized server. It would be effective to capture the real-time EPR operation to understand how actual users interact the system and what kind of applications are running on the server, and then to rebuild it on the scenarios of stress testing.

5. Conclusions

This study presented practical measures for server sizing that usually comprised burdensome process in implementing TCC. The scenario-based stress testing needed to be improved in terms of performance estimation of the centralized server, while the actual data obtained from a hospital where TCC was introduced showed that it contributed to steady operation of the TCC system.

References

[1] D. Schlosser, et al, Performance comparison of windows-based thin-client architectures, *In Proceedings of the Telecommunication Networks and Applications Conference* (2007), 197–202.
[2] J. Nieh, et al, A Comparison of Thin-Client Computing Architectures, *Technical Report CUCS-022-00 Department of Computer Science, Columbia University, November,* (2000)
[3] J. Nieh, et al, Measuring the Multimedia Performance of Server-Based Computing, *In Proceedings of the 10th International Workshop on Network and Operating System Support for Digital Audio and Video* (2000), 55–64
[4] A. Brian, et al, Technical and Architectural Issues in Deploying Electronic Health Records (EHRs) over the WWW, *Stud Health Tech Inform* **143** (2009), 93–98.
[5] S. Kuwata, et al, Oshidori-Net: Connecting regional EPR systems to achieve secure mutual reference with thin-client computing technology, *IFIP Advances in Information and Communication Technology,* **35** (2010), 82–89
[6] Y. Matsumura, et al, The Current State of the Operation Related Systems and Their Next Subjects, *Japan J Med Inf* **27** (2007), 157–167.
[7] S. Kuwata, et al, Effective Solutions in Introducing Server-Based Computing into Hospital Information System, *Stud Health Tech Inform* **143** (2009), 435–440.

International Perspectives in Health Informatics
E.M. Borycki et al. (Eds.)
IOS Press, 2011
© 2011 ITCH 2011 Steering Committee and IOS Press. All rights reserved.
doi:10.3233/978-1-60750-709-3-138

EHR Strategy: Top Down, Bottom Up or Middle Out?

Thomas C BOWDEN[a,1]

[a] *Chief Executive, HealthLink International Limited*

Abstract. Around the world a number of countries have made a concerted effort to embed Information and Communications Technology (ICT) within their health systems. It is widely acknowledged that the successful application of ICT to health systems can bring about significant benefits. A number of areas commonly singled out for improvement include: coordination of care; improved medication management; and streamlining the transfer of a patient's care from one healthcare provider to another. There are also perceived cost-benefits including reduced duplication of services and improved service utilization. Countries across the world have chosen many and varied paths to automating their health systems. Health systems are intrinsically very complicated and changing rapidly. Because they represent a high proportion of government expenditure, it is important to understand what is being achieved by each of the broad approaches that are being taken.

Keywords. EHR strategy, health-system integrator, summary care record.

Introduction

There is little disagreement that improving health systems is a high priority. An ageing population and workforce issues combine with concern from taxpayers, balking at the rapidly increasing cost of healthcare, to create enormous pressure for systemic improvement. Disappointingly, very few countries have to date established a dependable information management infrastructure that has delivered large scale service improvements or substantial cost savings.

One group of countries including Australia, Canada and the United Kingdom has focused upon development of nationally run systems, albeit in some cases partially devolved to their states or provinces. Another group of smaller countries, Denmark, New Zealand and Holland, has encouraged private sector organizations to develop and sell information services under controlled conditions. We are now at a very interesting point; one at which we can see the results achieved by a range of differing strategies. It is timely to attempt to assess which emerging trends provide useful guidance in the development of national EHR strategy.

1. The Devil's in the Detail – the UK National Programme Examined

Countries the world over are wrestling with the question of whether and how to share electronic health records. Canada, Australia and the United Kingdom are all believed to

---

[1] Corresponding Author: Tom Bowden, Chief Executive, HealthLink International Limited, PO Box 9920, Newmarket, Auckland, New Zealand, 1149; Email: tombowden@healthlink.net

have spent sums of in excess of US$1 billion dollars (in the case of the UK, many times this amount) and none of them has much to show for it. Only the United Kingdom has comprehensively reviewed progress to date.

Because of the very large amount of money invested in the NHS's National Programme for Health Information Technology (NPfIT), an amount reportedly approaching £13 billion, the government decided to undertake a series of reviews. The NHS appointed Dr Trisha Greenhalgh OBE, Professor of General Practice at University College, London, to head a team to review both the Summary Care Record (SCR) project and Healthspace, the personal electronic health record system providing patients with online access to their personal information held within their SCR.

Professor Greenhalgh's 223 page review *The Devil's in the Detail* [1] found that the SCR and Healthspace programmes were showing only modest benefits for the amount of money invested. The review called into question some of the fundamental premises upon which the projects were based.

It is particularly concerning that, after 13 years and expenditure of nearly £13 billion, the NPfIT has shown such limited usefulness. However, although Professor Greenhalgh's report is very recent and the report's critics have barely had a chance to respond, it does seem that some worthwhile insights can already be drawn:

1. There is likely to be merit in making the records of people with chronic illnesses and medication readily accessible to a number of interested parties. Availability of a SCR is a useful resource for that purpose.

2. There appears to be relatively little value in making a SCR accessible for most 'run of the mill' patients.

3. Clinical staff are generally suspicious of the completeness and accuracy of information they are getting from a shared record. This is creating an apparent reluctance to refer to it. Clinical staff appear especially reluctant to view the SCR as a single source of truth.

4. The cost of developing and maintaining a shared record system of a reasonable quality is substantial, to the extent that there are simply not enough IT literate clinical staff to make such systems available and to maintain them to a satisfactory level.

5. The public have continuing concerns over the privacy of their information. The effect that protracted debate has on the public's trust in the health system is as yet unknown. Whether or not heightened awareness of the SCR will influence members of the public to distance themselves from healthcare providers such as general practitioners remains to be seen.

Unfortunately the NPfIT's effort to effect large scale transformation of the UK health system faced many of the problems that often confront tasks of this magnitude. Professors Cresswell and Sheikh, from the Centre for Population Health Sciences, University of Edinburgh, have made the following comments on the problems encountered and the underlying reasons for them:

"The history of large- scale information technology (IT) projects is littered with examples of failure and this is also true of many healthcare settings. A central reason underpinning many of these failures is that IT initiatives are often politically rather than clinically motivated, resulting in disenfranchisement of healthcare professionals and other key stakeholders from the outset. Once a policy decision has been taken, the lack of appreciation of and attention to the socio-cultural implications of new

developments on patterns of working and organisational processes is a further recipe for disaster."[2]

While the British health system seems to have made limited discernable progress, other countries/jurisdictions are doing well with far less elaborate and expensive approaches to addressing the problem. The US is not a poster-child for healthcare nor for health IT, but there are some examples of excellence including Kaiser Permanente a large health insurer which enables its members to connect to their electronic health records via a 'patient portal' that is similar in concept to the NHS' Healthspace. Kaiser Permanente's patients are using this facility extensively. This indicates that by allowing some degree of choice and flexibility as to system design, governments are far more likely to be successful in their efforts to encourage the use of individual electronic health records.

2. Public Private Partnerships are Working

Countries such as Holland, Denmark and New Zealand are making incremental progress at much lower cost than their counterparts in Canada, the U.K. and Australia. Rather than trying to re-engineer their health system to put in place a comprehensive set of electronic health records, each of these countries has opted for an incremental 'bottom up' approach to electronic health record development.

Denmark, Holland and New Zealand have made some progress in this area by encouraging the evolution of *'Health-system Integrators'*. These are highly focused organisations capable of designing, overseeing and supporting the exchange of clinical information and the integration of the end-user systems.

The *Health-system Integrator (HSI)* is a specialised company whose job it is to determine what is required and then to make it happen, in a manner that healthcare providers will find truly useful day in and day out. An HSI's role is also to enable clinical computer systems to exchange patient information in an interoperable, seamless, dependable and well-supported manner. Software development, integration with EMR (electronic medical records) system vendors' products and provision of user training are just some of the tasks that an HSI needs to execute successfully to make eHealth useful at a grass-roots level. Exchange of information must be underpinned by a wide range of highly disciplined activities, including product testing and readily accessible and well-managed customer support.

At a strategic level the hallmarks of a successful *Health-system Integrator* are: specialised expertise; active promotion of standards compliance; and a track-record of continuous innovation. Countries that have encouraged adoption of this market paradigm have found it to be an effective means to implement new and useful technologies for the exchange of clinical information between computer systems used across their health sectors.

The Danish, Dutch and New Zealand governments have each encouraged the development of market-driven initiatives by private sector organizations. These organisations work toward execution of a national strategy and are content to be constrained by national and international standards. In each of these countries there has been an enormous upsurge of eHealth development. International studies (Commonwealth Fund reports, OECD studies) demonstrate that these countries have made far more progress in delivering eHealth than have countries following centrally mandated approaches.

Evolution rather than revolution is the key. In Denmark almost every routine healthcare transaction is automated. In New Zealand web-services based electronic referrals and referred services ordering are widespread, as they are in Holland. *HSI* companies in both countries have been steadily building their capabilities since 1993-4. Recently they have begun working together to share technology. In Holland, the growth of electronic services has been dramatic; *Topicus Health* is one of the fastest growing companies in the country and has recently commenced offering services in nearby Belgium.

3. New Zealand is Making Real Progress

In New Zealand, there is a hefty emphasis on primary care. Three HSI organisations were set up in 1994 in response to government's request to industry to develop specialised services for the sector. Fifteen years on New Zealand's general practices use a wide range of eHealth services including the exchange of 50 million messages annually. Just as in Denmark, New Zealand's primary care practices exchange electronic information with a large number of organisations throughout the sector. A typical New Zealand medical practice exchanges information electronically with between 50 and 60 other parties in any given month. Now, building upon a sound foundation of core electronic messaging services, New Zealand's general practices are beginning to use web services based technology for online hospital referrals and radiology/ pathology service ordering. Many more new and useful services are currently being planned or developed.

4. A National IT System from the Middle Out?

There is an emerging view that rather than focusing upon the minute details of interconnection and trying to develop and run IT projects themselves, governments should focus upon overall health system strategy and policy. Enlightened governments everywhere are now looking at how best to foster and encourage investment in and development of an open and dynamic Health-system Integration marketplace. In his paper *'Building a National Health IT System from the Middle Out'* Professor Enrico Coiera, from the Centre for Health Informatics, Institute for Health Innovation, University of New South Wales, Sydney, Australia argues:

"The top-down approach of many national programs for healthcare information technology (IT) may be at the heart of their current problems. The medical-industrial complex loves a big procurement, and the contracts do not get much bigger than for building nation-scale health information systems (NHIS)". [3]

Professor Coiera asks whether we really need government embedded in the process of IT implementation, something with which it so clearly and routinely struggles. Professor Coiera also poses the question of whether government should not instead be concentrating upon simplifying policy rules, given that it is policy in which they are expert?

Professor Coiera argues in favour of a 'middle-out' approach, one that acknowledges that government and providers all have different starting points, goals, and resources. He foresees an approach in which Government does not mandate immediate standards compliance, but helps fund the development process. He believes that when the public interest is strong, government has a key role to provide support and incentives that encourage clinical providers to acquire systems that are technically or functionally compliant, and to pursue innovations that keep their systems compliant over time.

Other international experts agree with the broad thrust of Professor Coiera's argument. The United Kingdom based King's Fund is starting to promote *"Polysystem Theory"*, under which there is recognition of the complex and evolving environment of a 'polysystem'. *Polysystem Theory* eschews prescriptive and dictatorial approaches in favour of clearly defined objectives; a minimum set of hard and fast rules/boundaries; and effective incentives and disincentives; all of which are underpinned by strong leadership, supported by periodic reviews informed by commentary, constant feedback and comparisons from all stakeholders. According to Polysystem Theory successful achievement of complex change projects necessitates clear agreement on what needs to be achieved to accomplish system change but plenty of flexibility as to how it is approached.

5. Conclusion

Starkly different policy options have been chosen by health systems around the world. The marked contrasts and widely disparate results should provide excellent research opportunities for policy-makers and indeed all those with an interest in information technology and its application to transformation of health systems. Ideally, researchers will question their own beliefs and ponder upon what might be the best policy frameworks to strive for within their own environments.

References

[1] T. Greenhalgh, K. Stramer, T. Bratan, E. Byrne, J. Russell, S. Hinder, H. Potts, "The Devil's in the Detail: Final report of the independent evaluation of the Summary Care Record and HealthSpace programmes." (2010) London: *University College London*
    https://www.ucl.ac.uk/news/scriefullreport.pdf
[2] Informatics in Primary Care http://www.radcliffe-oxford.com/journals/j12_informatics_in_primary_care
[3] E. Coiera, "Building a National Health IT System from the Middle Out" *JAMIA* **16** (2009), 271-273

International Perspectives in Health Informatics
E.M. Borycki et al. (Eds.)
IOS Press, 2011

doi:10.3233/978-1-60750-709-3-143

143

Beyond Individual Patient Care: Enhanced Use of EMR Data in a Primary Care Setting

Marianne TOLAR[a,1] , Ellen BALKA[a]

[a] *School of Communication, Simon Fraser University, Burnaby,*
British Columbia, Canada

Abstract. With the introduction of electronic medical record (EMR) systems into the primary care sector the collected data become available for purposes beyond individual patient care, i.e. chronic disease management, prevention and clinical performance evaluation. However EMR systems are primarily designed to support clinical tasks, and physicians focus on the treatment of individual patients. In this paper we follow the path of a community health centre (CHC), tracking the changes that came about with the secondary usage of EMR data, and presenting some of the lessons learned.

Keywords. electronic medical records, primary care, secondary use of data, prevention, chronic disease management, case study, action research

Introduction

In recent years, the introduction of EMRs into primary care settings has captured the attention of practitioners, policy makers, payors, and patients. One of the potential benefits of the use of EMR systems across multiple settings and institutions is the "capability to mine vast amounts of structured medical record data" [1, p.71] for the evaluation of the effectiveness of clinical care or the surveillance of diseases. However, the focus of current EMR systems is on individual patient care. Changes would have to be introduced to "ensure that clinical data could be reused for public health purposes ... [and] ... to expand the clinical data model to collect and process new types of data" [2, p. 399]. An interoperable infrastructure is a prerequisite to achieve these goals, the development of a uniform, standardized terminology being one of the major barriers [3].

In this paper we track some of the difficulties of data generation back to the clinical care context. We follow a community health centre (CHC) in their use of practice searches as part of the advanced functionality of an EMR system to support multiple goals, including prevention and management of chronic diseases.

---

[1] Corresponding Author: Marianne Tolar, Simon Fraser University, School of Communication, 8888 University Drive, Burnaby BC, Canada V5A 1S6; E-mail: mtolar@sfu.ca.

1. Methods: Action Research

The case study is undertaken within an action-research framework. Designed to bridge the gap between theory, research, and practice [4], action research generates research about a social system while trying to change it [5]. Action research is particularly well suited to research aimed at problem solving and improvement [6]. Primary data collection consisted of extensive observation and informal interviews that focused on documenting issues the clinicians and medical office assistants (MOAs) encountered in their use of the EMR system. An ethnographic approach was taken because it often provides "a much better means of anticipating the dynamic effects on work organization" [6, p.21]. In a concluding round of data collection interviews with the clinical and administrative staff were conducted.

In her role as participant observer the researcher took on the tasks of IT support. She helped personnel at the clinic understand and figure out problems with the software, not only in terms of the secondary usage of data, but also more generally troubleshooting any difficulties with the IT system [7]. The researcher was present at the CHC for nine days a month on average, over a period of nine months. Extensive field notes were taken reporting on the issues encountered and the communication between the involved actors.

The analysis in this paper draws back on the data collected by the researcher between August 2008 and April 2009, as well as on interviews conducted in September and October 2010 with four out of the six doctors working at the CHC, the clinical pharmacist, and the nurse practitioner.

2. The Case: Using an EMR system in a Community Health Centre (CHC)

The CHC has been using their current EMR system since its initial implementation in 2004 which is reported on elsewhere [8]. It supports the storage and retrieval of administrative and clinical information, the documentation of patient encounters, as well as scheduling of appointments and billing. At the time of this research the clinic had already established a high level of routine in the use of the system. They had gradually taken up some of the more enhanced functionality of the EMR system like automatic alerts and reminders, built-in checklists, and flow-sheets for patient education. While many of the smaller changes were just informally realized, the clinic followed a PDSA (Plan – Do – Study – Act) approach for some of the major initiatives that had been implemented in reaction to the evaluated data. This allowed them to try, assess, and adapt or discard changes in a focused but versatile manner.

3. Results: Introducing a New Paradigm of Using EMR Data

3.1. Systematic Feedback: Practice Searches

Practice searches allow EMR users to search through the clinics' patient population for patients with specified attributes (e.g., all female patients over 50 years of age who have not had a pap test done in the last 12 months). In the CHC the practice searches are used for different purposes:

Chronic disease management: Results from practice searches are used in regular sessions called "CDM huddles". In these sessions the clinical pharmacist and/or the nurse practitioner huddle with the clinicians individually and go through lists of their chronic disease patients identifying those who need special attention and coordinating according follow-up tasks like arranging for outstanding lab tests.

Screening and prevention: Potential chronic disease patients are identified through practice searches. They are also used to screen patients for preventative or regular checkups like colorectal testing or mammograms.

Reporting: The practice searches are used to support the generation of reports that are requested by varied stakeholders, for example to enhance the administration of flu shots by providing estimates for future needs.

Tracking performance: Finally, the clinic has set up what they refer to as a "quality dashboard" that allows them to monitor their performance in terms of chronic disease management, screening and hospitalization. Practice searches are run regularly to track changes in quality indicators, e.g. according to guidelines for diabetes care. Their development over times is visualized in graphs that show for each of the doctors their own numbers as well as the clinic's average and a target value as defined by the health authorities (who are the payors).

3.2. Lessons Learned: Setting Up and Implementing Initiatives

The practice searches afford the systematic identification of areas for service quality improvement. However to actually have this information available and make use of it some preconditions have to be fulfilled:

Identification of focus and implementation of initiatives: The practice searches allow for a wide range of indicators for the quality of care to be evaluated. To be effective in actually changing practice, initiatives have to be introduced to follow up on the areas that are identified as needing improvement. This might include calling patients in or handing out information. As this adds additional tasks to an already busy work day of doctors and MOAs it is crucial to decide on specific areas to focus on. As one of the doctors emphasizes, it has to become part of the everyday workflow to be sustained.

Software functionality and knowledge of software: Once a focus is chosen the practice searches have to be set up accordingly. To be able to do so, knowledge of the range of functionality offered by the software is necessary to map it with the aims of the clinic. This includes finding out what searches are possible within the software, and identifying problems in the availability of data. As this again imposes additional tasks, it was important for the clinic to have a person with ample IT knowledge to develop an understanding of the software that would allow them to delegate these tasks. As mentioned by the clinical pharmacist "That was the joy of having [the researcher]: I asked her for the search, and she built it." Another obvious however crucial point is the reliability of the software. It happened that practice searches had to be set up anew after updates of the software, leading to frustration on part of the personnel at the CHC, and leaving them with the feeling of wasted effort.

Testing and tailoring: While the initial setup of the practice searches can be done by IT support, input from clinicians is needed to test them and check the results for their accuracy. The doctors do this by going through the lists of patients produced by the practice searches and by comparing them to what they know about their patients, identifying those who are either missing or should be included on the lists. Other means of checking are the patient lists generated by the CDM toolkit or the billing codes entered into another part of the EMR. In a next step the reason for wrong or incomplete data has to be tracked down. One of the doctors explains: "… and there is all sorts of nuances that an IT person wouldn't understand clinically. […] So for instance, doing mammograms you have to put in an exclusion for women who have had [bi-lateral] vasectomies. So you are just kind of refining the searches, looking at the different clinical situations. Or maybe there is two or three ways of labeling a specific disease process, so you have to label it consistently amongst all your clinicians and use the same ICD9 code." Of course, to be available it also has to be ensured that diagnoses are entered into the problem list in the first place.

Designated personnel and resources: IT support has already been mentioned as a precondition for the efficient use of practice searches. Another important resource is the personnel that is responsible to perform the practice searches, collect the data on a regular basis, and communicate the results back to the clinic or individual doctors. At the CHC these tasks are carried out by the clinical pharmacist together with the nurse practitioner, who both have a designated part of their weekly schedules to work on CDM coordination.

4. Discussion

In the adoption of the EMR to make enhanced use of patient data, new paradigms of care are emerging. We are moving, away from the mere focus on individual patient care to include an awareness of larger populations, and more systematic feedback on specific groups of patients. In the case study presented here we have seen that physicians found the CDM huddles especially helpful to regularly check up on their chronic disease patients. The quality dashboard was appreciated as a means to keep aware of preventative and screening initiatives that the clinic has chosen to focus on.

It is important to note however that data are not automatically available only because an EMR system is in use. In the case of the CHC practice searches were provided as an enhanced functionality of the EMR software. They had to be specifically set up, tested and tailored to the needs of the clinic. The quality of the data that can be retrieved depends heavily on the coding and classification system that is used. Also as pointed out by others much of the information that GPs need to treat patients is found "between the lines" in free-text fields which makes it inaccessible for automatic retrieval [9]. The context of the production of data, i.e. clinicians documenting patient encounters or prescribing medication and ordering examinations, is different from the context in which these same data are used to derive information about the whole patient population or the clinic performance. The information has to be disentangled, and this disentangling entails work [10].

The effort had to be coordinated within the whole team of the CHC. Additional tasks included not only the administration of practice searches, but also for doctors and MOAs following up with patients for checkups or providing information. As a group, the clinic had to determine which areas of focus to address for prevention, patient management or monitoring. Their choices were influenced by a combination of incentive structures and accepted wisdom in the form of practice guidelines.

5. Conclusion

Realizing the goals that EMRs have been introduced to meet related to secondary use of patient data can be challenging for clinics. The tools used and the information entered have to be accommodated as to allow for the grooming of patient populations. Our research suggests that once EMRs are introduced, there is a period during which staff first struggle to integrate them into their daily practices. The use of advanced features such as practice searches occurs once an EMR implementation has reached a degree of maturity, when software bugs and hardware problems related to the initial implementation have been solved, and practitioners and office staff have integrated basic functions of the EMR into daily practice. It was only at this point that staff in the clinical setting we studied were able to begin using practice searches on a regular basis, and it was through their initial attempts to use these features that they became aware of the need to alter work practices (e.g., by introducing greater uniformity in coding). Our work [7] suggests that utilization of advanced features of EMRs to support secondary use of data creates a need for additional technical support and coordinative functions, however because the use of advanced EMR features remains in its infancy, it is not yet clear how best to meet such needs.

References

[1]   P. G. Goldschmidt. HIT and MIS: implications of health information technology and medical information systems. *Commun ACM.* **48**(10) (2005), 68-74.
[2]   R. Kukafka, J. S. Ancker, C. Chan, J. Chelico, S. Khan, S. Mortoti, K. Natarajan, K. Presley, K. Stephens. Redesigning electronic health record systems to support public health. *J Biomed Inform.* **40**(4) (2007), 398-409.
[3]   A. L. Rector. Clinical terminology: Why is it so hard? *Methods Inf Med.* **38**(4-5) (1999), 239-252.
[4]   I. M. Holter, D. Schwartz-Barcott. Action research: What is it? How has it been used and how can it be used in nursing? *J Adv Nurs.* **18**(2) (1993), 298-304.
[5]   E. Hart, M. Bond. *Action Research for Health and Social Care: A Guide to Practice.* Buckingham UK: Open University Press; 1995. 244p.
[6]   K. Bodker, F. Kensing, J. Simonson J. *Participatory IT Design: Designing for Business and Workplace Realities.* Cambridge MA: MIT Press; 2004. 355p.
[7]   M. Tolar, E. Balka. Infrastructure in the Making: The Case of an EMR System in a General Practice Setting. CD ROM *Proceedings of AHIC.* Kitchener, Ontario, Canada: 2010.
[8]   N. Boulus. *A Journey Into the Hidden Lives of Electronic Medical Records (EMRs): Action Research in the Making.* PhD thesis, School of Communication, Simon Fraser University, Spring 2010.
[9]   M. A. Johansen, J. Scholl, P. Hasvold, G. Ellingsen, J. G. Bellika. "Garbage In, Garbage Out" – Extracting Disease Surveillance Data from EPR Systems in Primary Care. *Proceedings of CSCW.* San Diego, California, USA: 2008: 525-534.
[10] M. Berg, E. Goorman. The contextual nature of medical information. *Int J Med Inform.* **56**(1): (1999), 51-60.

Acknowledgments

The work presented was carried out within the project "Knowledge to Action: Supporting Continuity of Care and Practice", financed by the Canadian Institutes of Health Research and Canada Health Infoway. Our thanks go to the researcher who collected the data in participant observations, as well as to all the personnel at the CHC, who provided access to the field and their time for interviews, and are a pleasure to collaborate with.

International Perspectives in Health Informatics
E.M. Borycki et al. (Eds.)
IOS Press, 2011
© 2011 ITCH 2011 Steering Committee and IOS Press. All rights reserved.
doi:10.3233/978-1-60750-709-3-148

e-Health Promises and Challenges: Some Ethical Considerations

Eike-Henner W. KLUGE[a, 1]

[a] *University of Victoria, Victoria, British Columbia, Canada*

Abstract. eHealth is a cost-effective and efficient way of providing health care to patients who would otherwise be excluded or underserviced. However, eHealth also presents a series of ethical and legal challenges which, if not met before its implementation, can undermine its success. Among other things, privacy, consent and liability are implicated, as are changes in the health care professional-patient relationship and in the role of health informatics professionals. Legacy systems and interoperability present further challenges, and outsourcing may pose special problems. This paper highlights some of these issues and outlines their implications.

Keywords. eHealth, ethics, privacy, consent, liability

Introduction

The delivery of health care has always been profoundly influenced by technological developments and innovations.[1] Certainly, this is true of modern health care whether it be in medicine or nursing, surgery or diagnostics, imaging or pharmacology. Indeed, it has been argued that modern health care professionals are obsessed with technology and rush to apply innovations like children who cannot wait to try out a new toy [2, 3] and that eHealth in particular is implicated.

Of course such a sweeping view of eHealth may be unfair. If its proponents are to be believed, eHealth has the potential for overcoming barriers of geography [4], professional availability [5], limitations of transportation and infrastructure [6], and even problems caused by socioeconomic disparity. Moreover, it holds the promise of maximizing effectiveness and efficiency at the lowest possible cost without seriously interfering in patients' lives. Arguably, therefore, eHealth is not an instance of the technological imperative but the considerate choice of responsible health care planners. Nevertheless, eHealth comes with a number of potentially serious challenges. These are not insurmountable. However, they should be addressed and solved prior to implementation lest downstream difficulties undermine what otherwise would be a beneficial development.

---

[1] Corresponding Author: Eike-Henner W. Kluge, University of Victoria. Victoria, BC, Canada, V8W 3P4; E-mail: ekluge@uvic.ca.

1. Technical Reliability and Appropriateness

To begin with, eHealth presents obvious technical issues. Device safety and standardization are clearly implicated,[7] as is the ability to ensure data integrity and reliability, and the power to gather and communicate data accurately with appropriate back-up measures to guard against malfunction or interruption.[8] Moreover, from a human perspective the technology's ability to provide accurate and appropriate patient data without constant technical supervision is essential, since otherwise eHealth could easily devolve into an intolerable intrusion into patient lives, sacrificing quality-of-life on the altar of efficiency. [9]

2. Interoperability, Legacy Systems and Quality Assurance

As well, since eHealth is not a stand-alone modality but intended to complement existing modalities, it has to integrate seamlessly into whatever is in place. This means that technical interoperability with existing health systems in all their aspects, including legacy systems, is essential. Failure in this regard will undermine its effectiveness and may have serious legal consequences. Moreover, interoperability goes beyond the institutional hospital-based setting. Since patients travel and interact with physicians and health care providers who are not hospital based, interoperability must be construed in the widest possible terms.

Furthermore, given the rapid changes in ICT, diagnostic technology etc. there lies a duty, rooted in the fiduciary nature of the health care provider-patient relationship, to ensure that eHealth systems contain appropriate measures to ensure a seamless legacy structure within themselves so as to integrate their own protocols and components with previous versions as these become obsolete and are replaced. Consequently, even more so than with any other method of delivering health care, eHealth is not a modality that is complete and can be "forgotten" once it is in place.

Finally, as a new service modality, eHealth is subject to close scrutiny regarding appropriateness, safety and the like. The need for interoperability, however, makes it highly likely that such scrutiny will expand beyond the immediate context of eHealth itself to include the existing health care structures, so that operational flaws can be correctly identified as belonging either to the existing structures, to eHealth itself or to their interface, and that appropriate corrective action can be taken. Therefore, while quality assessment is part of normal quality management, the introduction of eHealth may well accelerate this process. The financial costs of introducing eHealth may therefore go beyond the direct costs associated with its implementation.

3. Privacy, Data Ownership and Unique Patient Identifiers

Privacy concerns also acquire a new dimension. By and large, national laws and international conventions (such as the European Union Directive 96/46/EC) stipulate that health care professionals and institutions have a duty to protect the confidentiality of patient data to the best of their ability, and that breaches in this regard should be communicated to the subjects of the data in due time and in an appropriate manner.[10] Various techniques and measures have been developed to achieve this end, and while privacy breaches do occur, they are relatively infrequent and are usually the result of professional malfeasance or inaction.

eHealth changes this situation because it introduces patients and their home environment into the mix. Privacy measures developed for institutional contexts may be neither possible nor appropriate in the home setting, yet privacy requirements remain. Care must therefore be taken that appropriate adjustments or additions in the relevant protocols are made to accommodate the differences in locale and human interactions, and that it is clear whose obligations extend how far and under what circumstances.

Information ownership and control may also present serious issues. Thus, in some jurisdictions information in patient records belongs to the patients and, except for carefully delimited circumstances, may not be accessed, manipulated or communicated without patient consent. In other jurisdictions this is not the case. Here, ownership and/or control lie entirely in the hands of health care providers and patient access to information about themselves is at the former's discretion and may be selective. With the globalization of telemedicine and eHealth, this may become problematic. Some jurisdictions - the European Union again is the most obvious example - have attempted to deal with this issue through regulatory provisions and by quasi-legislative means. [10] However, these still allow national laws and rules to predominate in critical and troublesome cases and thus effectively leave unresolved the question of which laws and standards apply. While treaties may address the issue between different countries, they leave unresolved the question of what rules apply for global eHealth where members of health care teams may not be in jurisdictions that are part of a particular treaty process.

Moreover, eHealth is impossible without electronic health records (EHRs). These must be linkable on an as-needed basis so that the correct diagnosis can be made and the right intervention given to the right patient at the right time. This is impossible without unique patient identifiers (UPIs). While some jurisdictions have introduced UPIs, ethical and legal concerns have been raised about them, specifically in regard to such issues as possible "function creep" in their usage. [11]

Finally, eHealth may involve a changing group of diverse professionals who may never come in contact with the patients. EHRs, therefore, become central in no merely accidental sense. Data suggest that this may threaten patients' perception of themselves as persons, and raise the fear of becoming re-defined as mere sets of data distributed among a variety of data banks and subject to purely administrative considerations, where rights are trumped by efficiency and responsibilities are shrugged off for the sake of for the sake of administrative ease and profit. [9]

4. Outsourcing and its Associated Problems

Another parameter that may deserve attention is outsourcing. Specifically, since little technology is developed in-house and even national players are often incapable of providing it and the associated services at an acceptable price, there is the temptation to ameliorate costs by outsourcing [12, 13]

This may be problematic if the relevant corporations are headquartered or located in countries with security and privacy laws that differ from those of the eHealth providers. For instance, US-based corporations are subject to the *USA Patriot Act* [14].

This makes it impossible for them to guarantee that the records or data in their possession (including the base codes for their operating systems) will not be accessible to US intelligence agencies without the procedural safeguards that may be mandated in the eHealth provider's jurisdiction.[14] As the case of Maximus BC (which was contracted to provide health record records services for British Columbia and whose parent company is in the US) illustrates, dealing with this issue may transcend the resources and mandates of eHealth providers because it may require the passage of appropriate legislation.[15] This raises privacy concerns to a whole new plateau.[15]

Finally, since eHealth requires intensive monitoring and fast turn-around times but trained staff is scarce or unavailable on a constant basis, there may be the temptation to turn to international medical diagnostic and consultative service providers. This has already happened in other contexts. Radiographs originating in Chicago have been read in Bangalore [16] or Zurich [17], billings originating in Berlin or Mexico City have become outsourced to Bloomington [18] or Chennai, etc.[19]. This raises the question whether eHealth providers who outsource such services have enforceable mechanisms to ensure that distant parties providing the services will abide by at-home laws and can effectively be held responsible for professional errors.

5. Liability and Patients as Co-Deliverers of Health Care

In traditional health care, data that underlie health care decision-making are developed by health care professionals, and control of data gathering and manipulation lies in the hands of the professionals and their staff. Data-related mistakes or misadventures, therefore, are purely a matter of professional care, diligence and competence. With eHealth, patients become participants in the data generation process when data gathering and transmission is not entirely automated through indwelling telemetry etc.[2-22]. This introduces the possibility of patient error either in measuring or on reporting values. Even when the process is automatic, patients may accidentally interfere with measurement or with the transmission process, resulting in misadventure. Liability apportionment therefore assumes a new dimension that is further complicated when significant others are involved and the issue of their co-responsibility arises.

There are, of course, legal precedents from other areas of health care when patients contribute to negative outcomes. However, these are grounded in the traditional model of the health care professional-patient relationship. It assumes that the delivery of care involves a direct patient-professional encounter, that the patient's contribution to the functioning of the techniques and technologies is minimal, and that the reliability of instrument-based patient data is independent of patient skills. eHealth changes this picture. Accordingly, it is doubtful that eHealth providers can rely on traditional approaches to liability. The development of new consent and liability models acknowledging the expanded agency patient (and/or significant others) therefore seems a prudent precondition before implementing eHealth.

Finally, eHealth also requires the development of appropriate patient-training modules. Failure to do so may well amount to professional and/or institutional negligence. [9]

6. Conclusion

eHealth presents the promise of rationalizing health expenditures by limiting institutional admissions and interventions to truly appropriate cases.[9] However, eHealth also poses challenges that are more than merely technical in nature. These include value-issues that go to the very nature of health care, to the nature of the health care provider-patient relationship, and they involve issues such as informed consent, privacy and liability. Moreover, eHealth presents human challenges. Data show that while some patients welcome eHealth as evidence of concern for patient well-being, others reject it as an unacceptable medicalization of the home environment and as an intolerable intrusion into their homes and private lives.[9] None of these issues detract from eHealth's promise of cost-effectiveness and efficiency. However, this promise should not be allowed to obscure the fact that the challenges posed by eHealth are multi-dimensional and should be addressed prior to its implementation.

References

[1]   B. Hoffman, Is there a technological imperative in health care? *Int J Tech Assess H Care* **18** (2002), 675-689.
[2]   A. J. Hanson, *The idea of progress and the goals of medicine. In M.J. Hanson and D. Callahan, The goals of medicine: The forgotten issues in health care reform*, Georgetown University Press, Washington, DC, 137-151, 1999.
[3]   S. Wolf, B. B. Berle, *The technological imperative in medicine*, Plenum Press, New York, 1981.
[4]   R. M. Wachter, The "dis-location" of U.S. medicine — the implications of medical outsourcing, *New Eng J Med* **354** (2006), 661-5.
[5]   L. H. Schwamm, E. S. Rosenthal, A. Hirshberg, P. W. Schaefer, E. A. Little, J. C. Kvedar, I. Petkovska, W. J. Koroshetz, S. R. Levine, Virtual TeleStroke support for the emergency department evaluation of acute stroke, *Acad Emerg Med* **11** (2004), 1193-1197.
[6]   D. Blumenthal, Stimulating the adoption of health information technology, *New Eng J Med,* **360** (2009), 1477.
[7]   S. Kokolakis, D. Gritzalis, S. Katsikas, Why we need standardisation in healthcare security, *Stud Health Tech Inf* **69** (2002), 229-37.
[8]   S. Pavlopoulos, A. Anagnostaki, D. Koutsouris, A. Lymberis, P. Levene, M. Reynolds, N. Geordiadis, C. Lambrinoudakis, D. Gritzalis, Vital signs monitoring from home with open systems, *Stud Health Tech Inf* **77** (2000), 1141-5.
[9]   K. Tran, J. Polisena, D. Coyle, K. Coyle, E-H. Kluge, K. Cimon, S. McGill, H. Noorani, K. Palmer, R. Scott, *Home telehealth for chronic disease management*, Canadian Agency for Drugs and Technologies in Health, Ottawa, 2008.
[10] EU Directive 94/56 EC Article 4, Article 8.4, Article 13:1, etc. updated in EU Directive 2002/58.
[11] M. Metherell, Security fears may delay e-health reforms until after election, *Sidney Morning Herald*, [Cited on 2010 March 22] Available from: http://www.smh.com.au/technology/technology-news/security-fears-may-delay-ehealth-reforms-until-after-election-20100321-qo72.html
[12] N. Sanjiv, J. D. Singh, R. M. Wachter, Perspectives on medical outsourcing and telemedicine — Rough edges in a flat world? *New Eng J Med* **358** (2008), 1622-162.
[13] F. Levy, A. Goelman, K-H Yu, Paging Dr. Gupta: Radiology as a case study in sending skilled jobs offshore, *Milken Institute Review* **2** (2006), 64-72.
[14] *Uniting and Strengthening America by Providing Appropriate Tools Required to Intercept and Obstruct Terrorism Act* (HR 3162) §215.
[15] British Columbia Office of the Information and Privacy Commissioner, Privacy and the USA Patriot Act: Implications for British Columbia Public Sector Outsourcing; [Cited on 2010 April 19] Available from: http://www.oipc.bc.ca/sector_public/archives/usa_patriot_act/pdfs/report/privacy-final.pdf

[16]   A. Kalyanpur, V. P. Neklesa, D. T. Pham, H. P. Forman, S. T. Stein, J. A. Brink, Implementation of an international teleradiology staffing model, *Radiology* **232** (2004), 415-9.

[17]   Steinbrook R, The age of teleradiology, *New Eng J Med* **357** (2007), 5-7.

[18]   Outsource Management Group Available from: http://www.outsourcemedicalbilling.com/.

[19]   Senter Soft Technologies, [Cited on 2009 April 17] Chennai, Available from: http://www.sentersoftech.com/business-process-medical.html.

[20]   R. Bellazzi, S. Montani, A. Riva, M. Stefanelli, Web-based telemedicine systems for home-care: technical issues and experiences, *Comp Meth Prog Biomed* **64** (2001), 175-87.

[21]   A. Dittmar, F. Axisa, G. Delhomme, C. Gehin, New concepts and technologies in home care and ambulatory monitoring, *Stud Health Tech Inf* **108** (2004), 9-35.

[22]   N. Oudshoorn, Diagnosis at a distance: The invisible work of patients and healthcare professionals in cardiac telemonitoring technology, *Soc Health Illness* **30** (2008), 272-88.

Health Informatics Initiatives in Developing Countries

International Perspectives in Health Informatics
E.M. Borycki et al. (Eds.)
IOS Press, 2011
doi:10.3233/978-1-60750-709-3-157

Monitoring of Congenital Anomalies in Developing Countries: A Pilot Model in Iran

Saeed DASTGIRI [a,1] , Yaghoub SHEIKHZADEH [b], Ali DASTGIRI [a]

[a] *Department of Community and Family Medicine, National Public Management Centre (NPMC), Tabriz, Iran*
[b] *Department of Health Information Science, University of Victoria, Victoria, British Columbia, Canada*

Abstract. Aims: This is an ongoing project aiming to establish a monitoring system of congenital anomalies in the Northwest of Iran, and to implement control and preventive tasks in the region. Methods: Our program covers about 15 000 births (average per year) in a defined area with about 350 cases (average per year) of congenital anomalies born in the region. The definition of the congenital anomalies is based on the standard coding system of the International Classification of Diseases according to the primary diagnosis of anomaly. Results: The program examines the rates and patterns of various types of congenital anomalies and looks for possible local causes and influencing factors in the population. This monitoring program provides a pilot model into the epidemiology and potential for prevention and control of congenital anomalies in the community level. Evaluation procedures are essential part of our program to monitor the effects of preventive services for congenital anomalies in order to identify and correct shortcomings. Conclusion: Our program provides some essential data as an epidemiological tool for local investigators, information for health service planners, clinicians and for genetic counselors. It may also help to identify regional interventions that could help to prevent and control congenital anomalies in the study population and similar areas.

Keywords. congenital anomalies, prevention, epidemiology, health information, control

Introduction

Occurrence of congenital anomalies varies between different countries ranging from 2 to 10 percent of births. Congenital anomalies are now making a proportionally greater contribution to ill health in childhood. They are a leading cause of perinatal mortality and childhood morbidity and disability in many countries [1-16]. The financial cost of treating children (mainly surgical correction) with birth defects, and the emotional effects and disruption of normal family life associated with deaths caused by

---
[1] Corresponding Author: Dr Saeed Dastgiri, Department of Community and Family Medicine School of Medicine, Tabriz University of Medical Sciences, Tabriz, Iran; Email: saeed.dastgiri@gmail.com.

congenital anomalies are also enormous for people in both developed and less developed countries.

The etiology of these disorders is still largely unknown. However, the prevention of these disorders is available in 60 percent of cases [17-18]. Genetic counseling and educational programs for high risk population are essential for success of any control program at the community level so that they can understand and accept the tenets of the preventive programs and be able to utilize it appropriately and to their advantage. Preventive strategies in developed countries have been shown as one of the contributing factors to the declining prevalence of congenital anomalies in the last few decades [19-20]. Such interventional programs should be considered by government and non-government organizations (including patient/parent support groups) in developing countries too.

Until recent years, there were no data available about the prevalence, etiology, and preventive strategies of congenital anomalies in the Northwest of Iran. Beginning from 2000, we carried out a research project on the epidemiology of congenital anomalies aiming to document the epidemiologic features of congenital anomalies in the Northwest of Iran as the baseline information to set up a regional population-based registry of birth defects [14, 21]. Our program was also presented and accepted in the 2006 annual meeting of International Clearinghouse for Birth Defects Surveillance and Research (ICBDSR) in Sweden, as a member of countries having an established registry for birth defects [21-22]. The program is now called Tabriz Registry of Congenital Anomalies (TRoCA).

1. Aims

The principal aims of our program are to establish a monitoring system of congenital anomalies in the Northwest of Iran, and to implement control and preventive tasks in the region. The TRoCA program examines the rates and patterns of various types of congenital anomalies and looks for possible local causes and influencing factors in infants diagnosed in maternity hospitals, children hospitals or genetic clinics. Application of this monitoring and surveillance program may provide a pilot model and insights into the epidemiology and potential for prevention and control of congenital anomalies in the whole region and in similar areas.

2. Design, Study Population, and Analysis

The TRoCA program was initiated in 2000. It is a hospital-based registry (located in the Alzahra University Hospital of Tabriz University of Medical Sciences) covering all births and children in the city of Tabriz. This city is one of the three major cities in the country and is the centre of East Azarbaijan Province. Infants diagnosed in three public maternity/children medical centers (Alzahra, Taleghani and Children hospitals) as having birth defects are covered in this program. These hospitals provide obstetric and gynecological services in the study population. The program covers 15 000 births (average per year) in the defined area with about 300 cases (average per year) of congenital anomalies born with one of the anomalies in this population.

The definition of the congenital anomalies for the purposes of the program is based on the standard coding system of the International Classification of Diseases (ICD) and British Pediatric Association [23]. Thus, the subjects comprised all births registered and notified to those hospitals and medical centers with a primary diagnosis under one of the following headings: nervous system anomalies, genito-urinary tract and kidney defects, anomalies of limb, chromosomal anomalies, cleft lip with/without palate, congenital heart disease, musculoskeletal and connective tissue anomalies, digestive system anomalies, eye and ear anomalies and other anomalies.

All infants are routinely examined by a gynecologist, obstetrician or neonatologist at birth and hospital discharge. The examinations include assessment of general health, maturity and congenital anomalies. General epidemiological data and basic characteristic information are collected for all births. Information is also gathered for mothers of all malformed infants. Other women giving births in those hospitals with normal newborns might be, in case, considered as matched control groups for research purposes.

Information is collected using the standard data form of European Registration of Congenital Anomalies (EUROCAT) for congenital anomalies [16]. This form is routinely used in all European countries participating in the EUROCAT surveillance program of congenital anomalies. The parents or accompanying adults are asked to provide basic information required on the form. Technical information is filled on the form using diagnostic records of each subject. Data are anonymised at source of data collection to keep personal information private. More details of the organization and performance of the TRoCA can be found elsewhere [24].

3. Epidemiological Findings

Total prevalence of congenital anomalies was 1.7 per 100 births between 2000 and 2008. Genito-urinary tract and kidney defects, anomalies of nervous system, and limb anomalies accounted proportionally for more than 68% of anomalies in the region. There was an increasing trend in the prevalence of congenital anomalies in the study area from 2000 (1.05 per 100 births) to 2008 (2.45 per 100 births).

This time trend was not however significant using linear regression statistical analysis where the dependent variable was the prevalence of congenital anomalies and the predictor was the birth year from 2000 to 2008 ($P = 0.07$).

4. Applications

TRoCA provides some essential data and identifies local interventions that could help to prevent and control congenital anomalies in the study population. Some of these interventions may be specific to the study population and similar areas, whilst others may have more general applications.

Moreover, TRoCA may also help health care system for affected families who need, and an epidemiological tool for local investigators, information for health service planners, clinicians and for genetic counselors.

5. Monitoring and Evaluation

Evaluation procedures are essential part of our program to monitor effects of preventive services for congenital anomalies in order to identify and correct shortcomings. Fortunately, using our current registry of congenital anomalies, we can monitor the number of new cases in the coverage area. Patients can then be followed up to assess the extent to which the educational interventions have been taken into account and to evaluate the amount and quality of the prevention information provided to other family members. Using the registry data, prenatal diagnosis services can also be assessed by birth prevalence rate of affected individuals, the choices that couples (at risk) make with respect to using prenatal diagnosis, the rate of prenatal diagnosis performed, the rate of births of children with avoidable conditions, and the rate of medical termination of pregnancies due to fatal defects.

Acknowledgements

Authors wish to thank Dr Mohammad Heidarzadeh, Miss Akram Tajahmad, Mrs Elham Rezaian, Mr Heidar Fathizadeh, Ms Mina Noorbakhsh, Ms Neda Poodratchi, Ms Zahra Altafi and our colleagues at Alzahra, Taleghani and Children hospitals of Tabriz University of Medical Sciences for their assistance on data collection and project management. We also thank Ministry of Health and Medical Education (Neonatal Unit) and Tabriz University of Medical Sciences for funding this project.

References

[1] C.M. Druschel, J.P. Hughes, C. Olsen, Mortality among infants with congenital malformations, New York State, 1983 to 1988, *Pub Health Rep* 111 (1996), 359–365.
[2] E. Powell-Griner, A. Woolbright, Trends in infant deaths from congenital anomalies: results from England and Wales, Scotland, Sweden and the United States, *Int J Epidemio* 19 (1990), 391–398.
[3] M. Gatt, A*nnual Congenital Anomalies Report in Malta*, Department of Health Information, Guardamangia, Malta, 2002.
[4] M.M. Thein, D. Koh, K.L. Tan, H.P. Lee, Y.Y. Yip, C.Y. Tye, W.O. Phoon, Descriptive profile of birth defects among live births in Singapore, *Teratology* 46 (1992), 277–284.
[5] L.I. Al-Gazali, R. Alwash, Y.M. Abdulrazzaq, United Arab Emirates: Communities and community genetics, *Comm Gen* 8 (2005), 186–196.
[6] K. C. Johnson, J. Rouleau, Temporal trends in Canadian birth defects birth prevalence, 1979–1993, *Can J Public Health* 88 (1997), 169–176.
[7] International Clearinghouse for Birth Defects Monitoring Systems, *Annual Report 2005: with data for 2003*, International Clearinghouse for Birth Defects Monitoring Systems (ICBDSR), Roma, Italy, 2005.
[8] P. A. Baird, Prenatal screening and the reduction of birth defects in populations, *Comm Gen* 2 (1999), 9–17.
[9] J. Mulinare, L.Y. Wong, H.Q. Gu, J.D. Erickson, A population-based birth defects surveillance system in the People's Republic of China, *Paed Peri Epid* 17 (2003), 287–293.
[10] R.E. Stevenson, W.P. Allen, G.S. Pai, R. Best, L.H. Seaver, J. Dean, S. Thompson, Decline in prevalence of neural tube defects in a high risk region of the United States, *Paed* 106 (2000), 677–683.
[11] H. Hamamy, A. Alwan, Hereditary disorders in the Eastern Mediterranean Region, *Bull World Health Org* 72 (1994), 145–154.
[12] S. Dastgiri, D.H. Stone, C. Le-Ha, W.H. Gilmour, Prevalence and secular trend of congenital anomalies in Glasgow, U.K, *Arch Dis Childhood* 86 (2002), 257-263.

[13] C. Bower, E. Rudy, A. Ryan, Cosgrove P., *Report of the Birth Defects Registry of Western Australia*, King Edward Memorial, Hospital Women's and Children's Health Service, Subiaco, Australia, 2004.

[14] S. Dastgiri, S. Imani, L. Kalankesh, M. Barzeghar, M. Heidarzadeh, Congenital anomalies in Iran: A cross-sectional study on 1574 cases in the north-west of country, *Child: Care, Health and Development* **33** (2007), 257–261.

[15] C. Bower, S. Eades, J. Payne, H. D'Antoine, F.J. Stanley, Trends in neural tube defects in Western Australia in indigenous and non-indigenous populations, *Paed Peri Epidemio* **18** (2004), 277–280.

[16] EUROCAT Working Group, available at: <http://www.ihe.be/eurocat>, 2007.

[17] A.E. Czeizel, Prevention of congenital anomalies by periconceptional multivitamin supplementation, *BMJ* **306** (1993), 1645–1648.

[18] A.E. Czeizel, Z. Intody, B. Modell, What proportion of congenital anomalies can be prevented? *BMJ* **306** (1993), 499-503.

[19] World Health Organization, *Community Approaches to the Control of Hereditary Diseases*, Report of a WHO advisory group, World Health Organization, Geneva, Switzerland, 1985.

[20] World Health Organization, *Control of Hereditary Diseases*, Report of a WHO scientific group, World Health Organization, Geneva, Switzerland, 1996.

[21] Tabriz Registry of Congenital Anomalies, available at: <http://www.tbzmed.ac.ir/troca>, 2007.

[22] International Clearinghouse for Birth Defects Surveillance and Research, available: <http://www.icbdsr.org>, 2007.

[23] British Paediatric Association, *British Paediatric Association Classification of Disease*, 1979.

[24] S. Dastgiri, L. Kalankesh, M. Heidarzadehe, A. Tajahmade, E. Rezaiane, A new registry of congenital anomalies in Iran, *J Reg Manage* **37** (2010), 9–27.

International Perspectives in Health Informatics
E.M. Borycki et al. (Eds.)
IOS Press, 2011
© 2011 ITCH 2011 Steering Committee and IOS Press. All rights reserved.
doi:10.3233/978-1-60750-709-3-162

Economics of Health Informatics in Developing Countries

Ronald J. HÉBERT [1]
Heron Technology Corp.

Abstract. Health Informatics (HI) has become a world wide issue since 2005 when the WHO Health Metrics Network (HMN) was formed to encourage all of the developing countries (151) to get started in eHealth. Prior to this HMN initiative the only countries with HI in place were the developed countries (40) and a few developing countries (Jamaica, Malaysia, etc.) that were just getting started in HI with a very limited number of applications compared to the developed countries. This paper suggests that much of the experience in HI gained in the developed countries can be shared with the developing countries as 'lessons learnt' – as long as the issue of economics is kept front and foremost in the planning.

Keywords. developing countries, health informatics, health economics

Introduction

Under the HMN initiative over 100 developing countries were provided with modest grants to conduct surveys of their HI situation, to confirm for all involved that in fact there were limited systems in place, even on a manual paper-based basis in most countries. More recently the Global Fund for HIV/AIDS, TB and Malaria has allocated about US$1.5 billion for Health Systems Strengthening (HSS), which includes HI.

The current Information Technology and Communications in Health (ITCH) conference aspires to share information among attendees and industry on ICT in developing countries.

"Health Informatics: International Perspectives will provide a unique opportunity to focus on international comparisons. Major lessons will be there to be learnt by both developed and developing communities as health informatics becomes ever more central to the organization and delivery of healthcare across the globe."

1. Big Questions

Let's explore some of the big questions for HI in developing country public health:
(a) Why are all of the developed countries fairly well established in HI?

---

[1] Author: Ron Hébert, Heron Technology Corp , Markham, ON, Canada   email   ronh@herontech.com

(b) Why have all of the developing countries not even started in HI?
(c) Are there some international comparisons available?
(d) What lessons have been learnt?
Answers to some of the big questions in HI will follow in the next section.

1.1. Why Are All of the Developed Countries well Established in HI?

Economics! The main reason is that the developed countries can afford to implement HI, even when major mistakes are made, along the path to ultimate success in the years ahead. It is obvious from experiences in commercial business activities that computerization brings many benefits not available from manual paper-based systems, and that these benefits are also delivered on a cost-effective basis. The same rationale applies to HI. In the 1960s and 1970s when the developed countries started into HI there was no HI software, hardware was extremely expensive relative to clerical costs, and there were no known best practices to draw upon. After 40 years of experience the developed countries have learnt a lot and now do have many lessons to share with the international community of 151 developing countries just now starting into HI.

1.2. Why Have All of the Developing Countries not Even Started in HI?

Economics! This is clearly the most identifiable single factor that differentiates the developed countries from the developing countries. A developing country by definition has an annual GDP per capita of less than US$10,000. A specific example to demonstrate this difference can be shown in a mid-range developing country – Jamaica – when compared to Canada, one of the 40 developed countries. Canada has an annual GDP per capita of $38,440 whereas Jamaica has an annual GDP per capita of $3,900, demonstrating a distinct differential in spending capability ($10 to $1). When looking closely at the public health sector, we see an even more dramatic differential with Canada spending about $3,800 annually on public health per capita, compared to Jamaica's $156 annually on public health per capita (24 to 1).

We know from experience in Canada that health budgets are constantly under great pressure, and that HI in particular is under even greater pressure, for not all HI expenditures demonstrate a clear payback for funds spent in the eyes of the taxpayer. Imagine then how much more difficult it must be to allocate public funds for HI in developing countries. If the HI costs in Jamaica were the same on a per capita basis as in Canada, then it would cost 23 times more per capita for HI in this country selected as an example. Jamaica is relatively well off compared to most African countries where the annual per capita public health spending is often in the range of $10 to $20.

1.3. Are There Some International Comparisons Available?

Yes, there are some comparisons available, however on a very limited scale, since only a very few developing countries have even attempted to start to computerize their health sectors. Since economics is at the heart of success, or failure, let's look at some comparisons that are based on economics.

An example with which the author is familiar is the implementation of a Patient Administration System (PAS) in Jamaica (1997 to now). As noted, if the costs of this PAS were the same as in Canada – where it was developed – it would not be sustainable in Jamaica, and would have ceased operation a long time ago. A close examination of the one-time and on-going costs of the Heron PAS in 13 large hospitals and clinics of Jamaica reveals that the annual per capita cost of the PAS is about US$0.81. This compares to about US$12.00 per capita for a PAS in Canada, as deduced from the 2009 study done by Branham Research of Ottawa. This ratio of 1 to 15 permits the PAS to actually remain sustainable in an environment where the annual per capita health spending, compared to Canada, is in the ratio of 1 to 24.

Even though a PAS is the first module to be implemented on the clinical side, Jamaica has not had the financial resources to move on to the many other clinical modules desired (Pharmacy; Diagnostic Imaging; Laboratory; Dietary, etc.) in the hospitals as would be found in the hospitals of all of the developed countries. However, the PAS in Jamaica has permitted the Minister of Health (John Junor) to state that Jamaica benefits from an 'evidence-based' health system, and the CDC says Jamaica IT could be a world 'model'.

1.4. What Lessons Have Been Learnt?

Many lessons have been learnt, however these lessons could not be expected to be known to the key government officials, or taken very seriously by their   paid 'consultants'.

2. The Main Lessons Learnt

The bottom line answer is that HI is a very complex matter – in the same category as 'Reverse- Engineer the Brain'[2]. The following are some of the main lessons learned.

2.1. Get Started!

Unfortunately, since this is a very complex matter almost all of the 151 developing countries have yet to even 'start'. It is essential to start thereby enabling the officials within the country to begin to understand the challenging path that must be travelled during the coming years. Once started, progress can be made slowly.

2.2. Where to Start?

On the clinical side a country should start with a PAS (Patient Administration System) which manages all encounters and the identity of the patient – at least at the local hospital level. On the financial side the General Ledger module should be implemented to manage the budget at the hospital and overall country level.

2.3. Economics?

Since this matter is at the heart of success – or failure – it is very important that every component of the HI implementation be at the lowest cost possible. Some of the lessons learnt in this regard are:

- Lay out an implementation plan that costs no more that 1% of the annual health budget, with all one-time costs (hardware; software; training; installation) being amortized over 10 years. Include local technical support.
- Use low cost desktop devices, such as 'thin-clients' and avoid devices that require any on-site technical support such as 'fat-client' PCs.
- Training should be on a group (5 to 10 hospitals) basis, and based on the 'train-the-trainer' approach. Use of the Internet with such software products as GoToMeeting will reduce travel costs and provide flexibility in training hours.
- Standardize all system components, particularly software and hardware.
- Utilize 'Open Source' software tools such as the license-free Linux operating system, and other Open Source tools to reduce license costs.

2.4. Patient mobility and UPI:

When HI began in the developed countries, little or no consideration was given to the fact that a patient might present at different hospitals which would, of course, require that his/her health records be available at each facility. Since we now recognize that during a patient's lifetime encounters will be made to many health facilities. Provision must be made in HI for this reality. The country, early on, should establish a Unique Patient Identifier (UPI) permitting patient mobility.

2.5. Consultants?

This is a serious issue for a developing country just starting into HI. Since there is usually limited, if any, local expertise in HI an external consultant that is knowledgeable in HI is an essential component in the development of a plan permitting the government to secure approval of the necessary funds. However, all too often the consultant is from a developed country and is not familiar with the basic economic differences in the per capita health budget of a developed/developing country. The reality is that most consultant HIS reports are not acted upon – as the underlying economic matters are not incorporated – and the report 'sits on the shelf'.

2.6. Go Slowly

All too often an external consultant presents a comprehensive HIS (Health Information System) implementation plan that may include upwards of 20 application software modules, to be implemented over 3 to 5 years. This approach will fail, and has always failed, yet consultants continue to present such an HIS approach on a short timeline, often for local political reasons. The HIS will fail for 2 main reasons:
- The costs will rapidly exceed the suggested 1% to 2% of health budget level
- The 'business process' of moving from a manual paper-based system to an HIS becomes completely overwhelming, particularly in the matter of integration between the various application software modules.

An example of a developing country that opted to implement an HIS in 1998, with the guidance of their retained consultant, is Limpopo province, South Africa. By 2002 the HIS had failed, at a loss of about US$50 million. This implementation is mentioned herewith since it is one of the rare instances where an ICT failure has been so thoroughly documented in a developing country. A report on this HIS failure was prepared by Health Systems Trust, a non-profit health overseer in South Africa. There are many lessons to be learnt from this failure noted by BMJ[3], and officials in developing countries looking at eHealth today may care to study this 'case study'.

2.7. Single vendor or Multi-vendors:

The single-vendor approach – application software modules from the same vendor - was historically popular in the developed countries, based mainly on the 'one-contract-to-sign' approach. Since the introduction of 'middleware' in the mid-1990s the earlier single-vendor approach has given way to the multi-vendor approach with application software being from many 'specialty' vendors, such as PAS from one vendor, Pharmacy from a different vendor, etc.

The multi-vendor approach is even more critical for developing countries that face an extended implementation timeframe, say over 30 years, compared to the developed countries that have much higher resource levels – financial and personnel.

Also, experience in Canada has shown that the success rate of staying in business by the 'specialty' vendors is much higher – at 90% - than for the single-vendors – at 17% - over the period of twenty years (1989 – 2009). Since a developing country will require many more years to implement an HIS than a developed country, the risk factor is far lower with the multi-vendor 'specialty' application software approach.

2.8. Programs Not 'Projects':

Some developing countries are of the opinion that there are certain advantages in writing their own application software modules ('projects'), as opposed to purchasing the application software modules from vendors (programs).

In the early days of HI in Canada, as well I am sure in the other developed countries, this sentiment held favour in many hospitals. One of the major problems with this approach is that there can be no up-front budget, nothing to continuously monitor, and in the end most IT projects become 'run-aways'. It is a dead concept.

2.9. 'Dangerous Enthusiasms':

This statement refers to the cause of many HI failures in all countries, and is particularly appropriate to the developing countries which are now trying to 'catch up' to the developed countries which are 30 years ahead in experience and have in-place systems that can be integrated to new application software modules.

The book 'Dangerous Enthusiasms'[4], by Robin Gauld and Shaun Goldfinch, outlines a number of massive HI failures in New Zealand, a developed country, which can, and did, recover from the many noted health sector failures. However, if HI failures on the same scale were to occur in a developing country the economic effect would be devastating for years to come.

3. References

[1] 'Advance HI' is 1 of the 14 'Grand Engineering Challenges of the 21st century' www.engineeringchallenges.org
[2] BMJ (British Medical Journal) provides an overview and links to the Health Systems Trust, South Africa, report on HIS in Limpopo

[3]   http://eprints.ucl.ac.uk/1987/1/860.pdf
[4]   'Dangerous Enthusiasms, E-Government Computer Failure and Information System Development', by Robin Gauld & Shaun Goldfinch, Otago University Press, 2006 (contains two chapters on health ICT)
[5]   http://www.otago.ac.nz/press/booksauthors/2006/dangerous_enthusiasms.html

International Perspectives in Health Informatics
E.M. Borycki et al. (Eds.)
IOS Press, 2011
© *2011 ITCH 2011 Steering Committee and IOS Press. All rights reserved.*
doi:10.3233/978-1-60750-709-3-168

An Online Method for Diagnosis of Difficult TB Cases for Developing Countries

Alvin MARCELO,[a,1] Zafar FATMI,[b] Paul Nimrod FIRAZA,[a] Shiraz SHAIKH,[b]
Alvin Joseph DANDAN,[a] Muhammad IRFAN,[b] Vaqar BARI[b], Richard E. SCOTT[c]

[a] *University of the Philippines, Manila, Philippines*
[b] *Aga Khan University, Karachi, Pakistan*
[c] *University of Calgary, Alberta, Canada*

Abstract. Optimal use of limited human, technical and financial resources is a major concern for tuberculosis (TB) control in developing nations. Further impediments include a lack of trained physicians, and logistical difficulties in arranging face-to-face (f-2-f) TB Diagnostic Committee (TBDC) consultations. Use of e-Health for virtual TBDCs (Internet and "iPath"), to address such issues is being studied in the Philippines and Pakistan. In Pakistan, radiological diagnosis of 88 sputum smear negative but suspected TB patients has been compared with the 'gold standards' (TB culture, and 2-month clinical follow up). Of 88 diagnostic decisions made by primary physicians at the spoke site and electronic TBDC (e-TBDC) at hub site, there was agreement in 71 cases and disagreement on 17 cases. The turn-around time (TAT; patient registration at spoke site for f-2-f diagnosis to receiving the electronic diagnosis), averaged 34.6 hours; ranging 9 minutes to 289.2 hours. Average TAT at the rural site (59.15 hours) was more than the urban site (15.9 hours). Comparison of e-TBDC and f-2-f diagnosis with the gold standards showed only slight differences. Using culture as the gold standard, e-TBDC decisions showed greater accuracy (sensitivity - 32.4%) as compared to f-2-f (27.6%); using 2-month clinical follow-up as the gold standard, f-2-f diagnosis showed slightly better improvement in patient symptoms and weight as compared to e-TBDC. In Philippines "iPath" was trialed and demonstrated that e-TBDCs have potential. Such groups could review cases, diagnose, and write comments remotely, reducing the diagnosis and treatment delay compared to usual care.

Keywords. telehealth, telemedicine, eHealth, tuberculosis, TB control, TBDC, electronic TBDC, Internet TBDC, iPath.

Introduction

Tuberculosis (TB) control remains a major problem for many developing nations, especially those with a weak health system and limited human, technical, and financial resources such as Pakistan and the Philippines.[1] Directly Observed Short Course (TB-DOTS) is the internationally recommended and cost effective strategy to detect and cure TB, with up to 95% cure rate even in the poorest countries. In addition, TB

---

[1] Corresponding author. Alvin B. Marcelo. UP Manila-National Telehealth Center, University of the Philippines, Manila, Philippines; email: alvin.marcelo@gmail.com

Diagnostic Committees (TBDC) was introduced in some countries to improve the accuracy of diagnosis. TBDCs are local face-to-face panels of clinicians who evaluate smear negative, but symptomatic TB cases whose x-rays show lesions suggestive of TB.[1] In most developing countries, trained physicians or chest specialists manage TB cases.

However, developing countries lack specialists and TBDC members in remote and rural areas, and also lack proper training in DOTS guidelines. This leads to an increasing burden of drug resistant TB (MDR) patients, and to a delay and incorrect diagnosis and treatment of TB patients. These challenges are amenable to telehealth solutions through establishing 'e-TBDCs' that meet through convenient electronic means, using time more efficiently, eliminating travel, and reducing related costs.

This study compared the accuracy and efficiency of an electronic method of diagnosing sputum negative clinically suspect TB patients to the conventional face-to-face (f-2-f) method, using TB culture and 2-month follow-up visits as the gold standards in Pakistan. It also describes the strengths and weaknesses of "iPath" as a platform for telemedicine by the e-TBDC used in the Philippines.

1. Review of Related Literature

Tuberculosis, a curable disease, infects one third of the world's population and kills two million every year. Ten (10) of the 22 high-burden TB countries (including Pakistan at #6 and Philippines at #9) lie in Asia, where TB is the leading cause of death among infectious diseases. An estimated 1.3 million people died from TB in 2008. The highest number of deaths was in South-East Asia (34%), while the highest mortality per capita was in the Africa Region. [1,2] The WHO declared TB a public health emergency in 1993, and announced in 2007 that 60 per cent of TB cases worldwide are now detected, and most are cured. [3] However, despite signs that the epidemic may be slowing; major impediments to greater progress exist including inequitable access to diagnosis and treatment.

The Philippine National Tuberculosis Control Program (NTP) adopted the Public-Private Mix DOTS (PPMD) strategy to harmonize and synchronize TB services among public and private sectors and increase case detection. A typical TBDC is chaired by the NTP Medical Coordinator (public sector) with members from the public and private sectors - TB experts who represent various disciplines (mainly radiologists and internists). Currently, the TBDC is created at the province or city level, sometimes the district level. For the smear negative cases, this strategy reduces over-diagnosis, over-treatment, and drug wastage, and ensures that active cases are detected and provided with the appropriate anti-TB treatment. [1]

In a typical Philippine province, up to 50 TB cases are evaluated every month. [1] It takes two weeks to one month before a sputum negative but clinically positive patient is assessed by a TB diagnostic committee in a face-to-face meeting. Reasons include: 1. the inability of busy clinicians to engage and commit; 2. the very modest PhilHealth honorarium; 3. the lack of TB specialists [radiologists, infectious disease, and pulmonary medicine specialists]; 4. the urban based practice of these specialists; 5. and, lost opportunity costs (i.e. clinic time, travel expense) when participating in the TBDC (resulting in cases being pooled until a sufficient number require attention). [1]

In Pakistan, TBDOTS coverage was increased to 100% in public sector hospitals; but a large section of the population receives treatment from the private sector. Although TBDCs do not yet formally exist, Pakistan's NTP recently started PPMD to improve the coverage. While laudable, Pakistan still lacks trained physicians and chest specialists in remote and rural areas making telehealth (which could improve coverage of specialist whilst at the same time reducing the burden of disease [4]), attractive. A new system could be developed where specialists convene as an e-TBDC, allowing them to interact electronically at their convenience without the accompanying costs. [1]

One potential platform identified in the literature is "iPath", an open source (PHP-based), hybrid Web- and e-mail-based telehealth platform developed by Department of Pathology, University Hospital Basel (www.iPath.ch). It can be considered a content management system and a group-ware tool. Cases can be sent as e-mails with the case title as the subject of the e-mail, the clinical description as the main text and images attached as files. These e-mails are automatically processed by "iPath" into web pages and imported into a specified 'user group' according to the area of interest of the sender. "iPath" then stores these medical cases, with attached images and other documents, in closed, moderated user groups. Pages can be accessed by approved members of a specific user group to review cases, provide consultative comments, and participate in case discussion. [5,6,7] Members of a group can elect to receive automatic e-mail notification, to alert them to new cases or added comments. This electronic approach will pave the way in exploiting the full interactivity of the Internet, which allows rapid feedback and change to continuously mould information into a useful knowledge.[8]

2. Methodology

The electronic approach described above was applied in both Pakistan and the Philippines. The conventional f-2-f method differs in the composition of members in both countries. The conventional f-2-f method in Pakistan involves a single general practitioner providing routine care in TB Diagnostic Centers while in the Philippines, it is composed of TBDC members in the study site proper. In addition, the "iPath" software was tested in the Philippines only. The electronic and conventional radiological diagnosis of 88 TB sputum smear negative suspects was compared with the TB culture report and a 2-month clinical follow up.

In Pakistan (Figure 1), digitized chest X-rays (CXR) were sent by e-mail from

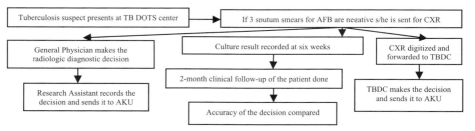

Figure 1. Flow Diagram of electronic TB Diagnosis vs. Face to Face in Pakistan

remote TB diagnostic centers in Gambat (a suburban town) and Orangi (a rural area) to the e-TBDC (a Radiologist and Pulmonologist) at an urban health care center (Aga Khan University (AKU)) for expert consultation. Images were taken by digital camera and uploaded to a computer. A digital form with a brief clinical history was attached with the X-ray and sent through email.

The e-TBDC doctors recorded their decisions in digital format and sent it to the research team. The decisions of the e-TBDC were compared to the 'conventional TBDC' and with the 'Gold standards'. The 2-month clinical follow up assesses deterioration or improvement in the symptoms and weight of the patient to judge the accuracy of the original diagnosis. The turn-around time (TAT; registration to decision) was measured for both electronic and conventional processes.

In the Philippines, cases from two areas (Pasay City and Capiz province) were randomly chosen and read by e-TBDC members from the other location (cases of Pasay City were uploaded (Figure 2) and reviewed by the TBDC members in Capiz province, and vice versa). The conventional (f-2-f) decisions of a particular TBDC were then compared to the 'on-line' decisions made by the other TBDC for the same cases, and to the culture results. The collected data includes the referral form (containing patient's history, physical examination findings), sputum AFB results, sputum culture results, x-rays, electronic results and face to face decisions.

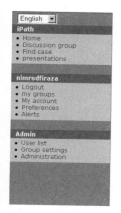
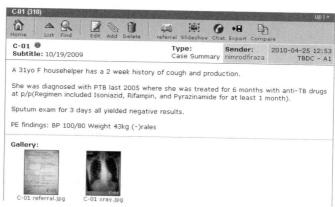

Figure 2. Sample Case summary with Digitized TBDC form and X-ray plate

3. Results

A total of 88 cases were enrolled at two sites (Orangi and Gambat) in Pakistan. The mean age of the enrolled participants was 37.6 (SD =19.7) years (56.8 % males). Mean weight of enrolled participants was 45.7 (SD =10.1) kg. The most frequently reported symptoms in TB suspects included cough greater than 3 weeks (92%), low grade fever (77.3%), weight loss (68.2%), and blood stained sputum (43.2%). A previous history of close contact of TB was noted in 39.8%, and only 8% had history of previous TB infection. Of the 88 diagnostic decisions made by the electronic TBDC (e-TBDC), there was agreement with the conventional TBDC in 71 cases (80.6%) and disagreement in 17 cases (19.38%).

The TAT data showed the average delay in waiting for a TBDC result compared to face-to-face result was almost one and a half days (34.6 hours; range 9 minutes to 289.2 hours (almost 12 days)). The average delay at the Gambat *rural* site (59.15 hours) was more than for the Orangi *urban* site (15.9 hours).

So far, the 2-month follow-up has been completed for 49 participants in Pakistan. Comparison of the f-2-f TBDC and e-TBDC diagnosis to the 2 gold standards of the study showed almost similar results with slight differences. Comparison of the culture results showed e-TBDC decisions to be slightly more sensitive (32.4% positive) as compared to f-2-f TBDC (27.6% positive). In contrast, the 2-month clinical follow-up results showed better improvement in symptoms and weight of the patients diagnosed by the f-2-f TBDC as compared to the e-TBDC.

The e-TBDC members in Pakistan showed satisfaction with the quality of images, were at complete ease in making diagnostic decisions, and never requested repeat X-rays. In addition, the response of the e-TBDC was quick, often returning their decisions the very same day.

Use of "iPath" as a platform for e-TBDC in the Philippines was also satisfactorily demonstrated. Strengths included its ability to store TB cases with attached images such as x-rays and referral forms and other documents into a closed user group. These 'private' groups can review cases, diagnose, and write comments. In addition, they can subscribe to receive automatic e-mail notification, e.g. when a new comment is added to one of their cases or a new case is entered into a group. Weaknesses encountered while using "iPath" included authentication issues, existing program bugs, inaccessibility without Internet access, and use of uncommon icons to represent new comments (red X mark which usually means a warning or an error) and new cases which use eyes (usual icon is an asterisk or bold letters as in Gmail or Yahoo).

At this moment there are already 50 cases uploaded in "iPath". The TB culture results are still pending for most of the cases. In the coming months once the cases are completed, further analysis of the accuracy and efficiency will be measured.

4. Discussion

Internet availability is rapidly increasing in developing countries, and using information technology for virtual expert opinion is a feasible option where specialists are unavailable. The results of this study provide evidence that e-TBDC's using digitized images for radiologic diagnosis of TB are an effective method in developing countries like Pakistan and Philippines. Preliminary data analysis shows that e-diagnosis is as effective as face to face diagnosis, as judged by the culture result (Gold standard), and that e-TBDC diagnosis was more sensitive as compared to f-2-f diagnosis. Furthermore, e-TBDC diagnosis was more specific, when compared with both the 'Gold standards' (culture and 2-month follow-up), being able to rule out non-TB patients. The technical strength of "iPath" is being a Web-based application akin to a content management and a group-ware tool. This allows virtual access anywhere through Internet connectivity. This also allows remote moderating, to assign other users to the group and to delete erroneous data, obviating the need for central administration. The vetting of e-TBDC (prior to authentication) might be discouraging, and some of the bugs might discourage TBDC members. Other limitations experienced were the frequent need to check emails or login to "iPath" (for notifications), and instability of the platform. Furthermore some e-TBDC members showed resistance to viewing slides on a computer screen, had difficulty accessing the platform, or were reluctant to ask a moderator for help. These issues resulted in reduced logins and response to case notifications from the site. In addition, the platform is currently dependent on a single host-server without back-up should it crash, and the uploading of images was noted to be slow which led to erroneous or repeated attempts to upload images.

5. Conclusion

TBDOTS has been universally proven to be an effective strategy for control of TB. Improving coverage of TBDOTS programs and correct diagnosis in remote and rural areas is a key to a successful control of TB in developing countries. This study demonstrates an innovative telehealth solution for diagnosis of sputum smear negative suspect TB patients through e-TBDC support in rural, remote, even urban areas where consultants are unavailable. The use of "iPath" for hosting e-TBDCs is a potential alternative to the current practice of face-to-face TBDCs. Since "iPath" is written in an open source web language (PHP) that can be embedded in HTML (hypertext markup language), it can create customized forms for structured responses that make it more efficient to use, easily understood, and standardized for TBDC use. It would also save costs on travelling, paper use, and time because e-TBDC data can be easily accessed using the web. This platform will also reduce difficulties related to storage and retrieval by preventing the loss of data, inadvertent loss or destruction of x-ray films, and faster access to stored data and results. By using this telehealth solution, TBDC members can interact electronically at their convenience, improve TB-DOTS coverage, and reduce delay in diagnosis related to the conventional process. From a clinical perspective, the latter is very important; the shorter the period a TB patient is left untreated, the shorter the exposure of the family and the community to the bacilli, and the more efficient the TB control program is.

References

[1] A.B. Marcelo, Z. Fatmi, R E Scott, S Khoja, Online TB Diagnosis (SS-ve) to Improve Case Detection In the TB-Dots Program; *Global Telemedicine and eHealth updates; Knowledge Sources, Med-e-Tel* **2** (2009) 508-510.

[2] Annual TB report 2006. NTP Pakistan available at: www.ntp.gov.pk

[3] World Health Organization. Global tuberculosis control: Surveillance, Planning, Financing. *WHO report 2007*. Geneva; 2007.

[4] Johnston K, Kennedy C, Murdoch I, Taylor P, Cook C. The cost-effectiveness of technology transfer using telemedicine. *Health Policy Plan.* **19** (2004), 302–9.

[5] Brauchli K, O'Mahony D, Banach L, Oberholzer M. iPath: A Telemedicine Platform to Support Health Providers in Low Resource Settings. *The Journal on Information Technology in Healthcare* **3**(4) (2005) 227–235.

[6] Blunier, Mark. iPath User Manual. 06.05.2004. Pp. 1-22. Telemedicine Platform iPath: http://telepath.patho.unibas.ch.. Swiss Tropical Institute. Date Accessed June 4, 2010. http://www.cred.ro/cd_capitalisation/FILEADMIN/USER_UPLOAD/BILDER/SCIH_CD/RONEONA T/TELEMEDICINE/USER_MANUAL_FOR_IPATH_V2.PDF

[7] iPath User Manual. Printer Friendly Version. By Kurt - Posted on May 5th, 2006. Date Accessed June 4, 2010. http://iPath.ch/site/book/export/html/452

[8] Edejer, Tessa. Disseminating health information in developing countries: the role of the internet. *BMJ* **321** (2000) 797–800.

International Perspectives in Health Informatics
E.M. Borycki et al. (Eds.)
IOS Press, 2011
© *2011 ITCH 2011 Steering Committee and IOS Press. All rights reserved.*
doi:10.3233/978-1-60750-709-3-174

Developing a Medical Records System at the Ola During Children's Hospital, Freetown, Sierra Leone

John DAWSON [a,1], Matthew CLARK [b], Liz PELOSO [c]

[a] *School of Health Information Science, University of Victoria, Victoria, British Columbia, Canada*
[b] *Honorary Research Fellow, University of Leicester Medical School, Leicester, UK Chairman of the Board of Directors, Welbodi Partnership, Cambridge ,UK*
[c] *Senior Lead, National Health Practice, Deloitte, Toronto, ON*

Abstract. The development of a paper based medical record system and the corresponding database at the Ola During Children's Hospital, Freetown, Sierra Leone are described. This project took place within an extremely resource constrained setting, through the partnership of local and international collaborators. The key factors which define the project are incremental progress, the intent to migrate the data to OpenMRS to ensure its sustainability and building local capacity for database management.

Keywords. database, developing countries, openMRS.

Introduction

Research into the cost-effectiveness of hospitals in the developing world is difficult. Hospitals that are grossly under-resourced often lack the administrative capacity to accurately collect and manage sufficient data. This is particularly so at the Ola During Children's Hospital (ODCH), located in the densely populated and impoverished eastern part of Freetown, Sierra Leone. It is the country's only specialized paediatric facility and serves more than 11,000 patients each year. The hospital's chaotic medical records system fails to capture sufficient details about patients to provide continuity of care or to serve as a clinical, management or research tool.

Sierra Leone still has the highest child mortality rate in the world and has made little progress towards Millennium Development Goal number 4 (the reduction of child mortality by 75% by the year 2050) [1]. The international community has pledged tens of millions of dollars to improve the situation. Thus far the hospital has been largely

---

[1] Corresponding Author: John Dawson, 6969 Talbot Trail, R. R. # 1, Blenheim, ON, Canada, N0P 1A0, Canada; E-mail: johndawson@sympatico.ca.

overlooked by this international community, and unless it has a robust medical records system to evaluate both the efficacy and cost-effectiveness of donor investments, it will continue to be so. This paper describes the ongoing efforts in the development of such a system. As subsequent sections will illustrate, the hallmark of this effort is the planned migration from a simple but manageable database solution to OpenMRS, a more sophisticated and widely implemented open source medical records platform. Equally important is the recognition that this goal can only be achieved through incremental progress that recognizes the site's existing and evolving capacity to implement and maintain changes.

Although perhaps an extreme example, the situation in Sierra Leone is not unique. Thus although the intent is to provide a long term, sustainable solution for ODCH, ideally the lessons learned should apply to and be able to be leveraged by other countries facing similar challenges.   To ensure our objectives of sustainability and transferrable lessons were attainable, we consulted with Health Metrics Network professionals already working in Sierra Leone on a number of health data management initiatives. This early collaboration and planning advice allowed us to select solutions that would be both relevant and appropriate for the long term. An implementation strategy was developed that involved incremental steps that would easily transition to the data structures and architectures that were part of the long term vision.   The need to develop local capacity for the ongoing operation and development of the system was also deemed essential.

1. The Need for Improved Paper Medical Records

The paper-based part of an electronic patient record system is crucial. A medical records system will only ever be as accurate as the data recorded by the clinicians. ODCH had no forms for systematically documenting clinical data. Blank exercise books, similar to those used by primary schools, were used to record patient information. The degree of detail recorded was largely determined by the individual clinician and varied widely.   A clinical forms package was developed and implementation began during a three month period while a physician (MC) from the Welbodi Partnership (WP) was onsite at ODCH.   When designing the forms it was essential to have substantial input from local doctors. It was crucial for doctors to understand why the forms are important and to feel a sense of shared ownership.   The forms capture key information about the patient including basic demographics, social background, duration of symptoms, diagnosis, treatment and outcomes. These forms were intended to encourage medical staff to develop a rigorous clinical approach, standardize their documentation, and to facilitate data entry by medical records staff. The forms package is based on that used by the paediatric emergency unit at Kenyatta National Hospital, Nairobi.   It was refined after a number of consultations with the clinical staff at ODCH.   Initially, it was tested for a one month period before undergoing further refinement in response to feedback from staff. Dr. Tamra Abiodun, an experienced pediatrician and director of postgraduate training at ODCH, has further refined the forms to reflect more current clinical practice.   The first page of the package is completed by the nursing staff in triage and includes basic demographics and vital signs while the medical staff use the remaining forms to record clinical findings, diagnoses and medications.

A major challenge in implementing the new forms package was engaging the non medical staff. The new package is more expensive to print and initally the hospital was reluctant to take on an extra expense. The ongoing challenge is to ensure that there is always an adequte supply of forms available when patients arrive. Similarly, due to the expense, the hospital management is reluctatnt to leave a large supply of forms for use outside of office hours. Likewise, the correct paper work for children who die very early in their admission is not always complete. We are continuing to work with the hospital management team to improve the availability and use of the forms package.

2. Development of the Medical Records Database

Prior to the development and implementation of the clinical forms package, it was apparent that a computerized medical record system would be needed to efficiently and effectively utilize the information recorded by clinicians. The initial requirements were threefold: (1) to produce an electronic discharge summary containing salient details of a patient's previous visit(s); (2) to facilitate locating a patient's existing paper medical records for return visits; (3) to aggregate patient data for statistical reports needed by hospital management and for submission to the Ministry of Health and Sanitation's (MoH) district office. As ODCH did not have the expertise to develop and coordinate database implementation the WP enlisted the help of a foreign volunteer (JD). MC and additional WP volunteers who were onsite consulted with the developer by e-mail to enable remote development of the database.

The technical and human resources for implementing and maintaining a database were extremely limited. One standalone desktop PC and one notebook computer were available. Internet connectivity was extremely slow and available intermittently. The Microsoft Office^{TM} suite (including MS-Access™) is standard on all MoH computers. A college level IT graduate worked in the health records department. He was a proficient MS-Excel user, had basic familiarity with MS-Access but no database development experience. Foreign WP volunteers with some knowledge of MS-Access and MS-Excel were on site for varying periods of time.

Based on the limitations noted above, MS-Access™ was chosen for database development and the first phase of implementation. The rationale for this choice involved several factors. No additional funds were required to purchase MS-Access™. Staff and volunteers at ODCH had at least some familiarity with it. Query creation is relatively simple as are minor form modifications. For training purposes, a non-production copy of the medical records system will provide the health records IT graduate with an in depth understanding of the system and illustrate the principles of relational database design. Recognizing and building upon the limited database expertise at ODCH enlists the staff as active participants in the system's development and ongoing operation. This is essential to improve local ownership, buy-in and capacity.

3. Planned Migration to OpenMRS

From its inception the MS-Access™ database developed at ODCH was intended to be an interim solution. The developer recognizes that MS-Access™ has limited scalability, both in terms of capacity and performance. At the present time the site's poor Internet connectivity precludes the use of a web based OpenMRS client with a central server and it lacks the hardware and technical expertise required to support a local client-server installation. Accordingly, a development and migration plan to OpenMRS has been formulated as illustrated in Figure 1.

OpenMRS is an established open source medical record system *platform* which has been successfully implemented at 125 clinical and research sites worldwide [2-4]. The use of OpenMRS has several advantages. It is free of charge. It can be customized to suit an organization's needs without programming and is supported by a large community of developers and implementers. It can be integrated with other health information systems. In this regard, a pilot project is currently underway in Sierra Leone which allows aggregated data from OpenMRS to be linked with data repositories at MoH health district and national levels [5]. These benefits will bolster the sustainability of the medical records system at ODCH.

The most significant step in the migration to OpenMRS involves splitting it into two components. The front end (user facing) portion will remain in MS-Access™ in order to leverage existing user experience and training. The back end (database tables) will be converted to MySQL, a much more robust and scalable database system which is also used as the backend for OpenMRS. In addition the architecture of the MS-Access™ database will be progressively aligned with OpenMRS. The look and feel of the MS-Access™ user interface will be replicated within OpenMRS.

4. Challenges

There is a need for continuous quality improvement to ensure the accuracy and completeness of data collection. Data entry continues to occur in the medical records department, after a patient has been discharged. This presents a problem in terms of missing data. For example, in the absence of even a rudimentary paper admission-discharge-transfer system, medical records staff are often not informed of patient discharges, resulting in the inflation of statistical measures such as "days of care".

The fact that many patients' actual dates of birth are unknown and cannot be reliably determined presents another challenge, requiring the inclusion of an "age estimated" database field. It is not uncommon for many patients to have the same estimated date of birth and identical names, requiring additional search parameters and scrutiny to locate a patient's record.

The need for efficient data management became even more evident when Sierra Leone's Ministry of Health and Sanitation began providing free health care to pregnant and breast feeding women and children under age 5 in April, 2010 [6]. Previously parents were required to pay a consultation fee of Le15,000 ($3.50), making care unaffordable to many in a country where the average per capita income is $320 [7]. Following the introduction of free health care, the number of patients increased from 40-50 per day to 120-150 per day [8].

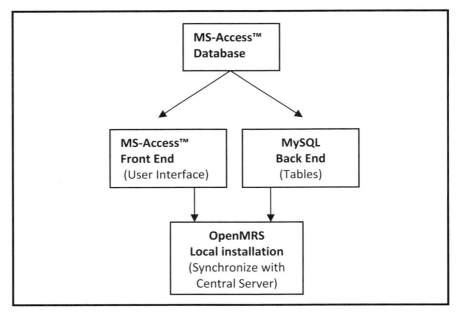

Figure 1. Planned migration path from MS-Access™ database to OpenMRS

5. Next Steps

In future the database will be expanded to capture progressively more content from the clinical clerking package. Prior to each expansion, it is critical that the data integrity is assured through ongoing quality review. Initially data will continue to be used primarily in aggregate form. This assists the hospital in meeting its internal and external reporting requirements, and is especially important for maintaining and increasing funding. At present the opportunity to integrate database output (either in paper or electronic form) with real time clinical processes is extremely limited. This barrier will also need to be addressed through incremental changes in clinical workflow and the fostering of an institutional culture that values the collection and effective utilization of patient information. The database can be used to monitor the impact of a variety of possible interventions. These range from small donations of equipment such as pulse oximeters or laboratory equipment, to much more expensive schemes such as improving staff remuneration and eliminating user fees. At a community level cluster trials could be used to investigate the impact of health education programs on accessing hospital care for sick children. The accomplishments noted above have been achieved through the combined efforts of ODCH and resources provided by international collaborators. These resources have been effectively utilized through the onsite coordination provided by several team members from the WP. In keeping with ODCH's resource constrained environment, this project continues to rely heavily on the contributions of volunteers.

For the database to be sustainable over the long term there must be a gradual transition from reliance on foreign expertise to that which is developed locally. It is intended that the IT graduate working in the health records department will eventually assume responsibility for the database's ongoing operation and development. This will require a considerable amount of training which will be provided by the developer. The amount of training which can be accomplished remotely versus provided on site remains to be seen. Other candidates for this level of training must also be identified to ensure that the long term operation of the database is compromised by over dependence on a single staff member. The current developer will continue to provide oversight and consultation for issues which cannot be resolved locally and to ensure that the database continues to evolve in ways that are consistent with the goal of its eventual migration to OpenMRS.

6. Conclusions

Over the course of approximately one year and in the complete absence of any previous systematic clinical data collection methods, we have demonstrated that it is possible to establish a paper based medical record system, and to develop and implement a corresponding medical records database using MS-Access™. The key descriptor of these achievements has and will continue to be *incremental progress*. The planned migration to OpenMRS is equally important. Without it the database would be destined to become yet another unsustainable "health data silo", an unfortunate circumstance which has occurred in other developing countries [9].

We have shown that through a sustained partnership between local and international collaborators (contributing their expertise both on site and remotely) projects such as this are indeed possible, even within an extremely resource constrained environment.

References

[1] UNICEF, *Sierra Leone Multiple Indicator Cluster Survey 2005, Final Report,* Statistics Sierra Leone and UNICEF-Sierra Leone, 2005.
[2] B.W. Mamlin, P.G. Biondich, B.A. Wolfe, H. Fraser, D. Jazayeri, C. Allen, J. Mirinda, W.M. Tierney, Cooking up an open source EMR for developing countries: OpenMRS—A recipe for successful collaboration, *AMIA Annual Symposium Proceedings* (2006), 529-523.
[3] H.S.F. Fraser, P. Biondich, D. Moodley, S. Choi, B.W. Mamlin, P. Szolovits, Implementing electronic medical record systems in developing countries, *Informatics in Primary Care* **13** (2005), 83-95.
[4] OpenMRS, *Where in the World?* available at: http://openmrs.org/about/locations/, last accessed October 14, 2010.
[5] Health Metrics Network, *Enabling HIS Integration and Data Interoperability - a Pilot Case in Sierra Leone,* HMN Weekly Highlight, 30 April 2010, available at: http://www.who.int/healthmetrics/news/weekly_highlights/his_integration_and_data_interoperability_in _sierra_leone/en/index.html, last accessed June 29, 2009.
[6] UNICEF, *Sierra Leone Announces Free Health Care for Mothers and Children,* At a Glance: Sierra Leone, 27 April 2010, available at: http://www.unicef.org/childsurvival/sierraleone_53435.html, last accessed June 29, 2009.
[7] World Bank, *Sierra Leone at a Glance,* available at: http://devdata.worldbank.org/AAG/sle_aag.pdf, last accessed June 29, 2009.
[8] A. Paul, *The Welbodi Partnership,* personal communication, 11 May 2010.
[9] H.C. Kimaro, J.L. Nhampossa, Analyzing the problem of unsustainable health information systems in less-developed economies: Case studies from Tanzania and Mozambique, *Information Technology for Development* **11**:3 (2005), 273-298.

Healthcare Modeling and Simulation

International Perspectives in Health Informatics
E.M. Borycki et al. (Eds.)
IOS Press, 2011
© 2011 ITCH 2011 Steering Committee and IOS Press. All rights reserved.
doi:10.3233/978-1-60750-709-3-183

Making Eco-Friendly Transportation Safer: Developing Computer-based Simulations to Assess of the Impacts of Bicycle Accident Prevention Interventions on Healthcare Utilization

Christian JUHRA[a], Elizabeth M. BORYCKI [b], Andre W. KUSHNIRUK [b],
Jim ANDERSON [c], Marilyn ANDERSON [d]

[a] *Department of Trauma-, Hand- and Reconstructive Surgery,
University Hospital Münster, Germany*
[b] *School of Health Information Science, University of Victoria,
Victoria, British Columbia, Canada*
[c] *Purdue University, West Lafayette, Indiana, USA*
[d] *Anderson Consulting, West Lafayette, Indiana, USA*

Abstract. Computer-based modeling and simulations are becoming increasingly used for applications in health and safety. In this paper we describe a multi-phase project aimed at modeling bicycle accidents in Munster, Germany. The work involved a first phase of collecting empirical data on accident rates and severity. In the second phase a computer-based simulation model of bicycle accidents was created, using data from phase one to identify relevant parameters in the model. Finally, initial results from running the model are described that will be used to inform decision making regarding safety initiatives.

Keywords. computer-based simulation, bicycle accidents, computer-based modeling, healthcare utilization, health informatics, patient safety, accident prevention

Introduction

Globally, there are significant changes occurring in society. Worldwide citizens are choosing to use more environmentally friendly forms of transportation (such as bicycle use) to reduce their dependence on fossil fuels while at the same time improving their personal fitness. Although this shift has a number of positive benefits, there are also societal costs such as increases in the number of trauma-related injuries leading to death and disability. Government policy makers and healthcare administrators need to understand the implications of these societal changes upon healthcare service utilization (e.g. hospital and physician visits). Such knowledge supports these decision-makers in developing laws, policies, and plans that can address these emergent healthcare needs (i.e. bicycle accident related traumas). One method that can be used to support decision making is computer-based modeling and simulation of the future impacts of such decisions. Computer-based modeling and simulation has been used to support decision-making in a variety of health related areas. The purpose of this paper will be to describe a methodology for developing computer-based simulation models that describe: (1) the costs of current bicycle usage upon trauma-related injuries and deaths and (2) the impact of introducing new helmet legislation on costs.

1. Background

Münster is a German town with a population of 273,000 people. In 2009 bicycles were the primary method of transportation. Bicycles were used more often (i.e. 37.8%) than cars (36.4%). Bicycles are used around 450,000 times each day. In 1982 bicycles were used 270,000 times a day. The rise in bicycle use has also led to an increase in the number of bicycle accidents. In 2009, the Münster police were called to 690 bicycle accidents where a cyclist was injured. During the same time period, all patients that were admitted to an emergency unit, in one of the six hospitals in Münster, were anonymously reported to the Münster Bicycle Study. Within a year, 2,153 patients suffered from an injury caused by a bicycle accident (i.e. nearly triple the number of accidents known to the police).

2. Methods and Results

2.1. Phase One: Bicycle Accident Survey

Between February 2009 and January 2010, data on bicycle accidents leading to injuries were collected by the Police of Münster and the emergency units of Münster's six hospitals. Researchers systematically acquired data from the Police and hospitals and combined the data. It must be noted that simultaneous and comprehensive data collections were necessary as the police are not always called and not every bicycle accident results in injury. The data were collected from three different sources: voluntary patient reports, police accident reports, and hospital health records. 2,153 patients were included in the study. For each of these patients, a patient, hospital or police record or any combination of these existed in our database. 1,410 patient and 1,529 hospital records were included in the database. In total, 1,767 patients were treated at a hospital. 386 people did not go to a hospital. 3 people died in a bicycle accident. During the same period, 650 bicycle accidents where individuals were injured were recorded by police. Following this, every injury was classified according to type [strain, fracture, bruise (i.e. no open wound), open wound, brain injury] and localization. Each patient could have multiple injuries and the same injuries could be classified into multiple types. An open fracture was thus classified as a fracture and an open wound.

Looking at reasons for hospital admission, traumatic brain injuries were the leading cause. However, the largest resource consumption was attributed to fractures of the upper extremities with major surgery (see Table 2).

Localization	Strain	Fracture	Bruise	Open wound	Brain Injury
Abdomen			14	8	
Pelvis		7	87	19	
Head (excl. Face)		9	83	85	101
Face	1	62	54	192	
Upper Extremity	97	203	327	202	
Chest		26	94	15	
Lower Extremity	88	70	329	186	
Spine	52	23	31	13	

Table 1. Types and Localization of Injuries

DRG	Number	Description (simplified)	Costs
B80Z	39	Traumatic Brain Injury	31.668,00 €
I21Z	21	Fracture of Upper Extremity with Major Surgery	55.272,00 €
J65B	12	Soft Tissue Damage, Open Wounds	9.744,00 €
I57C	9	Lower Extremitiy Fractures with Minor Surgery	25.956,00 €
I13B	8	Lower Extremity Fracture with Major Surgery	33.600,00 €

Table 2. Reasons for Hospital Admission (Top-5)

Using costs associated with accidents as provided by the German Road Agency (BASt) [1], a total burden to society summing up to 28,349,749 Euro was caused by bicycle accidents in a year in the city of Münster. Among these, 1 death and 39 hospital admissions were caused by traumatic brain injury alone, summing up to a total cost to society of 4,565,376 Euro. While bicycle accidents pose a burden to the injured individual and society, regular bicycle use does have a positive effect. Using the Health Economic Assessment Tool provided by the WHO [2], the present value of the mean annual benefit of bicycle use in Münster was 77,063,000 Euro. However, a 10% drop in bicycle use would decrease this benefit by nearly 7 million Euros. Since there is evidence that the introduction of bicycle helmet laws would lead to a decrease in bicycle usage, the potential negative effects may outweigh the positive. Even if a bicycle helmet law could prevent all brain injuries and would at the same time prevent 10% of former bicycle users from continuing their bicycle usage, it would have a negative burden to society of nearly 3 million Euros.

2.2. Phase Two: Development of a Computer-based Simulation Model of Accidents

The development of a computer-based simulation model of bicycle accidents was carried out in a series of sequential steps. In step one, three experts with backgrounds in trauma medicine, health services administration, nursing and systems analysis reviewed the empirical data from phase one. The experts conducted a round table discussion where they reviewed the results from phase one data and developed a list of key simulation parameters (i.e. variables related to bicycle accidents that would need to be modeled in a computer-based simulation). Examples simulation parameters included: age, sex, type of bicycle used, type of protection used. The baseline values for parameters (e.g. rates of differing types of accidents) were arrived at from reviews of phase one data and the relevant evidence-based research on bicycle accidents. In step two, the experts generated a list of potential types of interventions from the relevant literature and empirical data (from phase one) that that could be employed to reduce the number of bicycle accidents and severity of the injuries resulting from those accidents (i.e. interventions aimed at reducing death and disability). Some examples include: educational interventions, implementation of bicycle helmet laws and modifications to the environment (e.g. introduction of bicycle lanes). In step three, the experts reviewed the empirical data from phase one and the evidence-based literature and developed a list of key output variables (i.e. variables that would be measured or assessed to evaluate the impact of potential interventions) in three key areas: (1) death and disability, (2) health service utilization, and (3) number and severity or accidents. In step four, the resultant model was implemented using the Stella© simulation package, [3] and is shown in Figure 1. The model depicts bicycle accidents and their consequences over a period of one year. The number of accidents that result in patients being treated at the hospital was estimated. Based on the cost of the five top hospital admissions shown in Table 2 the total annual cost in Euros can be calculated.

2.2.1. Running the Initial Simulation Model

The graph below (see Graph 1) provides estimates of the annual cost of bicycle injuries under current policies as well as the projected cost under a policy that would require riders to wear helmets (see Graph 2). The model estimates that this policy would reduce the annual number of injuries requiring hospital treatment by 219 and reduce the cost by 4,300,241 Euros annually primarily by significantly reducing traumatic brain injuries.

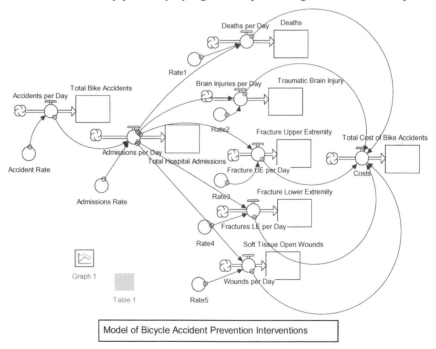

Figure 1. Initial Stella Simulation Model

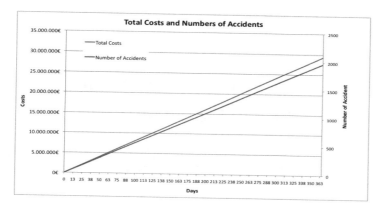

Graph 1: Estimate of Annual Costs Based on Current Injuries

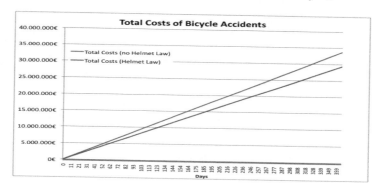

Graph 2: Estimate of Annual Costs Based on Helmet Law

3. Conclusions

Bicycling is an environmentally friendly way of travelling short distances while at the same time improving ones health. As such, it should be promoted by policy makers. There is a need to make cycling safer, but making cycling safer can have wanted and unwanted effects. Simulations can be used to assess the impacts of interventions aimed at making cycling safer. Further simulations will be developed to inform policymaker decision making involving bicycle safety, injury reduction and health system costs.

References

[1]   Unfallkosten nach BASt [Cited on 2110 May 29] Available from:
        http://www.bast.de/cln_015/nn_40694/DE/Publikationen/Infos/2007-2006/02-2006.html
[2]   Available from: http://www.euro.who.int/en/what-we-do/health-topics/environmental-health/Transport-and-health/publications2/pre-2009/health-economic-assessment-tool-heat-for-cycling.-user-guide-2008
[3]   A. W. Kushniruk, E. Borycki, J. Anderson, M. Anderson, Combining two forms of simulations to predict the potential impact of interface design on technology-induced error in healthcare. *Proceedings of the 17th Annual International Conference* on Health Science Simulations, Ottawa, Canada, 2008.

International Perspectives in Health Informatics
E.M. Borycki et al. (Eds.)
IOS Press, 2011
© 2011 ITCH 2011 Steering Committee and IOS Press. All rights reserved.
doi:10.3233/978-1-60750-709-3-188

Model Human Behavior: Don't Constrain It!

H. Dominic COVVEY, Donald D. COWAN, Paulo ALENCAR, William MALYK, Joel SO, D. HENRIQUES, Shirley FENTON
University of Waterloo, Waterloo, Ontario, Canada

Abstract. Healthcare processes are complex and highly variable from day to day. Healthcare process execution can be affected by any participant in a process, including clinicians, the patient, and the patient's family, as well as environmental factors such as clinician, staff, facility and equipment availability, and patient clinical status. However, only a few solutions exist that enable computer support for a process to address the full complexity and variability of healthcare processes. We have re-conceptualized workflow and developed an innovative process representation and execution framework based on concepts from software engineering, machine learning, complexity, and database management. This new framework frees processes to track human behavior, thereby releasing us from the constraints of past methods. Our approach is also serving as a new architecture for software systems.

Keywords. workflow, adaptable information systems, process management

Introduction

Many of our existing computer-based systems and applications, by their very nature, tightly constrain human behavior. For a brief phase, during the set-up and implementation of a system, in most systems a degree of adaptation to the local environment is possible. However, once this adaptation has been implemented, it effectively freezes the work processes into a state that is virtually invariant, frustrating our need for adaptivity to changing situations. Over the last few years there has been increasing recognition of the importance of the requirement for the support of flexible, adaptable processes if systems are to be truly successful and address the needs of their users. In particular, it has become clear that systems must synergistically align with and support the constantly varying nature of human workflow. In this article we will use the terms 'workflow' and 'processes' interchangeably, as well as considering clinical and operational processes similarly.

Furthermore, while it is recognized that healthcare processes are complex, little has been written about the fact that health care satisfies the formal definition of a complex system, exhibiting characteristics such as having many interacting agents and objects whose behavior is affected by feedback and that adapt to their histories, a system that is influenced by its environment, that appears to be 'alive' as it evolves, that exhibits emergent phenomena that arise without a central controller, and a 'system' that comprises a complex mix of ordered and disordered behavior, with parts acting at the edge of chaos [1].

Although much has been done on the representation of workflow in business settings, the representation of workflow in highly dynamic settings, like health care, has remained a challenge until now. Complex dynamic environments are characteristic of health care. They typically involve considerable human interaction resulting in a high degree of variability. Healthcare settings have many decision makers, kinds of decisions, events and a multitude of reactive, subsidiary workflows that often require a quick revision of the course of action. Operational and treatment protocols attempt to regularize workflow, but the needs of care, the great variety of situations and individuals' decisions, the exigencies of the moment (such as equipment failure), and the nature of human beings frustrate attempts at regularization, often resulting in protocols being labeled as "rigid" or "cookbook medicine" and hence being abandoned. While event sequences in healthcare processes may abide by loose constraints, they are largely non-deterministic. Therefore, it is difficult, if not impossible, to prescribe fully healthcare workflow. Instead, workflow must be dynamic, self-adapting and evolving at execution-time to match the dynamicity of the environment.

Traditional workflow representation and execution technology, by its very static nature, supports a finite set of scenarios. In fact, traditional workflow is understood to support, at best, the union of atomic workflow patterns described by van der Aalst [2]. Available workflow platforms that support these patterns are often incomplete, unsatisfactory, or even non-existent. In fact, no single commercial product supports all listed patterns [2]. We have developed a new way of representing and guiding healthcare processes that is able to address workflow variability and complexity. This work has provided enhanced ability to model and guide human behavior, minimizing the need to constrain it.

1. On the Concept of Dynamic Workflow

To begin, we must define exactly what "dynamic workflow" means. First, we distinguish the notion of workflow scenario (the real-world environment and processes; what is actually happening) from workflow application (the computer-encoded form of a workflow scenario; a computer model of reality):

By separating application from scenario, we can see that workflow scenarios range from static at one extreme to dynamic at the other. In static scenarios, all instances of scenario execution are substantially similar, both in terms of the work performed (the goals: "what" and "why") and the specifics involved (the "who", "when", "where" and "how"). In dynamic scenarios, on the other hand, each instance of scenario execution addresses the same work goals, but the specifics of each instance vary from instance to instance. A workflow scenario is (highly) dynamic when there is a (high) degree of instance to instance variability and unpredictability (in tasks, sequence, actors, etc.), to achieve the same work.

Traditional workflow technologies adequately support classic "prescribed"/pre-defined workflow applications: workflow is prescribed at design-time to model a static scenario that, at run-time, is supported by the prescribed workflow application. Dynamic workflow applications, on the other hand, must dynamically assemble the workflow at run-time, in response to the dynamic scenario being modeled.

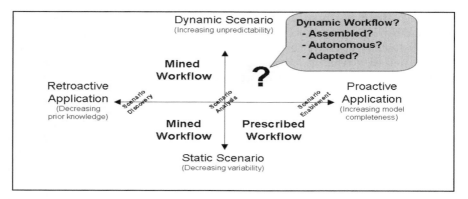

Figure 1. Overlay of Applications and Scenarios

To rationalize the workflow problem space further, we note that workflow applications can be divided into two classes: Proactive workflow: the workflow application is proactively applied to scenario execution, and the application relies on design-time completeness for run-time efficacy – anything undefined at design-time becomes a run-time exception. Examples are workflow automation, workflow facilitation – scenario enablement workflow applications that are proactive in nature. Retroactive workflow: the workflow application is retroactively realized from scenario execution, the application relies on run-time analysis for next-iteration design-time efficacy – anything not captured during run-time will be omitted at next design-time, and the workflow is only clear after-the-fact. Examples include workflow mining, workflow reengineering – scenario discovery workflow applications that are retroactive in nature. Some workflow applications reside between these extremes. Examples include workflow-based decision support systems (e.g., Careflows), process tracking, process diagnostics, and workflow simulation.

An overlay of the workflow application spectrum atop the workflow scenario spectrum provides a clear view of the workflow problem space as shown in Figure 1.

This overlay of concepts reveals a relationship between workflow scenario and workflow application and suggests that prescribed workflow and mined workflow (both achievable by traditional workflow technologies) can address much of the workflow problem space. However, the upper-right quadrant (proactive workflow application in dynamic workflow scenarios) cannot be addressed by traditional workflow technologies. We define dynamic workflow (application) as a class of proactive workflow applications that use techniques beyond those of traditional workflow (i.e., prescription and mining) to enable or model highly dynamic workflow scenarios. We also suggest that dynamic workflow must be implemented by techniques such as run-time workflow assembly, autonomous workflow inference, or adaptive workflow.

2. Clarifying Dynamicity

In order to clarify the concept of dynamic workflow, consider the following: (1) static/prescribed workflows are characteristic of many commercial processes: the workflow (e.g., actions, actors, objects and sequencing) can be completely described and the pre-defined workflow will be executed similarly for each occurrence of a transaction; (2) static workflows are easy to represent and execute as they have few variations and no unpredicted exceptions; (3) dynamic workflows, characteristic of health care, will adapt and vary according to the situation and, although there are instance-to-instances similarities, the sequence of actions, the facilities/equipment used, and the agents participating will change in response to an emergency, the patient's clinical response, clinician intra-workflow insights, etc.; (4) dynamic workflows are challenging to represent as the workflow is a record of how the process was performed as well as guiding it. For this reason we say that dynamic workflows are historical records of what was at the time decided and done. Workflow descriptions can provide a bound on the workflow, but not a rigid definition of processes. Looking at workflow this way enables the efficient coupling of humans with computer-guided processes, reducing or eliminating the perception of protocol rigidity.

3. Representing and Executing Dynamic Workflow

Workflow is usually described by connecting services or tasks in a programmatic format such as a workflow language, flowchart or other sequencing mechanism. Thus, prescribing a workflow in a dynamic environment could require a protocol or "program" of immense complexity as one tries to ensure that all possible choices and their sequencing are captured in advance.

The approach used in our research to capture workflow and include dynamic services and context, and which has been used to describe over 40 service-oriented information systems [3], is based on the work by Jackson and Twaddl [4]. Workflow is represented using an entity-relationship (E-R) model [5] which is then transformed into a relational database. Thus, the control structure and all information about services are captured in a data structure that can be easily modified and then either compiled or interpreted into a workflow "program."

3.1. Entities

Following Jackson/Twaddle, the first step in producing an E-R workflow representation is to develop a data model in terms of entities that are central to the description of the business processes. In a medical laboratory context the data model could consists of entities such as admissions-clerk, patient, physician, test-order, etc. These entities have corresponding entries in the lab database.

3.2. Lifecycles, Stages and Services

Each entity in an operational information system has an associated "lifecycle". Each lifecycle goes through a number of sequential stages, each stage containing a number of services/tasks applied to the entity. A simple example of a lifecycle is the movement of a patient through the admission stage, to the testing stage and finally to the diagnosis stage. These stages can be divided into sub-stages. The lifecycle for the patient ends as he/she is discharged or passed on to a new lifecycle for further intervention. Services can be executed sequentially, conditionally, or repeatedly. Parallel execution is also possible through the splitting/fork and merging/join of services. Although stages cannot be skipped, they can contain a skip-this-stage task, e.g., if a patient does not complete the admission stage, then skip-this-stage would be executed in all subsequent stages. Services/tasks are interdependent: the application of one service may have to await the completion of services in other stages or lifecycles associated with other entities.

Generally, services are interconnected through control flow (sequence, condition, repetition, fork and join). However, it is possible to introduce dynamic services into the model that can be chosen based on the current situation. These dynamic services are chosen as the workflow progresses and the situation is determined. For example, there may be several devices that could provide a needed testing service. The choice of device could occur dynamically, based on variables such as machine or operator availability.

3.3. Workflow as an E-R and Database Model

Workflow lifecycles, stages, services and interdependencies can be represented by an E-R model. E-R models can be further mapped into a relational database where the concepts in the system (entity, lifecycle, stage and service) and the relationships among them each correspond to a table. Each entity has one corresponding lifecycle (1:1); each lifecycle can have multiple stages (1:n) and each stage can have multiple services (1:n). The relationships among the services can further be annotated to include sequence (pre-conditions and post-conditions), choice, repetition, fork and join. Pre-conditions and post-conditions can be used with dynamic services to specify services that must be performed before or after the selected service.

Thus, workflow is represented as a data-structure, a significant innovation. Code related to a service can be stored in the database as an embedded procedure. A data structure makes it possible to present the entire process graphically, supporting visualization.

The relationship between lifecycles, stages, and services in a workflow can be modified by changing a data structure rather than a program structure. Modifying workflow is therefore easier, because the abstractions corresponding to the workflow or control structure are clearly identified. End-users can easily be shielded from these details using a visual interface. In addition, E-R models represented by XML-tagged structures enable the development of a declarative domain-specific language for describing workflow.

The declarative workflow representation can be trans-formed into other representations such as BPEL [6], UML [7] or XMI [8] through transformations defined in languages such as XSL/XSLT [9]. This approach has been demonstrated [10] where XML-based declarations for agents were transformed into code written in C. This workflow model associates services with entities through a workflow structure, and services are loosely coupled to each other and to the related entity.

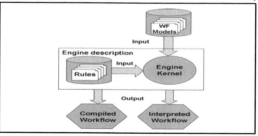

Figure 2: The workflow engine/machine

4. Making the Workflow Model into an Operational System

Workflow has now been converted to a data structure where the atomic service or task encapsulates the work to be done. The remainder of the data structure captures the relationships and dependencies among tasks. We now define a workflow machine or "engine" (compiler or interpreter) that is capable of traversing the workflow data structure in the proper sequence including dealing with dependencies. The machine processes (traverses) the data structure, interpreting or compiling the data in the structure into code which can then be launched.

The services can be manual, meaning there is a requirement for human intervention as in completing a form, or automatic as in processing a credit card payment. The workflow engine shown in Figure 2 is driven by a set of rules.

5. Workflow Engine for Dynamic Workflow

To address the representation of dynamic real world processes, we have designed an approach involving service selection and real-time composition of services into workflow instances (Figure 3). In this approach, we consider the activities within a workflow to be services. Example services include such activities as a receive-patient service, a register-patient service, a produce-report service, etc. These services are pre-defined and may themselves be composed of more granular services. These services can be provided by a services-server on request by the workflow generation engine. Services have pre-conditions (services that must be executed before this service) and post-conditions (services to be executed after this service).

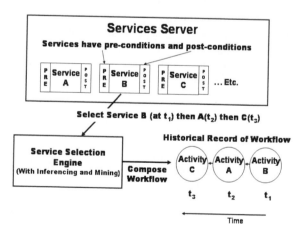

Figure 3. Service Selection and Workflow Composition

To choreograph these loosely-coupled services that comprise a workflow, a service selection unit is incorporated that can select services both statically (sequential prescription) and stochastically (by way of inference). An inference-engine based service selection mode selects services (the next activity in a workflow) based on the decisions of the participants in a workflow as well as on historical data collected from past instances (via mining). If a selected service indicates that it must be preceded by another service, this other service will be selected and executed, otherwise the first service will be executed, and so on. In this probabilistic model, services are selected at run-time based on three key criteria: available contextual knowledge of the current workflow instance, statistical knowledge collected and mined from previous workflow instances, and composition rules and constraints – a rules-engine. This rules-engine allows enforcement of service sequencing based on temporal dependencies, data availability, business rules, and role restrictions.

As mentioned, services can also be sequentially invoked, thus providing backwards compatibility with classic prescribed workflow models. A workflow instance continues selecting services (prescriptively and stochastically) until it has addressed all the required services to complete the process. In highly dynamic environments, workflows may possibly enter a state where the next appropriate activity is unknown and cannot be inferred. This may occur during times of process discovery or reengineering within an organization. To address this, we incorporate workflow mining services. A workflow mining service can record data from the current workflow instance and subsequently examine previous instances of whole workflows to guide the selection of services until participant decisions redirect the workflow. This forms a closed-loop feedback cycle with the inference-engine used for service selection.

6. Related Work

A number of approaches to the representation and realization of dynamic workflow have been proposed. As examples, workflow languages such as BPEL4WS [11], WSFL [12], and XLANG [13] have evolved. However, these solutions are limited in their ability to represent dynamicity and they do not consider context information as transition constraints of services. A situation-adaptable workflow system was described by Vieira and Rito-Silva [14] that can support service demands generated dynamically in a business process. This system can dynamically handle a user's requests using open-ended adaptation techniques. Our approach, however, also incorporates context and relies on context attributes to constrain service executions within a database-oriented realization.

7. Summary and Conclusions

It has become clear that classic, rigid workflows are too constraining to address the complexity and variability of workflows in healthcare environments. We have presented a framework for addressing the dynamic nature of healthcare workflows in a "computationally tractable" form, implementing a new understanding of dynamic workflow through the use of concepts from database theory, inference engines and service oriented architectures. This work, together with work in context informed workflow can be found in greater detail in the 2008 Business Process Management and Workflow Handbook [15].

Acknowledgements

This work has been support by NSERC Canada and Agfa.

References

[1]   N. Johnson, Simply Complexity: a clear guide to complexity theory. Oneworld Publications. 2007. ISBN 978-1-85168-630-8.
[2]   W. M. P. Van Der Aalst, A. H. M. Ter Hofstede, B. Kiepuszewski, A. P. Barros, Workflow Patterns. *Distributed and Parallel Databases*, **14(1)** (2003), 5-51.
[3]   D.D. Cowan et al. Software System Generation from an Enterprise Service Model. D.R. Cheriton School of Computer Science Report CS-2007-04. [Internet]. 2007. [cited 2009Dec.16]. Available from: http://www.cs.uwaterloo.ca/research/tr/2007/.
[4]   M. Jackson, G. Twaddle, Business Process Implementation: Building Workflow Systems. Addison-Wesley, 1997.
[5]   P.P.S. Chen, The entity-relationship model: toward a unified view of eata. ACM Transactions on Database Systems **1** (1976), 9-36.
[6]   Business Process Execution Language for Web Services version 1.1. [Internet]. 2003. [cited 2009 Dec 16]. Available from: http://www-128.ibm.com/developerworks/library/specification/ws-bpel/
[7]   J. Rumbaugh, I. Jacobson, G. Booch, The Unified Modeling language Reference Manual. Addison Wesley, (2004)
[8]   XML Metadata Interchange (XMI), v2.1.[Internet]. 2009. [cited 2009 Dec 16]. Available from: http://www.omg.org/technology/documents/formal/xmi.htm
[9]   Extensible Stylesheet Language (XSL) [Internet]. 2009. [cited 2009 Dec 16]. Available from: http://www.w3.org/Style/XSL/
[10]   P.S.C. Alencar, T. Oliveira, D.D. Cowan, D.W. Mulholland, Towards Monitored Data Consistency and Business Processing Based on Declarative Software Agents. Software Engineering for Large-Scale Multi-Agent Systems – Research Issues and Practical Applications. Garcia A, Lucena C, et al. (Eds), Lecture Notes in Computer Science (LNCS), 2603 (2003), 267-284.
[11]   T. Andrews, F. Curbera, Y. Golan, Business Process Execution Language for Web Services, BEA Systems, version 1.1., 2003.
[12]   F. Leymann, Web Services Flow Language (WSFL 1.0). IBM 2001.
[13]   S. Thatte. XLANG Web Services for Business Process Design. Microsoft Corporation 2001.
[14]   P. Vieira, A. Rito-Silva, Adaptive workflow management in WorkSCo, 16th International Workshop on Database and Expert Systems Applications (DEXA05) (2005), 640-645.
[15]   H.D. Covvey, D.D. Cowan, P. Alencar, W. Malyk, J. So, D. Henriques, S. Fenton S, The Representation of Dynamic, Context-Informed Workflow", In 2008 Business Process Management and Workflow Handbook, Workflow Management Coalition. Fisher L.,(2008)

196

International Perspectives in Health Informatics
E.M. Borycki et al. (Eds.)
IOS Press, 2011
doi:10.3233/978-1-60750-709-3-196

Waiting Time in Emergency Department by Simulation

Sima AJAMI [a, 1], Saeedeh KETABI [b],
Mohammad H. YARMOHAMMADIAN [c], Hosain BAGHERIAN [d]

[a] *Department of Health Information Technology Faculty of Medical Management &
Information Sciences, Isfahan University of Medical Sciences, Iran*
[b] *Department of Management, University of Isfahan, Isfahan, Iran*
[c] *Head of Health Management & Economics Research Center, Isfahan University of
Medical Sciences, Isfahan, Iran*
[d] *Isfahan Branch of Iran Legal Medicine Organization, Isfahan, Iran*

Abstract. The aim of research was to reduce waiting time at ED. Population
includes the patients who received services in ED. The arrival and service times in
different stations were collected for 663 patients. For data analysis, SPSS and
simulation technique were used. Results shows that add one intern to the Ear Nose
Throat (ENT) service makes the most reduction on the waiting time from 112.19
to 99.24 minutes. Health care managers, in the ED are usually physicians who are
not familiar with principals of management.

Keywords. emergency department, waiting time, simulation, scenario

1. Introduction

Emergency Department(ED) provides urgent clinical and Para-clinical care for patients
that injured in accidents and incidents. The injured patients need urgent treatment in
terms of according to their situation [1]. The results of different studies showed that
patient waiting time is one of the impressive factors on patient satisfaction. In a
research that titled "reasons of patient dissatisfaction at ED", finding showed main
reasons of dissatisfaction were waiting time 67% and absence of effective relationship
with patients by medical care staff 19% [2]. At recent years, patient waiting time in the
emergency process has had a great increase, for instance, in England waiting time was
increased to 4 hours and in Canada received to 2 hours [3]. Several studies in recent
years reveal that the number of people that visit ED has grown as in Canada to 14
million per year and in Britain to beyond 15 million in a year [4-6]. Simulations help
the management to optimize many factors such as work expenditure, patient waiting
time and number of personnel in ED [7]. In 2008, Statistics showed that
Ayatolahkashani Hospital, which is affiliated, with Isfahan Medical Sciences
University (IMSU) in Iran has 10 wards, 196 active beds, an average length of stay of
2.41 days, a bed occupancy of 70% and a turnover of 1.1 days. In addition, it has 30
beds in ED with 74 medical staff (26 nurses, 6 general practitioners, 2 anesthesiologists,

[1] Corresponding Author: Sima Ajami, Phone: 1-647-857-9770, Fax: 1-416-978-
7753, email: simajami@mie.utoronto.ca or simajami@yahoo.com

1 secretary, etc). The annual number of admissions to ED in 2006, 2007 and 2008 were 29446, 31735 and 32445 in respectively. The average daily admissions during the last three years were 81, 87, and 89 respectively. Regarding the particular situation of the hospital, due the high rate of emergency patients and their need to be admitted urgently, delay in servicing the patients not only increases dissatisfaction of health care render in hospital, but also causes delay in reception of new patients. Due to the long patient waiting times in ED and importance of minimizing costs and maximizing hospital resources productivity, it was felt necessary to study patient waiting time in ED services at by simulation technique.

2. Methods

This study was an analytical and cross-sectional study in which data were collected by forms, observation, and study of documentations. Isfahan city with a population of approximately 3,000, 000 has 22 hospitals. However, Alzahra Hospital and Ayatolahkashani Hospitals are the biggest emergency centers in the Isfahan province. Because of overcrowded and limitation of space and Medical personnel, researchers chose this hospital. Study population included the patients who received services in the Ayatolahkashani ED in May 2008. Researchers took permission from hospital administrators who encouraged personnel for cooperation. Then, research team interviewed with managers Medical personnel to know number of stations, personnel in stations, start and end time of personnel work in all stations in ED along with diagnostic wards (e.g. Laboratory, Radiology, Ultrasonography, and C-T Scan). Then, research team has drawn the flow work of patients' treatment process to receive diagnostic and care services in ED. For measuring waiting and service time, research team settled down in all stations related to ED's treatment process along with diagnostic wards (e.g. Laboratory, Radiology, Ultrasonography, and C-T Scan) during a two-week period in the spring 2008. Patients tracked by patient number wristband were worn after entering through ED door and research team recorded waiting and service time to measure their information in each station. Data included; current process, patients' wristband numbers, name of stations and duration of rendered service, time of arrival and departure to stations in Ayatolahkashani Hospital ED. In order to designing of patients arrival distribution of service time in different work stations data entered to SPSS, then type of distributions were identified via One-Sample Kolmogorov-Smirnov Test. Sample size of patients was based on number of patients who were treated in the previous year at the same time in Ayatolahkashani Hospital. In order to selection time of sampling that cover patient arrival pattern in different month of year one month in which patient arrival pattern was stable be selected and during it (May 2008) patient arrival time and patient service time in different stations and interval time. Finally, the required data of patient arrival time and patient service time in different stations for 663 patients during two weeks has been collected. Then, by using SPSS (Statistical Package for Social Science), distribution of patient arrival time and patient service along with related parameter in all stations were designed. After that, a simulation model for ED has been designed by simul8. Results from base model running and alternatives running were transferred to Excel software to analyze. The validity of model has been verified via comparison between actual data and the result of the simulation model. At the end, 20 alternative scenarios for reducing patient waiting time were suggested.

3. Results and Discussions

Results showed the stations that deliver services include; screen physician visit, admission, primary nurse, specialist visits (ENT, Orthopedic, and Neurosurgical), secondary nurse, Para-clinical (CT- Scan, Ultrasonography, Radiology, Laboratory) and tertiary nurse services at ED of Ayatolahkashani Hospital. Distribution of arriving time to ED was exponential with mean about 8.34 which indicated averagely seven people refer to ED.   According to findings, there were three type patients in ED; patient's type 1: These patients have life-threatening but treatable injuries requiring rapid medical attention that put on first priority than other types (Red). They use screen services, medical specialty services, nurses, Para-clinics and CPR (Cardio Pulmonary Resuscitation) services. Patients' type 2: They potentially have serious injuries, but are stable enough to wait a short while for medical treatment (Yellow). They move on similar path than type 1, except use of CPR service. The patients' type 3: They have minor injuries that can wait for longer periods for treatment and only uses nurse services and screen services (Green). From results, total percent of patient's type 1, 2 and 3 were 7, 50 and 43 respectively. Percent of patients' orthopedics, neurosurgical and ENT (Eye, Nose & Throat) services were 38, 30, and 11 respectively. Percent of patients whose didn't use any of these services and only use Para-clinics and screen services were 21. On the other hand, percent of patients in Laboratory, Radiology, CT-Scan and Ultrasonography services were 73, 65, 47 and 17 respectively. Distribution of services time in Radiology, ENT Intern and Resident were exponential and in other services were normal. Bottlenecks are stations which have maximum waiting time. As it can be seen from table 1, Laboratory Services, ENT Visit, and Orthopedic Visit were bottlenecks respectively. There were many factors corresponding to these delays and long waiting time but the most significant related to lack of efficient communications between different resident specialists. After designing model and running 1000 times, mean of waiting time and manpower idle time was earned (table 1 and 2). Table 1 illustrates that total mean of patient waiting time was 112.19 minutes in ED. The most and the least patient waiting times were 36.04 and 0.25 minutes in ENT and Admission services respectively.

Table1. Mean of Patient Waiting Time on Base Model

Stations of Services	Admission Process	Screen Physician Visit	Primary nurses'	Orthopedic Visit	Neurosurgical Visit	ENT Visit	Secondary Nurse Services	CT- Scan	Ultrasonography	Radiology	Laboratory	Tertiary Nurse
time	0.25	1.06	2.33	14.88	11.37	36.04	5.57	1.06	.78	5.85	20.17	11.30

The mean of the idle time of manpower in Para-clinical units (CT-Scan, Ultrasonography and Radiology) and admission unit were more than others. The least manpower idle time related to third nurse activity with 33.24 percent. After designing of base model and running it, mean waiting time and manpower idle time were obtained. Then 20 alternative solutions were suggested for reducing patients waiting time. According to stakeholder's viewpoint and hospital situations, alternative solutions were designed. These mainly related to improvement of processes' emergency care delivery and change number of manpower. After implementing alternatives, manpower idle time was designed. Then, in order to select the best alternative in ED and implement it successfully, researchers compared the results from running of any alternative in model with base model. Scenarios denote that we can reduce mean of care services time and waiting time for receiving care services with small changes in some stations. Findings of research that entitled "simulation in outpatient's services systems in Tehran educational and general hospitals" showed changing of physicians' visit-start-time in clinics can reduce patients' waiting time from 67.01 to 44.73 percent in minutes [8].

Stations	Admission	Screen Physician	First Nurses Activity	Orthopedics' Intern	Orthopedics' Resident	Neurosurgical Intern	Neurosurgical Resident	ENT Intern	ENT Resident	Second nurses activity	CT-Scan	Ultrasonography	Radiology	Lab	Third Nurses activity
Percent of Idle Time	63.84	60.48	54.54	45.16	42.66	50.5	45.66	46.94	48.28	42.73	79.98	87.19	64.51	38.22	33.24

Table 2. Percent of Manpower Idle Time in Stations of Services' Delivery

Many solutions have also been sought from operational changes by many researchers. The focus has been on patient flows, waiting times and throughput time in ED. Some of them focused, for their part, on fast-track solution or bed occupancy has been under examination [9]. Miller and colleagues proposed Grouping scenarios in the following hierarchy will be instrumental when executing scenarios and finding the best alternatives as follows: 1. Arrival volumes, 2. Inpatient beds, 3. Ratio of main ED and fast track beds, 4. Process improvements. Some solutions emphasized on number of manpower and equipments and some others on changing and improvement of processes and else on all factors [10]. Most of times, we can only improve processes and decrease waiting time without spending additional cost for human resources or institute new ward in ED. Findings in a study at Lancaster University in United Kingdom on ED performance by using simulation showed patients were actually triaged by 3 categories ("Minor", "Major" and "Life threatening"). The aim of triaging was to prioritize patients so that more severe cases are treated before less severe ones

[11]. In this research, also the results showed that general practitioners, interns, residents and specialists have multi-tasks in several places at Ayatolahkashani Hospital such as in operation room, different wards, and clinics that obviously decrease quality of care in ED. Research findings indicate that, in fact, unfortunately, doctors do not have tendency to do verity tasks and prefer to give more attention to their patients. In the other words, from our results, low experienced interns and residents were spending more time with patients and request more investigations and tests to make decisions for them. It is the opposite for experienced doctors that they are rapid in decision making. From our model, scenarios revealed that inexperienced doctors order more X-Ray and stem high congestion in Para-clinic departments. Because of mixing urgent patients with less severe patients to get Para-clinical services, severe patients have to wait to get their Para-clinical services (e.g. in CT-Scan).

4. Conclusions

Managers should learn scientific and simple methods to control and planning better. They should set up meetings to study and review flow works in ED at regular period.
In order to decrease waiting time in Para-clinical services, they should get to their services out of turn. Intern replace with general physician to decrease waiting time in ED. Hospital emergency Managers should inform online "Emergency Medical Services Center" about available bed that can better steer and distribute severe patients among other hospitals.

References

[1]   T. Abedi, F. Vaezzadeh, A. Baghbanian, F. Bahraini. *Hospital Administration*. Tehran: Gap Publication, 2003, [Book in Persian].
[2]   M. Q. Choyce, A. K. Maitra .Satisfaction with the Accident and Emergency Department, a Postal Survey of General Practitioners' Views. *J Accident Emerg Med*, **13** (1996), 280-282
[3]   Audit Commission .*Accident and Emergency, Review of National Findings*: October 2001.London: Audit Commission Publications: 2001.
[4]   T. Young, T. Eldabi .Simulating A & E Systems: More of the same or Lesson Learned. England: In *Proceedings of the 2006 OR Society Simulation Work Shop*. 2006.
[5]   Canadian Institute for Health Information. *Understanding emergency department wait time*. Ottawa Canada: 2005.
[6]   D. C. Lane, C. Monefeld, J. V. Rosenhead .Looking in the Wrong Place for Healthcare Improvements: a System Dynamics Study of an Accident and Emergency Department. *J Operation Res Soc* **51** 2000, 518–31.
[7]   F. Diyanatkhah, A. Shams, S. Riyazinia, D. Zargarisamani. A Comparative Study between Clinics and Para-clinics Emergency Services in Shariati Hospital from 2004 to 2006 in Isfahan [Thesis in Persian]. Isfahan Iran:A Industrial Management Institute, The Isfahan Branch, Equivalent Master Sciences Hospital Executive Management, 2007.
[8]   A. Aeenparast. Simulation in Outpatient's Services System; Model Proposing for Reducing Waiting Time for Outpatients in Tehran Educational and General Hospitals in 2005 [Thesis in Persian]. Tehran, Iran: Iran University of Medical Sciences, Faculty of Medical Informatics & Management; 2006.
[9]   T. Ruohonen, P. Neittaanmaki, J. Teittinen .Simulation Model for Improving the Operation of the Emergency Department of Special Health Care. In: *Proceedings of the 38th conference on winter simulation*. Monterey, California, USA: 2006. P: 453 – 458.
[10]   M. J. Miller, D. M. Ferrin, M. G. Messer .Fixing the Emergency Department: A Transformational Journey with EDSIM. In: *Proceedings of the 36th conference on winter simulation*, Washington, D.C, USA: 2004, Pages: 1988 - 1993.
[11]   M. Gunal, M. Pidd .Understanding Accident and Emergency Performance; Using Simulation. In: *Proceedings of the 38th conference on winter simulation*. Monterey, California, USA: 2006.

Human Computer Interaction

International Perspectives in Health Informatics
E.M. Borycki et al. (Eds.)
IOS Press, 2011
doi:10.3233/978-1-60750-709-3-203

Cognitive Analysis of a Medication Reconciliation Tool: Applying Laboratory and Naturalistic Approaches to System Evaluation

Andre W. KUSHNIRUK [1a], Susan L. SANTOS [b,c], George POURAKIS [d],
Jonathan R. NEBEKER [e], Kenneth S. BOOCKVAR [f,g,h]

[a] *School of Health Information Science, University of Victoria,*
Victoria, British Columbia, Canada
[b] *VA New Jersey Health Care System, East Orange, NJ*
[c] *Department of Health Education and Behavioral Science, University of Medicine &*
Dentistry of New Jersey, New Brunswick, NJ
[d] *Centers for Disease Control and Prevention*
[e] *VA Geriatrics Research, Education, and Clinical Center, Salt Lake City, UT*
[f] *Geriatrics Research, Education, and Clinical Center,*
James J. Peters Veterans Affairs Medical Center, Bronx, NY
[g] *Department of Geriatrics and Palliative Medicine, Mount Sinai School of Medicine, New York*
[h] *Jewish Home Lifecare, New York, NY*

Abstract. Adverse drug events can occur as a result of handoffs in patient care. To reduce the possibility of this occurring, the process of medication reconciliation (whereby the patient's medication history is compared to current and previous medications to ensure accuracy) is becoming recognized as becoming increasingly important. To address this, computerized medication reconciliation tools have been developed. This paper describes a combined approach to evaluating the impact of such a tool. The approach has included both an artificial laboratory-based evaluation component (involving observing subjects interacting with standardized patient cases), as well as a naturalistic condition (involving real patient cases). The results indicate that there are differences in the way that subjects interact with the medication reconciliation tool, with significant differences identified in the amount of time spent and accuracy of medication documentation between physician and pharmacist users.

Keywords. medication reconciliation, patient safety, cognitive analysis

Introduction

Studies of human-computer interaction in healthcare have applied a variety of approaches, varying from laboratory-based usability studies to naturalistic observation of users interacting with healthcare information systems for dealing with real patient cases. The different approaches have different advantages and disadvantages. In this

---

[1] Corresponding author: Dr. Andre Kushniruk; email: andrek@uvic.ca

paper we apply two different approaches to explore how physicians and pharmacists interact with a tool designed to reduce adverse drug events (ADEs) that can occur during handoffs. The objective was to gain an insight in the cognitive processes of users in interacting with such technology in dealing with both standardized cases (in a "laboratory" testing situation) as well as in dealing with a real patient case (in a "naturalistic" condition). Handoffs in patient care are critical points in healthcare where a variety of medication errors can occur [1]. At the root of this are possible discrepancies among prescriptions written at different times, by the same or different provider, changes in medication regimens, discontinuity of care and inadequate patient education. The potential for ADEs occurring as a result of handoffs led the Joint Commission (formerly the Joint Commission for Accreditation of Healthcare Organizations) in the United States to mandate in 2006 a process to reconcile medications across the continuum of care, a process known as medication reconciliation [2]. In the medication reconciliation process the provider accesses the patient's medication history and compares current medications with previous medications to ensure the lists are correct and consistent. In this paper we examine a decision support tool developed by the James J. Peters Veterans Affairs (Bronx, NY) to provide decision support for the process of medication reconciliation. The tool was developed in 2005 to comply with the Joint Commission's National Patient Safety Goal. To allow for integration with existing computer systems, the tool was embedded in the Veteran Affairs (VA) Computerized Patient Record System (CPRS) and allows users (physicians, pharmacists or other providers) to: (1) view the patient's outpatient medication use for the last 90 days from VA computerized pharmacy data, (2) view current VA inpatient orders, (3) record discrepancies between patient-reported medications and outpatient and inpatient medications in the VA computerized database (4) record diagnostic indications for and responses to these discrepancies.

The question of how to evaluate such a tool from a human-computer interaction (HCI) perspective is the focus of this paper. To this end we developed an evaluation plan that includes a cognitive analysis (CTA) of users interacting with the tool to complete medication reconciliation tasks using both artificial laboratory and naturalistic tasks to examine the interaction of users with the system to carry out medication reconciliation. The objective of this work was to assess the impact of the tool on the cognitive processing of the human users, as well as to provide practical impact to the designers of the tool to maximize its effectiveness. Previous work has considered evaluation of health related decision support in the context of either laboratory-based analyses or observational naturalistic studies [3]. The approach taken in this paper links both think-aloud methods and naturalistic recording and analysis in characterizing the cognitive impact of a medical decision support system on users' decision making and cognitive processes.

1. Methods

1.1. Subjects, Materials and Setting

7 internal house staff physicians and 5 staff pharmacists participated. The study took place in a quiet office, with a computer running a screen recording program (Hypercam©), with an external microphone plugged into the computer. The software tool being evaluated was a medication reconciliation decision support tool that was integrated with the VA's CPRS patient record system. Three standardized (i.e.

fictitious cases) were created that involved checking patient data for consistency of medications using the tool.

1.2. Procedure

In the laboratory-based condition subjects were asked to interact with the medication reconciliation tool and respond to the patient cases in checking to make sure that the patient's medications were correct. Subjects were asked to "think aloud", or verbalize their thoughts while doing this task. The computer screens were recorded using the screen recording software Hypercam©, along with the audio of the subjects' verbalizations. After completing the laboratory task, subjects were briefly interviewed about their experience in using the tool and any problems they may have encountered. This post-task semi-structured interview was audio taped. In a second condition (the naturalistic condition), the subjects were also asked to use the medication reconciliation tool in working on one or more real patient cases. In this naturalistic condition, subjects were instructed to verbalize their thoughts while doing the task. The subjects' verbalizations were audio recorded and notes were taken by the experimenters based on observation of the subjects' interaction with the medication reconciliation tool (e.g. notes about what screens they were on, and user problems in interacting with the tool).

2. Data Analysis

Data analysis first involved having the audio portion of both the laboratory and naturalistic conditions transcribed in their entirety. The computer screens and audio of the subjects' thinking aloud from the laboratory condition were coded using a program known as Transana © which allowed for the audio portion of the transcripts to be linked to the computer movie file of the actual user interactions with the medication reconciliation system. An initial video coding scheme was developed to guide the coding of the transcripts. Categories that were coded for included the following: (a) decision making activities (e.g. planning a medication, choosing a medication, etc.) (b) positive and negative comments about system features (c) strategies taken in doing medication reconciliation (d) information processes (e.g. making inferences, resolving ambiguity etc.) and (e) patient data review activities. The coding scheme was iteratively refined over a several month period. In addition, a number of sections of the data from the laboratory condition were coded by two coders to ensure a high degree of consistency (Kappa > .80). Data from the naturalistic condition (i.e. audio recordings and observational notes) were also analyzed using the coding scheme to identify issues and potential usability problems in interacting with the system. In addition, the time to complete tasks was recorded.

3. Results

The recordings of individual physicians and pharmacists interacting with the tool showed significant differences by profession in amount of time expended to complete medication reconciliation on a standardized, fictitious case, while using the computer template and interface used in actual practice (i.e. the laboratory condition). Five physicians took a mean of 8.1 minutes (s.d. 4.4; range 2.1-15.4) to complete the standardized case, whereas 4 pharmacists took 16.2 minutes (s.d. 4.8; range 6.3-25.1) to complete the same case (difference=8.1 minutes; p=.022 for comparison). The time difference was also correlated with better quality of documentation by pharmacists. As compared to the physicians who correctly documented the status of 8.6 medications on average in the medication reconciliation out of a possible 14, the pharmacists correctly documented the status of 11.3 medications on average for the same case (p=.05 for comparison). Pharmacists were also more likely to document the indication for each medication or medication change.

A difference in completion times of a larger magnitude, though not statistically significant, was also evident in our recording of physicians and pharmacists completing medication reconciliation on real cases in the course of actual practice (i.e. the naturalistic condition). Four physicians took a mean of 4.2 minutes (s.d. 2.1; range 1.3-7.4) to complete medication reconciliation on actual cases, whereas 5 pharmacists took a mean of 18.0 minutes (s.d. 8.6; range 6.3-25.1) (difference=13.8 minutes; p=.136 for comparison). Each hour of video data took several hours of time to be transcribed and coded using the video coding tool Transana©. An excerpt from a coded transcript of a pharmacist "thinking aloud" while interacting with the system (note the number in the excerpt refers to the time since the start of the task) in the naturalistic condition is shown below (also note that the same type of coding sheet was used for analyzing users' interaction with the tool in the laboratory condition):

Table 1. Coded Think-Aloud Transcript

Action/Verbalization	Strategy	Information Processing	Review	Comments
Subject: "... scroll down and see if I can find... they don't know what his meds are either... they started him on Seroquel 300. Ok new progress note"		Information ambiguity	Medication review (attention to dosage)	Patient and team don't know the exact meds: barrier to medrec
02:20 – [Select/Click: new progress note]				
Subject: "gotta search the patient. Reconciliation admission"	Strategy: medication reconciliation			Begins medrec after 2 minutes of patient review

In the above excerpt, we can see that the pharmacist subject first scrolls through the system to review the patient's medications, selects a new progress note and begins the process of medication reconciliation after 2 minutes of review. The qualitative analysis and coding of these recorded interactions across both the laboratory and naturalistic recordings, as well as the post-task semi-structured interviews, indicated a number of common themes including the following:

- Differences in strategies across subjects in how they carried out medication reconciliation -- with some subjects more extensively reviewing relevant documentation before beginning the medication reconciliation process, with others beginning the process much more rapidly.
- Differences across subjects in how subjects used the medrec tool and integrated it into their workflow.
- System and usability issues including the following: missing information on the status of medications, subjects' desiring the ability of the system to provide side by side comparisons of drug lists in the medrec template provided by the tool, and desire for a more esthetic medrec template.

- Perceived difficulty for physicians in finding the time to complete the medication reconciliation task given time available in their schedule.
- Differences across subjects in the time and effort expended and well as differences in the perceived importance and value of medication reconciliation.

4. Discussion

In this paper we have described an approach to evaluating a computerized medication reconciliation tool where we have employed both a laboratory-based and a naturalistic component to evaluation. The approaches were found to be complementary, with qualitative analyses of data from both parts of the study indicating that there were differences in the approach taken by subjects in interacting with the tool and carrying out the medication reconciliation process. The laboratory approach (involving presentation of standardized cases) allowed for statistical examination of these qualitative findings by allowing for direct comparison of the time taken by physicians and pharmacists and provided definitive evidence that for the same cases, there were significant differences between these two groups of subjects in the amount of time spent and accuracy of the documentation. Overall, the time spent on and participants' qualitative approach to the naturalistic cases was similar to the artificial cases, suggesting that the artificial cases adequately mimicked the naturalistic cases. At the same time, the pharmacists spent more time on the naturalistic cases than on the artificial cases, in contrast to the physicians, who spent significantly less time on the naturalistic cases than on the artificial ones. This finding implies that naturalistic observations are important for an accurate estimate of real staffing needs, and that discrepancies between naturalistic and artificial observations may differ depending on the profession. Coupled with the qualitative findings across both the laboratory and naturalistic conditions (regarding differences in time, effort, and perceived importance of medication reconciliation) the results of the study have argued for a more comprehensive introduction of the medrec tool to new users (i.e. emphasizing improved awareness of the importance of the medication reconciliation process, the medrec tool and providing further training on its use). System and usability issues raised by the study are being addressed as input to refinement of the tool and a subsequent round of focus groups (with both physicians and pharmacists) substantiated and extended the findings from the cognitive analysis reported in this paper. The work has general implications for conducting evaluations of health information systems, by showing that both artificial and real (naturalistic) testing can be successfully combined within a single study to be sure that the artificial condition closely approximates the naturalistic condition, and to arrive at a clearer assessment of the impact of decision support designed to improve patient safety.

References

[1] T. Alexander et al. Evaluation of an inpatient computerized medication reconciliation system. *JAMIA* 15(4) (2008), 449-452.
[2] B. Lesselroth et al. Design and implementation of a medication reconciliation kiosk. *JAMIA* 16 (2010), 300-304.
[3] E. Poon et al. Design and implementation of an application and associated services to support interdisciplinary medication reconciliation efforts at an integrated healthcare delivery network. *JAMIA* 13 (6), 581-592.

International Perspectives in Health Informatics
E.M. Borycki et al. (Eds.)
IOS Press, 2011
© 2011 ITCH 2011 Steering Committee and IOS Press. All rights reserved.
doi:10.3233/978-1-60750-709-3-208

Usability Analysis of the Tele-nursing Call Management Software at HealthLink BC

Simon A. S. HALL[a,b,1], Andre W. KUSHNIRUK[b], Elizabeth M. BORYCKI[b]
aHealthLink BC, Ministry of Health Services, British Columbia, Canada
bSchool of Health Information Science, University of Victoria, Victoria, British Columbia, Canada

Abstract. Usability engineering methods have been shown to be effective in identifying software problems that may lead to user operating inefficiencies, user errors, data encoding errors or far more serious health threatening consequences. This research project applied two complementary usability engineering analysis methods to a mature tele-nursing clinical call management software platform (a knowledgebase and an EMR product). Findings from the study revealed 100 discrete usability errors or problems. This research also introduced an adaptation of cognitive task analysis, with the development of a 'cognitive task screen-turn' analysis, which provided useful information about operating differences among users performing identical tasks that was particularly useful in revealing four unnecessary steps within the system.

Keywords. nursing informatics, usability engineering, tele-nursing, human-computer interaction, hybrid, electronic medical records, decision support systems

Introduction

Clinicians are increasingly being asked to use Information and Communication Technologies (ICT) in the practice and delivery of care. Automation in the form of ICTs and decision support software (DSS) is increasing each year. Limited availability of health human resources, cost factors, speed and quality are all factors that drive increasing automation in healthcare. Use of ICTs and DSSs has the potential to reduce the number of medical errors that occur through improved workflow, with automated reminders and alerts [1]. Research suggests it is also very important to be cognizant of the unexpected side effects that arise from using ICTs. Through evaluation we may learn more about these side effects. Tele-nurses face additional challenges, as there is no face to face contact with patients in their work. Nurses must build a picture of the patient through a process known as 'visualization work' (i.e. constructing a mental model of the caller) [2]. This absence of the patient focuses the tele-nurse on the supporting technologies to build a mental model of a patient. Research suggests that DSS may play a role in determining disposition due to this 'visualization work'. In previous work, DSS in telephone triage has involved public emergency calls for medical help [3], where lower acuity 9-1-1 calls were transferred to nurses who were using knowledge based systems to support nurse triage (i.e. either resolving the call, or

---

1 Corresponding Author. Simon Hall: simon.hall@healthlinkbc.ca

returning the call back to 9-1-1 for ambulance dispatch). This study investigated how task urgency and complexity affected decision making in a dynamic environment. In this paper we examine the usability of DSS and electronic medical records (EMRs) in supporting tele-nursing.

1. Usability Engineering Methods

There are two major methodological approaches that comprise usability engineering: inspection and testing [4]. Usability inspection is an approach that evaluates a software system on the basis of well-tested design principles such as visibility of system status, user control and freedom, consistency and standards, flexibility, and efficiency of use. This form of evaluation was first proposed by Nielsen in 1993 [4]. Using the inspection approach known as heuristic evaluation, one or more inspectors step through the system rating and identifying violations of heuristics. This approach differs substantially from simulated usability testing, as it evaluates the system agnostically. The approach can also be performed by almost anyone who is familiar with using computers, and is therefore not reliant on requiring the involvement of end-users (often very busy in clinical practice). This kind of evaluation is well suited to the design and build phases of a new application project, long before a system has been released to clients. In contrast, usability testing " involves gathering information about the actual process of using a system from representative users performing representative tasks"[5]. The results of this type of evaluation can be used to improve the features of a system prior to the completion its design or alternatively to assess the impact of fully implemented systems. These two approaches to usability engineering, when combined, can yield both complementary and unique results, due to their differing evaluative foci. As well, they can provide designers with valuable information about a system's usability that system owners and operators may have otherwise overlooked. In this paper we report on the usability of a tele-nursing call management system using both usability inspection and testing methods.

2. Methods

2.1. Subjects, Materials and Research Setting

Six registered nurses working at *HealthLink BC* participated in the study. The study took place at *HealthLink BC* which is a self-care/tele-nursing service staffed by Registered Nurses and other health care professionals accessible through 8-1-1 for the residents of BC. The software that was studied is used by tele-nurses as a call management software platform and consists of: (a) FC (i.e. a hybrid EMR), and (b) HWC (i.e. a DSS tool that provides clinical support algorithms and protocols to determine an appropriate response to client care needs).

2.2. Procedure

The research took place in two phases. In Phase One a heuristic evaluation was conducted by the first author of the FC and HWC applications. Nielsen's heuristics [4] were applied to assess usability problems with the applications. In Phase Two, where usability testing was conducted, subjects arrived at the call centre and were asked to complete two simulations. A research collaborator acted as a simulated caller and phoned in to the subject who received the call. The collaborator used two predefined scenarios (i.e. one routine: a caller with a headache, one complex: a caller with a burn). Nurse subjects were asked to respond to the calls. The computer screens of the application were video recorded using Camtasia©. The audio of the dialogue with the simulated caller was also recorded. At the end of each session, subjects were interviewed about their interactions with the system and asked to comment about key sequences that were video recorded using a cued-recall approach [5]. Analysis involved tabulating usability errors and problems identified from the heuristic evaluation, as well as transcribing and coding the video recorded interactions of subjects from the usability testing sessions (as described in the next section).

3. Results

3.1. Usability Inspection

A total of 53 errors in each of Nielsen's 10 heuristics (See Table 1) were recorded, with a substantially greater number of errors being reported with the FC (medical record) (n=42) system than with the HWC knowledge base (n=5), with only three attributable to interoperability issues (i.e. issues caused by differences between the two systems). There were no 'catastrophic' errors as defined by Nielsen, but unexpectedly, a high number of 'major usability' errors (n=7). 26 'minor' and 10 'cosmetic' usability errors were observed. For a production and maturing system, this is a significant count, and these errors were attended to with priority. It is also worthy to note, a high number of errors in rule #3 (i.e. "User control and freedom" were present).

Table 1. Error Count by Heuristic

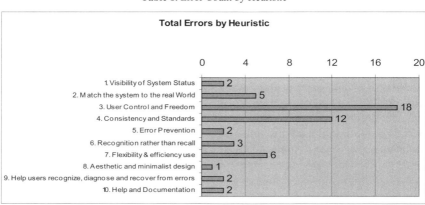

3.2. Usability Testing: Cued-Recall and Cognitive Task Screen Turn Analysis

Usability testing included the use of cued-recall and cognitive task screen turn analysis (CTSTA). Cued-recall analysis revealed 49 unique problems (i.e. 12 attributed to the HWC software, 28 to the FC software and seven to issues of interoperability). Results were discursive and textural. It should be noted that all nurses reached the same nursing triage dispositions.

Following this, CTSTA analysis was undertaken of the video recorded call data from the usability testing. CTSTA is a method we have developed where a screen-turn is defined as a user initiated request of the system to perform an action resulting in the display of a new screen of information. The recordings were analyzed to time-map screen-turns actioned by the tele-nurses in accomplishing cognitive tasks. Screen-turns can be grouped into cognitive tasks (or steps). The *HealthLink BC* Nursing Services' Quality Call Tool [6], was helpful in this analysis as it laid out eight key steps in a regular tele-nursing call. The major cognitive steps from this tool were reduced to four specific progress points: 1) **Identify** client 2) **Assess** client needs, 3) **Triage** and 4) **Chart** post call documentation.

Each nurse completed their simulated burn and headache calls with similar timings and screen turn counts, in each of the four cognitive steps. This was unexpected as the clinical complexity of a burn call in comparison to a headache call, would intuitively lead one to expect a longer call handle time. However, inter-nurse comparisons were substantially different. In the simulated headache call, the greatest inter-nurse time spread was during the 'Triage' task, with a high (Nurse 4 - 7min 16sec) being four minutes and eight seconds (4min 8sec) longer than the shortest (Nurse 1 - 3min 8sec). This may be partially explained by an unusually low 'Assess' time for Nurse 4, being suggestive that some client assessment continued in the 'Triage' step (i.e. Nurse 1 was cognitively assessing the caller from within HWC – not as trained). Another example was in the simulated Burn call during the 'Assess' task, with a high 4min 39sec call time (Nurse 2), and a low 46sec call time (Nurse 4). The difference in call time was three minutes and fifty three seconds (3min 53sec) longer. The overall length of the call was very nurse dependent. Nurse 6 was the fastest for both calls at 444 seconds (7mins 22secs) and 448 seconds (7mins 28secs), whereas the slowest call handle for the simulated burn was Nurse 5 at 731 seconds (12mins 11secs) and the simulated headache was Nurse 4 at 728 seconds (12mins 8secs). Further analysis linking the count of screen-turns was required to accomplish the four cognitive tasks. This work also proved valuable. Of most relevance was the identification of 'Unnecessary Screen-Turns'. An "unnecessary screen-turn" fails two of Neilsen's heuristics - #3 – User Control and Freedom, and #7 – Flexibility and Efficiency. Unnecessary screen turns occur when a user of a system has to pass through a screen in order to get to a desired screen. In this study four separate instances (observed in more than one simulated call) were noted for remediation.

A total of 105 unique problems/errors were documented within the combined system (i.e. FC and HWC). The FC system had more than three times the error occurrence than the HWC. Therefore, FC had the greatest opportunity for remediation (n=72) as compared to HWC (n=23). "Cued-recall" and "inspection" identified the presence of significantly greater errors with the FC than the HWC system. The area of 'interoperability' also reported a total of 10 errors, which may be remediated in either, or both products. A further analysis of error overlap between the two research methods was undertaken to validate the accuracy of the approaches in identifying common errors. Only 10 problems were identified during the cued recall related to errors detected during the heuristic inspection process. Conversely, only four of the errors reported during heuristic evaluation related to problems identified during the cued recall. This low correlation is interesting, and counterintuitive until one realizes that the systems (FC and HWC) have been in daily production use for many years (albeit with upgrades and enhancements throughout), and that nursing staff have already had sufficient time to become fully conversant with the many basic heuristic errors, learning to work around these errors in their skilled operation. This underlies the ability of users to adapt to usability problems and issues. While outside the scope of this study, further research is needed to determine the extent to which the usability of the software has an influence upon satisfaction or retention rates of nurses.

4. Conclusions

In the study reported in this paper, the authors found usability problems in what would be considered a mature system. Although there were errors identified during usability inspection, and testing, it was clear that users had learned to work around these errors. Although usability methods are often used for assessing systems in the development process, we have found through our research that these methods may also be highly applicable for identifying problems in mature systems. The results also served as a baseline usability assessment that has already been used to inform the development of a new release of the FC software, and this methodology is expected to be used iteratively through a number of cycles of future software upgrades. By establishing baseline data, measurable system improvements can be detected and reported. There is an additional opportunity to leverage 'Cognitive Task Analysis' to assist in training and possibly optimizing call handle times, but as much of call handle time is consumed in conversation with the caller, this observation (while clearly important to the *HealthLink BC* operations) is outside the scope of this software usability research. In June of 2010, *HealthLink BC* implemented a new release of FC that incorporated some 29 of the recommendations from the original research paper [7]. Plans are in place to repeat usability testing and inspection on this updated system, and evaluate the effectiveness of this software release.

References

[1] A. W. Kushniruk et al. Technology induced error and usability: The relationship between usability problems and prescription errors when using a handheld application *Int J Med Inf* **74**(7-8) (2005), 519-26.
[2] B. Edwards, Seeing is believing--picture building: a key component of telephone triage. *J Clin Nursing* **7**(1) (1998), 51-7.
[3] J. Leprohon, V. L. Patel, Decision-making strategies for telephone triage in emergency medical services. *Med Dec Making* **15**(3) (1995), 240-53.
[4] J. Neilsen, *Usability Engineering.* New York: Academic Press, 1993.
[5] V. L. Patel, A. W. Kushniruk, Interface design for health care environments: The role of cognitive science. Proceedings AMIA, 1998. *Annual Symposium* (1998) 29-37.
[6] BC-Nurseline, *Quality Call Tool.* Vancouver: HealthLinkBC: (2008) 6.
[7] S. Hall, *Usability analysis of the tele-nursing call management software at HealthLink BC.* Available from: School of Health Information Science, University of Victoria., 2009.

International Perspectives in Health Informatics
E.M. Borycki et al. (Eds.)
IOS Press, 2011

doi:10.3233/978-1-60750-709-3-213

Adapting Usability Testing Techniques to Gather User Requirements: An Illustrative Proposal

Paule BELLWOOD [a,1], Philipp NEUHAUS [b], Christian JUHRA [b]

[a] *School of Health Information Science, University of Victoria, Victoria, BC, Canada*
[b] *Münster University Hospital, Münster, Germany*

Abstract. Usability testing could greatly aid in gathering requirements for a system prior to its planning and design. An illustrative pilot usability study was carried out aiming to develop methodology for determining the functionality of the medical imaging software that is required to accurately assess medical images in emergency situations in a specific trauma department. Two individuals participated in the study. The proposed methodology for carrying out usability testing in a pre-planning and pre-development phase is illustrated in this proposal. The illustration showed that data collected in this manner may have a significant value. We, therefore, recommend a full pilot study to validate the findings.

Keywords. usability testing, requirement gathering

Introduction

Usability Testing (UT) is used to evaluate information systems. One approach to UT is testing systems that have already been developed and are fully functional. Another approach involves testing systems that are still going through the evaluation and requirements-refinement stages. When a Rapid Prototyping approach is used, prototypes or mock-ups are tested. Traditional UT occurs after the initial design or during the implementation stages of Systems Development Life Cycle (SDLC) [1,2]. The UT process can be adapted for every newly designed system that is being developed in order to prevent unusable systems and ensure that systems meet the requirements and needs of users and health care organizations [3]. However, selecting two or more sample systems that provide the user with partial or full capabilities, and adapting the current UT methods to determine the features of each system that the user favours or rejects may have an additional value when aiming to determine the features and capabilities the system in question should have. The testing of already existing systems followed by the identification of preferred and undesirable features in those systems may aid in creating a new system that meets all or most of user requirements.

---

[1] Corresponding Author: Paule Bellwood; E-mail: paulebw@uvic.ca.

1. Study Objectives, Setting, and Background

This paper describes an experimental pilot study and sets out to propose methodology for adapting UT techniques for systems pre-planning and pre-development phase by investigating the functionality of the medical imaging software that is required to properly assess medical images in emergency situations.

For illustrative purposes, the Onis 2.0 Free Edition and Sante DICOM Viewer Free were used [4,5]. There were two participants in this illustrative pilot study, both of whom were instructed to complete two scenarios with both viewers while "thinking aloud". The sessions were audio- and video-recorded using a camcorder, and the screens were captured using the Hypercam 2.0 software. The following hardware were used: (1) Samsung P210 Laptop (Screen: 12.1' TFT 1280 x 800 [WXGA]; Graphics: Intel GMA X4500 – 128 MB; Processor: Pentium® Dual-Core CPU T4200 @ 2.00 GHz; Installed Memory: 2.00 GB; System Type: 64-Bit; Operating System: Windows 7 Enterprise), (2) Canon Legria FS200 Camcorder, and (3) Velbon CX 686 Tripod.

2. Methodology

2.1. Subjects

In order to assess the methodology, two trauma surgeons from a large urban university trauma centre were asked to participate. Both participants had more than 4 years of experience in the field.

2.2. Procedure

Recording tools included a camcorder and a screen capture software. Initially, each subject was briefly informed about the purpose of the experiment. Each participant was given a demographic questionnaire and a questionnaire that asked about their experience with medical imaging software. The subjects were then given instructions and a task to complete with each viewer. Each participant was instructed to view x-rays of a woman's body or brain after a car accident using one of the two viewers under investigation, state the diagnosis, and suggest treatment. Successful completion of the task was considered to occur upon correct diagnosis and proposed treatment. The x-ray data was anonymous and obtained from one of the clinic's databases intended for training and research purposes. It contained actual images of a human body after a car accident. Each participant used one viewer to view the x-rays of the body, and another viewer to view the x-rays of the head. The subjects were instructed to "think aloud" and state their conclusions upon deciding on diagnosis. Users then were asked to answer questions indicating their satisfaction with the software and propose their recommendations.

2.3. Data Collection and Analysis

Since the underlying purpose of this experimental pilot study was not to evaluate a specific viewer but rather to find out what a viewer should support when diagnosing patients, and propose possible methodology for such studies, subjective metrics were recorded. The data on: (1) user feedback during the testing ("think aloud") and after the testing (answers and suggestions in questionnaires), and (2) the observation of the features in each viewer that the participants found confusing or difficult to use, were collected. In larger-scale testing environments with more users, the data could be analysed using Transana© or any other transcription and analysis software. Since this was an experimental pilot study with a limited number of participants aimed at proposing possible methodology for such types of studies, transcription software was not used. The gathered information was analysed directly by viewing the videos and noting user remarks, questions, and observations.

3. Results

3.1. Individual Results

The following two tables summarize detailed findings and recommendations from each user based on the scenario. In larger-scale studies, this part should be completed using Transana© or any other transcription and analysis software. Based on the results from individual findings, general recommendations may be proposed, summarizing and categorizing these results according to user comments.

Table 1. Scenario 1. The first CT-Scan is of a woman in her 50's shortly after a car accident. Please use the Onis 2.0 Free Edition software to make a diagnosis and suggest the treatment. Please "think aloud" while completing this task. When you have stated the diagnosis and treatment, please continue on to the next part and answer the questions about this software.

User	Sample Findings	Sample Recommendations/Comments
1	Troubles with the ZOOM function – took 50 seconds	User had to move the mouse while holding down one of its buttons. Having a scale bar on the screen that allows manual zoom without shortcuts would be more useful.
	The monitor was too small to be able to comfortably fit all 3 images on one screen.	Use a bigger monitor or keep the buttons/menus minimal.
	It took 8 minutes to diagnose.	The participant had not used the software previously.
2	Troubles finding the option for viewing split screens. Access to the feature is not clearly displayed.	In order to find this option, the user had to click the "View" menu and then "Split the current view". Since this option is desired for most DICOM viewers, it should be displayed more clearly on the initial screen.
	It took 5 minutes to diagnose	The participant had already used the software previously.

Table 2. Scenario 2. The second CT-Scan is of the same woman as in the previous example. Please use the Sante DICOM Viewer Free software to make a diagnosis and suggest the treatment. Please "think aloud" while completing this task. When you have stated the diagnosis and treatment, please continue on to the next part and answer the questions about this software.

User	Sample Findings	Sample Recommendations/Comments
1	No option for splitting the screens.	The option of splitting the screen and viewing different slices simultaneously is very helpful when diagnosing a patient. It should be available and displayed clearly on the screen.
	Difficulties finding the window level controls.	Even though the icon of window leveling was available on the screen, the user did not find it.
	Difficulties with undoing an action: the user changed the contrast of the picture, and could not undo the action.	This option or the option to access the initial unchanged picture should be made available.
2	The zooming option was difficult to use as it was too sensitive to mouse movements	Include the scale bar on the screen, so that the user could zoom in and out manually without using the mouse.
	It took 6.5 minutes to diagnose.	The participant had already used the software previously.

3.2. General Results

Once individual results were evaluated, it was concluded that the tasks were successfully completed using both viewers. Completing tasks with Sante DICOM Viewer Free, however, was more complicated and took more time due to the complexity of and lack of intuitiveness using the program. Table 3 summarizes major findings and considerations:

Table 3. Major Findings and Considerations

Software	Major issues	Solutions
Onis 2.0	Difficult to find the option for split screens, which allows to view the slices from 3 different positions simultaneously.	Icon and description on the initial screen which allows this feature.
Sante DICOM Viewer Free	There are too many icons and no explanations on the initial screen. This requires a user to be well trained with the software, which means that the program is not intuitive and is too complicated when making quick and accurate diagnosis.	The program should have only the main functions available, which should be clearly displayed both as icons and text on the main screen.

3.3. User Impressions and Final Recommendations

If this were a large scale study and it yielded similar results, the general conclusion that the users preferred Onis 2.0 Free Edition over Sante DICOM Viewer Free could have been drawn. In this particular pilot study, the aim was to experiment with the proposed methodology in attempting to find the features a system should have in specific situations that require rapid and accurate decision making. Given the limited user feedback, the following suggestions for a DICOM viewer serve as an example of the results that could be obtained from a larger-scale study. In the case of this specific study, we have concluded that the viewer should have the following options:

- Splitting the screens and viewing the images from different angles simultaneously
- Easily zooming in and out, and viewing the desired portion of the picture
- Window leveling
- The main screen of the viewer should not be occupied with too many icons and options (because that would make it difficult for the user to easily find the features)
- If the software has many features, they should be accessible under drop-down menus, and the icons on the main screen should aid in making quick and time-efficient diagnoses.

4. Discussion

Traditional UT methods address the need to test systems before the implementation or during the design phase of SDLC [1]. The same methodologies used in UT can be applied to the method of evaluating already existing systems and identifying the preferred features a system under study already has, or pointing out weaknesses that the future system should eliminate. The proposed methodology is a tool that allows end-users select parts of the system that they would like to use not only by asking them questions about the system, but also by allowing them to practically sort out the features they like or do not like. Certain features might not even occur to a user without the ability to see real examples and explore real cases. Users might have misconceived ideas about what a system should be capable of achieving when answering questions such as: "What would you like to be able to do with the system?" As a result of the proposed methodology, the observer is often able to notice more factors that influence the user decision making and that otherwise would likely not occur solely as a result of asking such questions. The observer can note the difficulties or frustrations with specific features or indicate features that the user would like to see in the final result. In all cases, however, this method can only be applied to system creation process based on previous systems available when selecting the features that users like. When creating new systems, the users can notice features that are lacking only if the system restricts them from successfully completing the tasks. If task completion is unrestricted, it will most likely not occur to the users to suggest a specific feature the new system should have.

5. Conclusion and Implications

The aim of this illustrative study was to determine whether adapting traditional UT methods to gather user requirements for a system, prior to its planning and design, can have a significant value. While the outcome of the study suggests that the proposed method may aid in gathering user requirements for a system in need, the validity of such outcome is challenged by the sample size. We, therefore, recommend a full pilot study with increased sample size to validate the methodology.

References

[1] A.W. Kushniruk, Evaluation in the design of health information systems: Application of approaches emerging from usability engineering. *Comp Bio Med* **32** (2002), 141–149.

[2] E.H. Shortliffe, J.J. Cimino, *Biomedical Informatics: Computer Applications in Health Care and Biomedicine*, Springer, New York, 2006.

[3] A.W. Kushniruk, V.L. Patel, Cognitive and usability engineering methods for the evaluation of clinical information systems. *J Biomed Inf* **37** (2004), 56-76.

[4] DigitalCore, Co.Ltd (2010). Accessed March 15, 2010 from http://www.onis-viewer.com/products.php?PHPSESSID=d8b8be62ce1ab5d7971e96edcb59547a

[5] Santesoft Medical Imaging Software (2010). Accessed March 15, 2010 from http://www.santesoft.com/dicom_viewer_free.html

International Perspectives in Health Informatics
E.M. Borycki et al. (Eds.)
IOS Press, 2011
© 2011 ITCH 2011 Steering Committee and IOS Press. All rights reserved.
doi:10.3233/978-1-60750-709-3-219

Usability Evaluation of a Pilot Implementation of the Electronic Clinical Transfusion Management System IT Specification for Blood Tracking

Kamran GOLCHIN[a], Philip GOOCH[a], Omid SHABESTARI[a]
Abdul ROUDSARI[a,b]
[a] *Centre for Health Informatics, School of Informatics, City University, London, UK*
[b] *School of Health Information Science, University of Victoria, Victoria, British Columbia, Canada*

Abstract. Safe working practices and patient safety are of critical importance in the administration of blood transfusion. While the use of information technology has been proposed to ensure the safety of this process, the usability of such systems has not previously been studied. We present the results of a usability evaluation of an electronic clinical transfusion management system being piloted by the National Health Service in England. A number of major usability problems were recorded, largely relating to unnecessary action, limiting user control and recovery from user error. Such problems can, however, be resolved by relatively minor changes to system functionality and design.

Keywords. blood transfusion, information technology, usability, user interface

Introduction

To ensure that the patients receive the right blood, safe working practices and patient safety are of critical importance in the administration of blood transfusion. In the UK, over a two-year period from October 1996, 191 incidences of ABO-incompatible blood transfusion were reported, of which three resulted in the patient's death [1].

In addition to continuous training and reporting incidences to related authorities, the use of information technology (IT) systems to improve safety by tracking blood from donors to recipients has been proposed. Barcodes and radio frequency identification (RFID) have been used to match patients with the right blood type and to ensure that the blood used is that which has been issued for the patient.

The effect on transfusion safety of such systems has previously been studied [2–7], but for an information system to be successfully deployed, and to be used in practice, it should meet defined standards of system usability. The design of the system's user interface (UI) is crucial in meeting these requirements.

This study considers the usability aspects of a blood tracking system being piloted by the National Health Service (NHS) in England. The system employs barcode and RFID technology, and uses automated tracking to maintain a complete record of blood products from donor to recipient.

1. Methodology

The study involved observation of 7 nursing staff in training sessions and 2 nurses in a live clinical setting on the two wards that were piloting the software. When evaluating use of a live hospital information system, selection of an evaluation technique that does not intrude on clinician workflow or that may inadvertently increase the risk of human error is crucial. The following two approaches were used:

Heuristic Evaluation aims to determine whether each element of a user interface follows established usability principles.[1] Heuristic evaluation was implemented using the 'Art criticism approach', in which an experienced critic in the field works with the system over a period and writes a review on the system's benefits and shortcomings [8].

Violations of heuristic principles can be classified according to their severity as follows[9]:

0 = No usability problem at all

1 = Cosmetic problem only: need not be fixed unless extra time is available

2 = Minor usability problem: fixing this should be given low priority

3 = Major usability problem: important to fix, so should be given high priority

4 = Usability catastrophe: imperative to fix this before product can be released

Sixteen heuristics were utilized in this study[2] and categorized according to their severity (considering their importance in the hospital environment). The most important principles (severity 3 and 4) are given below:

1. *User control and freedom*: if user makes a mistake, there should be a clear escape route, and the system also should support 'undo' and 'redo' functions (severity: 4).
2. *Help user recognize, diagnose, and recover from errors*: error messages should be expressed in natural language that precisely indicates the problem and suggests a solution (severity: 3).
3. *Remove unnecessary actions*: reducing the required time, number of clicks, and amount of effort to accomplish a task (severity: 3).
4. *Make interactions easy*: avoid making tasks and information difficult to see and perform, e.g. appropriate fonts and size of fonts and controls in the page (severity: 3).

Usability testing involves observing users while they work with the system in the field, with the focus on four areas of efficiency and performance, accuracy, recall, and emotional response. We implemented this technique using the 'professional review approach' over a series of site visits to carry out the usability evaluation while recording users' subjective experiences of the system's user interface and functionality.

---

[1] This method was first developed by Jakob Nielsen[10] on the basis of his expertise and years of experience in the field

[2] Although Nielsen's heuristics are the most widely used, other principles have also been developed, such as those of Gerhardt-Powals[11]. The principles 'Remove unnecessary actions' and 'Make interactions easy' were added by the researchers as they were specifically emphasized by the users during observation and interview.

2. Results

Heuristic evaluation: The application consists of different forms for each phase of the blood transfusion process (login, collect blood sample, begin transfusion, end transfusion, recording blood arrival and so on). For brevity, we report only problems of severity 3 and 4 here, with the corresponding section of the application.

1. **Remove unnecessary actions** (*severity: 3*)

- After clicking on the 'Print' button, the user needs to scan the patient's wristband. However, after scanning, the user has to click on the 'Print' button a second time (*collect blood sample*).
- The number of copies to be printed is set to 0 by default. As this value is never used, the user needs to change this value every time (*collect blood sample*).
- The functionality for recording vital signs is not used, so this step should be omitted instead of requiring users to skip it manually (*begin transfusion*; *end transfusion*).
- In the 'Enter transfusion status' dialog, the drop-down list has a single option, but the user still needs to select it to proceed. This step is unnecessary as the following screen prompts the user to record the end of the transfusion (*end transfusion*).
- After scanning their ID cards to log in to the system, users need to click the 'OK' button to continue with the login process. This is not consistent with the rest of the system and is an unnecessary action which could be removed (*log in screen*)

2. **Make interactions easy** (*severity: 3*)

- Choosing an item from the drop-down menus is difficult on touch screen monitors, as the dropdown list size is small in comparison to a typical user's finger tip. The dropdown list should be larger, or another control should be used for entering the number of copies required (*collect blood sample*; *end transfusion*)

3. **User control and freedom** (*severity: 4*)

- On the screen for selecting the number of labels to be printed, there is a 'Cancel' button below the drop-down list, which, instead of cancelling printing, forces the user to exit the program. As users might reasonably expect to click on a confirmation button below a drop-down list or other controls in a form, it is probable that a user may accidentally click on the 'Cancel' button (as it is the only button present), requiring them to start from the beginning (*collect blood sample*).
- If the user leaves the number of copies at 0 (the default), or if the user scans the printer before selecting the appropriate number, the system displays a prompt to select at least one copy. After the selection has been corrected and the user attempts to scan the printer again, the application repeatedly displays a message that it cannot communicate with the printer. At this point, there is no option other than selecting the 'No' button in response to the 'Try again' prompt, which returns the user to a screen with no option other than exiting the application (via the 'Cancel' button) and starting again from the beginning (*collect blood sample*).
- Currently there is no way to reprint a label should an error occur, forcing the phlebotomist to have to repeat the entire process – yet each of these attempts is logged in the system as a separate blood sampling (*collect blood sample*).
- At the system prompt 'Do you have more units to hang/fate for the same patient now?' clicking on the 'Yes' button requires the user to scan the barcode of the second bag. However, as there is no way to go back or undo this, if the 'Yes'

button was clicked in error the user has to exit the application (*begin transfusion*; *end transfusion*).

- In most cases, clicking the 'Cancel' button exits the application. By definition 'Cancel' should only cancel the most recent action, and return the user to the previous step; an 'Exit' button should be used for exiting the application. The current use of the 'Cancel' metaphor does not match the real world, and it also increases the risk of users making irreversible mistakes (*all parts of the application*).

4. **Help user recognize, diagnose, and recover from errors** (*severity: 4*)

- No appropriate error message is displayed if the user scans the incorrect barcode; the system provides no useful feedback or prompts (*collect blood sample*; *blood arrival*; *begin transfusion*; *end transfusion*)

Figure 1 presents a heuristic violation proportion chart, showing the number of violations for each heuristic principle. Figure 2 presents a severity proportion chart, showing the number of errors for each severity class. Of the 33 usability violations recorded, 14 (42%) were of severity 2 (minor usability problem), 12 (36%) were of severity 3 (major usability problem) and 6 (18%) were of severity 4 (usability catastrophe). The most frequent usability problems were related to the following usability principles:

User control and freedom: 6   instances,   of   severity   4
Remove unnecessary actions: 6   instances,   of   severity   3
Helps user recognize, diagnose and recover from errors: 4 instances, of severity 3

Usability Testing: Ten (30%) of the heuristic usability violations were validated by usability testing in both training and live environments. Of these, 4 were of severity 3 (major usability problem) and 6 were of severity 2 (minor usability problem). The most common problems were difficulty in working with drop down lists, and lack of helpful error messages, for example if the wrong barcode is scanned.

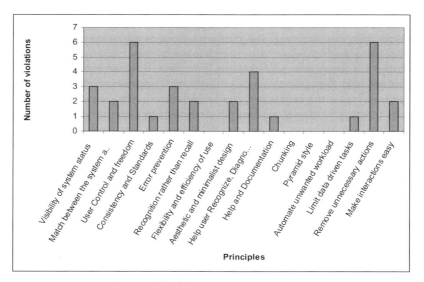

Figure 1. Heuristic violation proportion chart

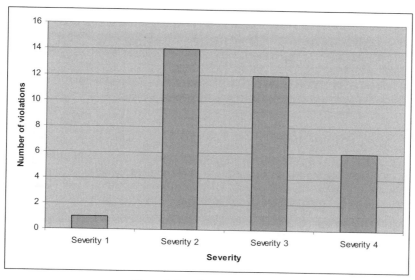

Figure 2. Severity proportion chart

3. Discussion

Some of the usability problems should be resolved as users become more familiar with the system (such as understanding why a problem occurs in cases where the system does not give an appropriate error message), although requiring learning and familiarity still violates the usability principle of *Recognition rather than recall.*

A number of changes were identified that should enhance the system's usability. Improved error messages, recovery from user error, and the ability to cancel or undo the last action would improve user control and freedom. Any default values should be the most frequently used value, or at least a non-zero value. Clearer 'checkpoint' stages that summarize the user's selections up to that point before final confirmation would provide a degree of confidence and certainty for the user, and decrease the risk of error.

4. Conclusion

The total number of major and catastrophic usability problems, combined with the large number of minor ones, suggests that the system should undergo a usability overhaul to address these before being rolled out on a large scale.

Overall the system benefits from a robust architecture and the user interface allows users to navigate the transfusion workflow adequately. Usability problems (particularly those of severity 3 and 4) make performing tasks more difficult and time consuming, which can increase the risk of human error. However, these problems can be resolved by relatively small changes either in the design of the forms or the application code behind them. This should lead to significant improvements in the user experience.

References

[1]   L.M. Williamson, S. Lowe, E.M. Love, H. Cohen, K. Soldan, D.B.L. McClelland, P. Skacel, J.A.J. Barbara, Serious hazards of transfusion (SHOT) initiative: analysis of the first two annual reports, *BMJ* **319** (1999), 16.

[2]   J.C. Chan, R.W. Chu, B.W. Young, F. Chan, C.C. Chow, W.C. Pang, C. Chan, S.H. Yeung, P.K. Chow, J. Lau, P.M. Leung, Use of an electronic barcode system for patient identification during blood transfusion: 3-year experience in a regional hospital, *Hong Kong Med J*. (2004), 166–71D.

[3]   C.L. Turner, A.C. Casbard, M.F. Murphy, Barcode technology: its role in increasing the safety of blood transfusion, *Transfusion*, (2003), 1200–9F.

[4]   M.F. Murphy, J.D.S. Kay, Barcode identification for transfusion safety, *Transfusion Med*, **11** (2004), 334–338.

[5]   L. Briggs, R. Davis, A. Gutierrez, M. Kopetsky, K. Young, R. Veeramani, RFID in the blood supply chain - increasing productivity, quality and patient safety, *JHIM*, **23** (2009), 54–63.

[6]   P. Pagliaro, R. Turdo, E. Capuzzo, Patients' positive identification systems, *Blood Transfus*. **7** (2009), 313–8.

[7]   A. Ohsaka, K. Abe, T. Ohsawa, N. Miyake, S. Sugita, I. Tojima, A computer-assisted transfusion management system and changed transfusion practices contribute to appropriate management of blood components, *Transfusion*. **48** (2008), 1730–8.

[8]   J. Wyatt, C. P. Friedman, *Evaluation methods in medical informatics*, Springer-Verlag, New York, N.Y., (2006), 34.

[9]   J. Nielsen, Severity Ratings for Usability Problems, [Internet], 2007, [cited 2010 Nov 15], available from: http://www.useit.com/papers/heuristic/severityrating.html

[10] J. Nielsen, Usability inspection methods, John Wiley & Sons, New York, NY, 1994.

[11] J. Gerhardt-Powals, Cognitive engineering principles for enhancing human-computer performance, *Int J Human-Computer Interact*, **8(2)** (1996), 189–211.

Initiatives in International Health Informatics

International Perspectives in Health Informatics
E.M. Borycki et al. (Eds.)
IOS Press, 2011
doi:10.3233/978-1-60750-709-3-227

227

POND4Kids: A Web-based Pediatric Cancer Database for Hospital-based Cancer Registration and Clinical Collaboration

Yuri QUINTANA[a], Aman N. PATEL[a] , Paula E. NAIDU[a], Scott C. HOWARD[a,b],
Federico A. ANTILLON[c], Raul C. RIBEIRO[a,b]

[a] *International Outreach Program, St. Jude Children's Research Hospital*
[b] *Department of Oncology, St. Jude Children's Research Hospital, Memphis, TN*
[c] *Unidad Nacional de Oncología Pediátrica, Guatemala City, Guatemala*

Abstract. The Pediatric Oncology Network Database, POND4Kids (www.pond4kids.org, POND), is an online, multilingual clinical database created for use by pediatric oncology units in countries with limited resources to meet various clinical data management needs including cancer registration, data collection and changes in treatment outcome. Established as a part of the International Outreach Program at St. Jude Children's Research Hospital in Memphis, Tennessee, POND aims to provide oncology units a tool to store patient data for easy retrieval and analysis and to achieve uniform data collection to facilitate meaningful comparison of information among centers. Currently, POND is being used to store clinical data on thousands of patients and measure their treatment improvement over a period of time. In 2009 POND included more than 100 pediatric oncology units; each has its own virtual private area. A case study of the UNOP Guatemala Clinic's use of POND is presented. On-going challenges at partner sites include inconsistent data collection methods, missing records, training for data managers, and slow or unreliable internet connections.

Keywords. cancer registry, pediatric oncology, international, collaboration, clinical improvement, clinical informatics, e-health.

Introduction

Established as a part of the St. Jude International Outreach Program, the Pediatric Oncology Network Database (www.pond4kids.org, POND) is an online, multilingual clinical database for supporting hospital-based cancer registration as well as data management for pediatric oncology treatment protocols. POND is used for cancer registration and analysis of protocol-based care in developing countries [1-3]. It facilitates collection of uniform data, their retrieval, and their analysis with the goal of improving care in individual cancer centers and collaborating groups.

This paper presents a technical overview of the system, an overview of the global usage of POND by international clinics, an example of a successful implementation of POND usage in a Guatemalan pediatric cancer unit, and some on-going challenges.

1. POND4Kids Overview

POND is implemented as a centralized web-based database that hosts multiple virtual sites, as shown in Figure 1. A common server is used to host the software, and data for each site are kept separate. POND was implemented using open source technologies (Linux, Apache, MySQL, PHP). POND provides a means for uniform data collection by providing checkboxes, calendar buttons, and pull down lists wherever appropriate. Standard reporting tools are provided, but custom reports are also available to address site-specific reporting needs. Survival curve and histogram charts are also provided.

Each virtual site has a site administrator who controls which users are added to the site and their access levels. A site administrator can share patient data in a de-identified format with an administrator at another POND site. The aim is to allow the data pertaining to a particular disease type to be shared among interested clinical investigators for research, quality improvement, and other types of analysis. Site administrators can create customized data entry forms, clinical protocol templates, and data entry workflows, all of which can be shared, if desired, with other POND sites via a common library.

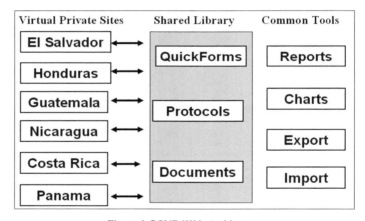

Figure 1. POND4Kids Architecture

2. Global Usage of POND4Kids by International Clinics

Currently POND is being been used by international pediatric oncology clinics to analyze clinical data on thousands of patients and to improve the delivery of treatments. In June 2010 there were 103 active POND sites of which 85 had entered records in the past 6 months. In the first 6 years of operation (2004–2010), the number of records entered in POND exceeded 34,090. International collaborations continued to grow with investigators on collaborative studies sharing their de-identified patient records (personal information such as names are never shared between sites) for collaborative studies. In 2010 the number of collaborations in which data were shared between POND sites increased to over 300, as shown in Figure 2.

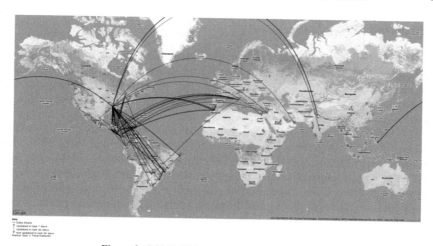

Figure 2. POND4Kids Data Sharing, as of July 1, 2010

3. Guatemala's Usage of POND4Kids

In Guatemala, a pediatric oncology clinic called Unidad Nacional de Oncología Pediátrica (UNOP) was established adjacent to the public pediatric hospital. Given the limited government resources to support a pediatric oncology program, a non-profit foundation called Fundación Ayúdame a Vivir was founded in May 1997 to provide the necessary resources for the proper maintenance, operation, and growth of UNOP as a center of excellence for treating pediatric cancer in Guatemala. Each year, about 400 children newly diagnosed with cancer are treated at UNOP. The 32 inpatient beds are fully occupied, and more than 70 patients receive care each day in the outpatient clinic. Survival rates for some types of cancer have increased from 28 percent to 70 percent, and the rate of abandonment of treatment has decreased, largely because Fundación Ayúdame a Vivir subsidizes the treatment for patients who cannot pay.

The use of POND by UNOP has grown consistently. Since 2004, the UNOP site has grown to include more than 3,700 patient records, as shown in Figure 3. The UNOP clinic has entered data for both current and past patients. As of July 1, 2010, UNOP POND site has 2,407 records of patients who are alive, and 1,327 of these records have had an update in the past year. Over the years the number of active data shares has increased as UNOP expands its collaborations with experts in specific disease specialties at other international pediatric centers.

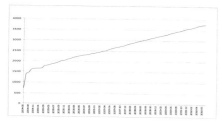

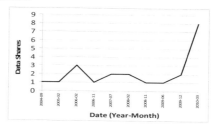

Figure 3a. Patient Records in the UNOP POND   **Figure 3b.** Data Shares from the UNOP POND

4. Discussion

POND provides clinical tools that fill an unmet need at many pediatric oncology hospitals, particularly those that have common protocols and wish to share information. There are several reasons for the success of POND at some sites, and there are barriers and failure factors at other sites. Challenges include training, cost, quality management, data access controls, access to clinical experts, and regular system improvements.

Availability of online training and support is one of the factors that has helped the deployment of POND but at times it can be difficult due to limited bandwidth and lack of Internet reliability. POND is sufficiently easy to use with minimal training for most users. Online help and training are available in English and Spanish. However, data managers need to have computer experience, and some may need additional supervision and guidance. A regional network of POND data managers was formed in Central America that allows for continued training, as well as mutual support and encouragement. Weekly online training meetings in English and Spanish offer support to data managers worldwide.

Cost is a major challenge for many sites. Funding for data managers at some sites enables those sites to have consistent data entry. Since 2004 a grant from the Pediatric Oncology Group of Ontario (Canada) and financial support from St. Jude Children's Research Hospital (Memphis, TN) have funded full-time data managers in several Central America countries. Other sites do not have sufficient funding to hire data managers, and the clinical staff does not have the time to enter records.

Data quality management programs are essential for clinical improvement. POND has online tools for report generation that yield data that can be used to monitor patient outcomes and identify areas in which improved care is needed [4]. However, these reports need to be regularly run and acted upon to improve areas of missing or incomplete data. There may also be a lack of standard operating procedures, inconsistent data collection methods, or missing paper records. More training and on-site audits could facilitate additional improvement in data quality and efficiency.

Security is an important part of any medical records system. The POND software resides in a dedicated server with a security firewall. Online tools allow users with administrator credentials to manage access to data by users of the site and to control sharing with external collaborators. Although the data are encrypted and password protected, some administrators are reluctant to store data outside their institution.

To obtain benefit from the data-sharing capabilities of POND, access to clinical experts is essential. In the case of UNOP there were sufficient external experts available to review clinical records and to provide suggestions for patient care or clinical data collection. Common treatment protocols used by pediatric oncology units in Central America were created in POND. Principal investigators of shared protocols have regular virtual meetings to review individual patients with complicated medical problems, protocol data, and administrative issues, and to develop strategies to improve clinical outcomes. These clinical meetings are held online on www.Cure4Kids.org, a web-based education and conferencing platform [5].

POND is upgraded regularly in response to feature-specific requests from users, such as calls for additional reporting tools. Once completed, upgrades are instantaneously and simultaneously available to all sites since they occur at the level of the server and are browser-independent. However, POND may not have all the functionality needed by a particular pediatric oncology unit, and so other tools may be required to complement POND. Some sites also suffer from slow or unreliable internet connections, and POND currently lacks offline functionality.

Despite these challenges, many sites in developing countries have been able to use POND to collect data for clinical improvement. The UNOP site is one of the most active POND sites, and its staff has been able to overcome many of the challenges related to funding, training and data management. Further efforts are still needed in the areas of standard operating procedures for data collection, data entry, data quality monitoring, and data analysis.

5. Conclusions

The POND4Kids initiative has shown that web-based technologies can assist countries with limited resources by enhancing the quantity and quality of clinical data and can support international clinical collaborations to facilitate protocol-based treatment for children with cancer. As a result, cancer centers in low-income countries can now effectively collect and analyze basic pediatric oncology data as a foundation for improved understanding of the occurrence of cancer in their area and the outcomes of their patients, with the ultimate goal of improving the survival of children with cancer. There is now an opportunity to expand the sharing of clinical protocols and quality improvement processes across many more regions and continents.

References

[1] S.C. Howard, M.L. Metzger, J.A. Wilimas, Y. Quintana, C.H. Pui, L.L. Robison, R.C. Ribeiro, Childhood cancer epidemiology in low-income countries. *Cancer* 2008;112:461-472.
[2] S.C. Howard, M. Marinoni, L. Castillo, M. Bonilla, G. Tognoni, F. Antillon, M.G. Valsecchi, C.H. Pui, R.C. Ribeiro, A. Sala, R.D. Barr, G. Masera, MISPHO Consortium. Improving outcomes for children with cancer in low income countries in Latin America. *Pediatr Blood Cancer* 2007;48:364-369.
[3] Valsecchi M, Steliarova-Foucher E. Cancer Registration in developing countries: luxury or necessity? *Lancet Oncol.* 2008;9:159-167.
[4] L. Ayoub, L. Fu, A. Pena, J.M. Sierra, P.C. Dominguez, C.H. Pui, Y. Quintana, A. Rodriguez, R.D. Barr, R.C. Ribeiro, M.L. Metzger, J.A. Wilimas, S.C. Howard. Implementation of a data management program in a pediatric cancer unit in a low income country. *Pediatr Blood Cancer* 2007;49:23-27.
[5] Y. Quintana, R. O'Brien, A. Patel, J. Becksfort, A. Shuler, A. Nambayan, D. Ogdon, G. Chantada, S.C. Howard, R.C. Ribeiro. Cure4Kids: Research challenges in the design of a website for global education and collaboration. *Information Design Journal (IDJ)* 2008;16: 243-249.

Acknowledgments
We thank Patricia Stephens for editorial assistance, The Pediatric Oncology Group of Ontario, Cancer Center Support (CORE) grant CA-21765 from the National Cancer Institute, and the American Lebanese Syrian Associated Charities (ALSAC).

International Perspectives in Health Informatics
E.M. Borycki et al. (Eds.)
IOS Press, 2011
© 2011 ITCH 2011 Steering Committee and IOS Press. All rights reserved.
doi:10.3233/978-1-60750-709-3-232

Occurrence Detection and Selection Procedures in Healthcare Facilities: A Comparison Across Canada and Brazil

Plinio P. MORITA[a], Catherine M. BURNS[a]

[a] *Department of Systems Design Engineering – University of Waterloo*

Abstract. Healthcare institutions face high levels of risk on a daily basis. Efforts have been made to address these risks and turn this complex environment into a safer environment for patients, staff, and visitors. However, healthcare institutions need more advanced risk management tools to achieve the safety levels currently seen in other industries. One of these potential tools is occurrence investigation systems. In order to be investigated, occurrences must be detected and selected for investigation, since not all institutions have enough resources to investigate all occurrences. A survey was conducted in healthcare institutions in Canada and Brazil to evaluate currently used risk management tools, the difficulties faced, and the possibilities for improvement. The findings include detectability difficulties, lack of resources, lack of support, and insufficient staff involvement.

Keywords. investigation, occurrences, detection, adverse events.

Introduction

Risks are an inherent feature of any environment and different tools have been used to manage them. Some industries have developed a wide variety of techniques and are currently in the vanguard of the risk management technology [1]. Several safety tools developed by military researchers have been widely adapted by the healthcare industry [2], being healthcare a high-risk service if compared to other industries [3,4].

In order to improve a risk-prone system it is necessary to investigate occurrences to gain more information about what has happened. Investigation procedures can be conducted using one of several available methodologies [5]. Occurrence awareness is best facilitated by the existence of an occurrence detection system. Without a strong detection system, many of the occurrences in the facility will go unnoticed and will not be investigated. An occurrence detection system consists of any tool available that has been designed with the intent of making the risk management team or investigation team aware of these occurrences. These detection systems can be differentiated as "active" and "passive". In a passive system, a notification process is available to the users and anybody can report an occurrence. These systems rely on the proactivity of the users and the development of a healthy safety culture [3,6] to generate adequate occurrence reports. The development of a safety culture improves investigations by both providing more resources and improving the engagement of the staff in the investigation process. In contrast, an active system consists of individuals searching the institution for occurrences to be investigated. Classifying occurrences and deciding which ones should be investigated is just as important as detecting them [7]. Normally institutions make such decisions based on a combination of several factors such as risk levels, regulatory obligations, legal consequences, financial outcomes, and public impact [1-2].

This project was conducted with the objective of assessing the currently used occurrence detection and occurrence selection methodologies in healthcare institutions, with a main purpose of increasing patient safety in healthcare facilities. We hypothesize that in Canada we will find institutions with inadequate occurrence detection systems, yet likely stronger systems than in Brazil. The comparison between Canada and Brazil is interesting because it provides information about two countries with different healthcare and legal systems and therefore different obligations to safety.

1. Material and Methods

This research project consisted of a survey that would allow the evaluation of the currently employed occurrence detection and selection methodologies. It was sent to several clinical engineers and members of risk management groups in healthcare institutions in both Canada and Brazil. This survey was divided into four main categories: questions about demographics and contact information, general questions about the investigation system, questions about the occurrence detection system, and questions about the occurrence selection system. The analysis is presented along with the data.

2. Results and Discussion

Demographic results – This part of the survey consisted of questions regarding the name and location of the hospital. From the 9 collected responses, 5 were from Brazilian hospitals and 4 were from Canadian hospitals.

General questions results – The survey indicated that only 11.0% of the participants did not have access to an investigation system. Regarding the types of occurrences currently investigated, 100.0% of the institutions that have an investigation system investigate near misses and incidents. Only 87.5% of these same facilities investigate accidents. Based on the literature in which institutions usually focus on occurrences with high levels of damage and public awareness, we had hypothesized that we would see a lower percentage of institutions investigating near misses and incidents [1,2], and a larger percentage of institutions investigating accidents. Since the results found were contrary to our hypothesis, it suggests that the participating institutions are aware of the importance of investigating near misses and incidents in addition to investigating accidents.

Occurrence detection results – The next topic we approached was whether the occurrence detection system used active or passive detection tools. The results show that 88.9% of all participants use passive detection tools and that only 22.2% of the participants use some sort of active occurrence detection tool. An interesting detail to provide here is that the two institutions that used active detection tools are located in Brazil. Since Canada has a more developed healthcare system [8], we had hypothesized that we would find a larger number of institutions with active detection systems in

Canada than in Brazil. Active detection systems increase the situation awareness of the institution regarding occurrences by increasing the number of perceived occurrences via the addition of channels through which information about an occurrence can reach the institution [9].

The participants were also asked which tools they use to detect occurrences. 66.7% of the participating institutions use a paper based occurrence notification system, 77.8% use an electronic occurrence notification system, 11.1% use an electronic occurrence detection system, 22.2% use occurrence scouting through the facility, and 11.1% use an electronic registry scouting system.

Since most institutions use only passive detection systems, the largest difficulty faced by the investigation system is underreporting. Some of the tools used by participants to encourage notification include: anonymity (11.1%), feedback about the notification (44.4%), training (55.6%), and safety programs promoting notification (77.8%). As part of encouraging notification, it is important to provide feedback about the investigation both to the person that made the notification and to the staff. Our results indicate that only 56% of the participating institutions provided such feedback to users. However, not receiving feedback can result in a lack of motivation to report future occurrences [1-2].

The passive detection systems discussed above can be separated into two different categories regarding their level of automation: non-automated notification systems which require the investigation team or the risk management team to check a database constantly for new occurrences. Automated notification systems are those that inform the investigation team as soon as an occurrence notification appears in the system. Automated notification systems would reduce the workload on the investigation team and the lag between the notification and the investigation, a lag that usually results in crucial information about the occurrence being lost [1,,2,5]. Only 33% of the participating institutions had automated occurrence notification systems, with more of these institutions in Canada than in Brazil. In Canada 50% of the institutions reported automated notification systems, while in Brazil only 20% reported automated systems. These numbers could reflect more developed risk management system in Canadian institutions.

Notification systems can differ on the amount of information they can gather, becoming more precise as more information is collected. A downside to more information is increased workload on the users, consequently reducing the number of notifications due to increased length of the notification form. This can be easily managed by the use of an electronic system with easy to fill forms. Participants were asked about the information collected by their notification system. 100% of the participating institutions collect information about the occurrence, 88.9% collect information about the people involved in the occurrence (such as doctors, nurses, patients, and family members), 77.8% collect information about the victims, 66.7% ask the user to categorize the occurrence (normally into near-misses, incidents, and accidents), and 66.7% collect information about the person making the notification.

The data presented in Figure 1 represents the results and is separated into responses from Brazil and Canada. It appears in the chart that the participating Canadian institutions collect a larger amount of information about occurrences than the participating Brazilian institutions.

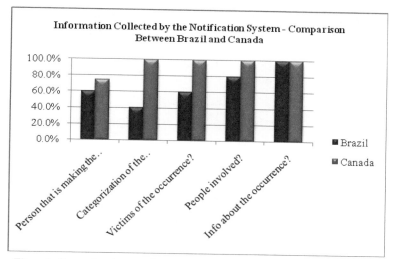

Figure 1. Comparison between Brazil and Canada: Amount of information collected by the notification system.

This increase in collected information likely reflects a more developed investigative culture in the participating Canadian hospitals since more detailed notifications provide information which can be used to better address risks. These results also show that notification systems still rely on the user categorization of occurrences. This can generate an unwanted variability in the categorization since people will have different perspectives and opinions about the same occurrence. Notification systems should collect information that allows the system to choose the category that occurrence belongs in. Of the participating institutions, 66.7% rely on categorization by the risk management team, 33.3% on categorization by the occurrence investigation team, and 44.4% on the person making the notification. None of the participating institutions have an automated categorization system.

Occurrence selection results – All institutions use a different set of criteria to decide which occurrences will be investigated. From the survey data collected, 77.8% of the participating institutions consider the damage level, 66.7% consider the frequency, 66.7% the regulatory obligations, 55.6% the financial outcomes, 44.4% the legal consequences, and 33.3% said that all occurrences should be investigated. These results show an interesting scenario in which not all institutions take into consideration regulatory requirements in decision-making. This can represent two different factors: either the lack of regulatory requirements or non-compliance to the existing requirements. This scenario can be better understood by separating the results into the two different participating countries. In Figure 2, it is possible to see that Canadian institutions take more factors into consideration when deciding which occurrences will be investigated. The differences between the healthcare and legal system in these two countries are replicated by these results, which reflect their different realities. The legal system in Brazil is not as effective as in Canada and very little legal action occurs regarding healthcare occurrences, while in Canada, doctors and hospitals can be prosecuted for malpractice or accidents.

One of the survey questions asked about the difficulties in choosing which occurrences should be investigated. The main difficulties described include: motivating people to notify risk management teams of all the occurrences, detectability issues, staff shortages, lag time between the notification and the investigation, inadequate resources to review and investigate each occurrence, and reliability of the information collected during interviews. These responses show a wide variety of issues that can be addressed by the development of a safety culture, increasing the situation awareness [9] about occurrences, and developing a better understanding of why notification does not occur for some events.

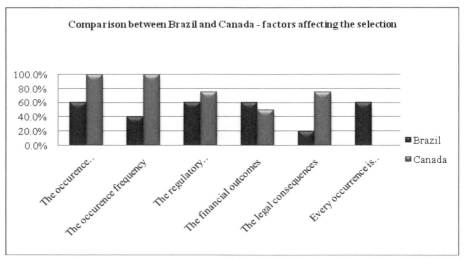

Figure 2. Comparison of factors affecting the selection of which occurrences should be investigated.

3. Conclusion

In the present study some expected difficulties were seen, but overall fewer problems were detected than were expected. These results also show that investigation teams still struggle with lack of adequate support and resources. The comparison between the two countries showed that the participating Canadian institutions have more developed risk management programs, with more complex notification systems, more selection factors, and better support for the notification. Contrary to our hypothesis, we found more institutions in Brazil, than in Canada, using active detection systems. One explanation for this peculiarity may be that the development of risk management programs in Brazil has been very strong in recent years. However, some of the results shown here might be a consequence of the small population size used in this study. Nonetheless, this preliminary research suggests that further investigation into this topic is warranted.

References

[1]   Center for Chemical Process Safety/AIChE. *Guidelines for Investigating Chemical Process Incidents.* New York; 2003.
[2]   P. P. Morita. Desenvolvimento de um Guia para Investigação de Incidentes em Ambientes de Saúde Baseado na Estrutura de Gerenciamento de Projetos. University of Campinas – UNICAMP, Campinas, Brazil; 2009.
[3]   V. F. Nieva, J. Sorra. Safety culture assessment: A tool for improving patient safety in healthcare organizations. *Qual Saf Health Care.* **12** Supplement 2: (2003), 17-23.

[4] R. L. Helmreich. On error management: Lessons from aviation. *BMJ (Clinical Research Ed.)*. **320**(7237) 2000, 781-785.

[5] P. P. Morita, C. M. Burns, S. J. Calil. The influence of strong recommendations, good incident reports and a monitoring system over an incident investigation system for healthcare facilities, In: *Human Factors and Ergonomics Society Annual Meeting Proceedings*. **53**(22) (2009), 1679-1683.

[6] P. P. Morita, S. J. Calil. The importance of a safety culture in healthcare facilities for the development of an incident investigation system, In: World Congress on Medical Physics and Biomedical Engineering (2009), 20-23.

[7] R. Berentsen, R. H. Holmboe. Incidents/accidents classification and reporting in statoil. *J. Hazard. Mater.* **111** (2004), 155-159.

[8] J. Epstein, R. Seitz, N. Dhingra, P. R. Ganz, A. Gharehbaghian, R. Spindel, et al. Role of regulatory agencies, *Biologicals*. **37**(2) (2009), 94-102.

[9] M. R. Endsley, D. J. Garland. *Situation Awareness: Analysis and Measurement*. New Jersey: Lawrence Erlbaum Associates; 2000.

International Perspectives in Health Informatics
E.M. Borycki et al. (Eds.)
IOS Press, 2011
© *2011 ITCH 2011 Steering Committee and IOS Press. All rights reserved.*
doi:10.3233/978-1-60750-709-3-238

National Strategies for Health Data Interoperability

Mu-Hsing KUO[a], Andre W. KUSHNIRUK[a], Elizabeth M. BORYCKI[a],
Chien-Yeh HSU[b], Chung-Liang LAI[c]

[a]*School of Health Information Science, University of Victoria,
Victoria, British Columbia, Canada*
[b] *Graduate Institute of Medical Informatics, Taipei Medical University*
[c] *Department of Health, Taichung Hospital, Taiwan*

Abstract. This paper compares the interoperability approaches of three countries: Taiwan, Denmark and Canada. The work maps out how various countries have addressed the interoperability problems as well as what factors affect decisions and the result, and in what manner. The key findings are as follows: (1) The federal government's ability to mandate standards affects choice of interoperability strategy; (2) E-Health status influences choice of interoperability strategy; (3) Differences in geography, population, and demographics affect the selection of national strategies towards interoperability.

Keywords. electronic health records, data interoperability, e-Health

Introduction

Worldwide, different countries have developed national level strategies to promote interoperability among EHRs [1]. These strategies have unique features that have been influenced by different aspects of each country's governments and technological development and culture. In this paper, the authors compare and contrast the strategies undertaken by three countries (*i.e.* Taiwan, Denmark and Canada) as they move towards developing interoperability between EHRs. A systematic review of the published literature was conducted. Data regarding the following aspects of each national strategy were collected: (a) federal government's governance power over healthcare organizations, (b) the current state of each country's e-health status, (c) the standards used in each country, (d) the data interoperability mechanisms used and (e) the benefits and drawbacks of each country's national approach.

1. National Level interoperability Approaches

In this section we examine national level interoperability approaches. Taiwan, Denmark and Canada are chosen as the study objects because all three countries have similar universal healthcare insurance policy of their own. This allows us to compare their national level health information interoperability strategies on the same basis. In addition, the three countries are located in different continents (Asia, Europe and North

America) and have different cultures. Differences in country's geography, population, demographics, healthcare system and health info-structure contribute in a major way to the feasibility of various approaches that ensure interoperability of EHR systems.

- *Taiwan's health data interoperability strategy*

Taiwan's national health information interoperability strategy is the Taiwan Electronic Medical Record Template (TMT) project. In 2007, the Department of Health (DoH), Executive Yuan, Taiwan determined to allocate about US$1 million to promote the TMT format in ten medical centres which collectively provide more than 10 million outpatient visits a year. TMT project aims to achieve a basis for building a portable, interoperable information infrastructure for EMR exchange in the country. The requirements for developing the TMT include: (1) minimal impact on the existing healthcare system; (2) easy implementation and deployment (3) compliant with Taiwan's current laws and regulations and (4) transformable to international standards. With this basic format template, it becomes feasible for people to check their own EMR within Taiwan [2].

- *Denmark's health data interoperability strategy*

Health information in Denmark is coordinated by MedCom, a private/public partnership established in 1994. MedCom is responsible for setting all of Denmark's standards related to health information. It is mandatory for each health region to use the standards established by MedCom and regions are regularly scrutinized to ensure that these standards are being followed [3]. Messages are transmitted across the Danish Healthcare Data Network (DHDN), a secure network connecting more than 5,000 different organizations and 100 different IT systems. The network is used by 97% of general practitioners, 74% of full time specialists, 100% of hospitals and pharmacies and 44% of local authorities. MedCom uses EDIFACT as the messaging standard for communicating between the primary and secondary sectors [4]. The actual exchange uses a point-to-point structure, wherein providers request information from other providers who each maintain their own databases. Due to interoperability assured by certified software, sender and receiver can respectively upload and download the messages into their own electronic record systems.

- *Canada's health data interoperability strategy*

Canada's main strategy and method for investment into the development, adoption and interoperability of electronic health is Canada Health Infoway (www.infoway-inforoute.ca). In July 2003, *Infoway* published the first version of EHR interoperable framework, the Electronic Health Record Solution Blueprint (*EHRS Blueprint*) [5]. It is a comprehensive and interactive document that describes the business and technical architecture of EHR solutions to be implemented across Canada. In the blueprint, *Infoway* promoted the use of common architecture and standards to ensure that systems can interoperate so that data can not only be shared over distance, but also read and understood. The common architecture is called EHR info-structure/EHR conceptual architecture.

EHRs are tied together by the Health Information Access Layer (HIAL), a set of Infoway-mandated specifications for integration, interoperability, privacy, security and other services. In general, each jurisdiction will have its own HIAL; they will follow a similar design and architecture and will use the same standards, although the vendors may be different. Therefore, patient health information is made available across different locations and jurisdictions by way of interconnecting EHR info-structure via the HIAL.

2. A Comparison of Three Countries' Strategies

In this section, we compare the interoperability strategies of three countries based on three criteria: healthcare systems, e-Health status, and information standards.

2.1. Healthcare Systems

All three countries adopted a universal healthcare insurance policy and are financed through public revenues. Although MedCom is a private/public partnership, the majority of its funding is from the public coffers. This means that each government has significant influence over policy since they provide funding. Whereas Denmark and Taiwan have the ability to implement policy nationally, MedCom and DOH-Taiwan have government authority to mandate interoperability standards. On the other hand, healthcare in Canada is for the most part under provincial jurisdiction. For Canada, this creates a situation where the federal government's primary influence in healthcare is through financial incentive, and its ability to implement a nation wide policy is through consensus building with and among the provinces and territories. Canada Health *Infoway* is forced to promote interoperability mechanisms through incentives, such as financial aid. In addition, the interoperability strategies that Canada promotes must meet the needs of each province, since they are the ultimate decision-making authorities. Currently, Canadian provinces/territories deliver care through regions in hospitals, community health agencies, primary care clinics, *etc*. They deliver locally and think locally. In addition, jurisdictions have made greater advances in health infostructure development, achieved more valued and visible e-health results, advanced their use of technology, and achieved better information for better health. So they might not desire a common EHR system or connect national initiatives (*Infoway*) with the local hospitals or doctors.

2.2. E-Health Status

Denmark and Taiwan have high EMR adoption rates and national level health infostructure in place. Therefore, it is less likely that data format/requirements and system structures will change dramatically over time[6]. For example, Taiwan's health smart cards are a significant investment, requiring the distribution of cards to every Taiwan resident, the purchasing of numerous card readers for every healthcare organization, and the provision of training for citizens and healthcare workers. This type of investment would not be possible if major changes were expected to occur to health information systems. Because of this, interoperability standards can be more rigid. Whereas Canada has a low rate of EMR adoption, it is likely that health information system structures and data format/requirements will evolve to facilitate greater EMR use. Therefore, the standards promoted by Canada Health Infoway need to have a certain amount of flexibility to allow for system growth and change.

2.3. Information Standards

Both MedCom and DOH-Taiwan have the ability to enforce exchange structures for their country's healthcare organizations and force healthcare organizations to adapt their clinical information systems to meet federal interoperability standards. In addition, because EMR adoption is high in both countries and because system structure will likely not change dramatically, they can implement exchange standards that are more rigid. For example, Taiwan proposed TMT for messaging Standards, and Denmark has developed the MedCom standard (EDIFACT and XML) for message handling between the systems. Canada focuses on common standards and architectures for interoperability, whilst the development of individual IT systems is done at the local/regional level [7, 8].

Canada's open source (e.g. the Reference Implementation Suite) and pre-certification mechanisms are less rigid and allow for each province to meet its unique needs while still maintaining interoperability. An open source strategy allows provinces to share their data structures. Pre-certification allows provinces' health care organizations to select from an assortment of vendors, all of which share common predefined interoperability mechanisms. It appears as though these flexible strategies were chosen because the Canadian federal government has no authority to mandate national standards. This means Canada Health Infoway can only encourage the use of standards, and they must meet every province's needs. Furthermore, low levels of EMR adoption likely means that system structures will change over time .

3. Conclusion

An interoperable EHR system that links clinics, hospitals, pharmacies and other points of care will help patients find information on classifications, treatments and waiting lists, and communicate directly with the healthcare services. This system also enables authorized health care providers timely access to their patients' comprehensive, up-to-date health information to support clinical decision making and integrated patient management across the continuum of care. This will help improve patients' access to health services, enhance the quality of care and safety, and result in efficiencies that save time and money.

However, there are many issues associated with the development of interoperable Electronic Health Records such as functional interoperability issue, data instance interoperability issue and metadata interoperability issue[9]. Many previous studies had proposed different methods in the attempt to conquer these problems. Interoperability methods can be categorized into point-to-point oriented model, standard oriented model and common-gateway model. Each has its benefits and limitations. On the national level EHR interoperability strategy, this study presented three countries' approaches to interoperability (Taiwan, Denmark and Canada). The key findings are as follows:

- *The federal government's ability to mandate standards affects choice of interoperability strategy*

The Denmark and Taiwan federal governments have the ability to mandate information technologies and standards for healthcare organizations. Therefore, it is feasible that both countries' implemented local standards such as TMT and EDIFACT in order to have a minimal impact on existing healthcare systems and meet their actual requirements. On the other hand, the Canadian federal government has no direct authority over most healthcare organizations. Thus, *Infoway* can only encourage the use of international standards and they must meet every province's or territory's needs.

- *E-Health status influences choice of interoperability strategy*

Denmark and Taiwan have high EMR adoption rates, have made greater advances in health info-structure development and achieved more valued and visible e-health results. Therefore, it is less likely that data format and system structures will change dramatically over time. As a result, both countries adopt more rigid terminology and message standard for data interoperability. While Canada has a low rate of EMR adoption, it has likelihood that health information system structures and data format will change in the future. Consequently, flexible standards such as SNOMED CT and HL7 are chosen that allow for the varying needs of each province and the changes to health information systems.

- *Differences in geography, population, and demographics affect the selection of national strategies towards interoperability*

Canada's populations are unevenly distributed through ten provinces and three territories (3.7 people/km^2), each with its own jurisdictional government. Taiwan and Denmark are much smaller countries with a much larger population density (638.5 people/km^2 and 127.8 people/km^2 respectively) when compared with Canada. Both countries have single health governance authority (Taiwan Ministry of Health and Danish Ministry of Health). These are probably also reasons that Canada adopted interoperability approach different from that of Denmark and Taiwan.

References

[1] HIMSS, Electronic Health Records: A Global Perspective. Healthcare Information and Management Systems Society (HIMSS), (2008). Retrieved June 20, 2010 from http://www.himss.org/content/files/200808_EHRGlobalPerspective_whitepaper.pdf
[2] W. S. Jian, C. Y. Hsu, T. H. Hao, H. C. Wen, M. H. Hsu, Y. L. Lee, Y. C. Li, P. Chang (2007) 'Building a portable data and information interoperability infrastructure - framework for a standard Taiwan Electronic Medical Record Template', *Comp Meth Prog Biomed* **88**(2),102-111.
[3] D. Protti, A Comparison of How Canada, England, and Denmark are Managing their Electronic Health Record Journeys, In A. W. Kushniruk & E. M. Borycki (Eds.) *Human, social, and organizational aspects of health information systems* (203-218). Hershey, Pennsylvania, USA: Medical Information Science Reference, 2008.
[4] K. Bernstein, M. Bruun-Rasmussen, S. Vingtoft, S. K. Andersen, C. Nohr, Modelling and implementing electronic health records in Denmark, Int J Med Inf **74** (2005) 213-220.
[5] D. Giokas, EHRS Blueprint: An Interoperable Framework. Canada Health Infoway, (2008). Retrieved June 24, 2010 from http://www.omg.org/news/meetings/workshops/HC-2008/15-06_Giokas.pdf
[6] D. Schrader, K. Mackie, M. Somlai, T. Sheaff, EHR Data Interoperability Mechanisms – A Comparison of Canada, Denmark and Taiwan's Strategies. HINF310 group project report, School of Health Information Science, University of Victoria, BC, Canada, 2009.
[7] D. Giokas, EHRS Blueprint: An Interoperable Framework. Canada Health Infoway, (2008). Retrieved June 24, 2010 from http://www.omg.org/news/meetings/workshops/HC-2008/15-06_Giokas.pdf
[8] Socialstyrelsen, National IT strategies – Denmark, England and Canada, (2009). Retrieved June 25, 2010 from http://www.socialstyrelsen.se/Lists/Artikelkatalog/Attachments/8374/2009-126-152_2009126152.pdf
[9] M. H. Kuo, HINF310 lecture note-week 5, http://web.uvic.ca/~h310/, 2010

International Perspectives in Health Informatics
E.M. Borycki et al. (Eds.)
IOS Press, 2011
doi:10.3233/978-1-60750-709-3-243

Applying a Methodological Approach for a Telecare Solution in Saudi Arabia

Khulud ALKADI[a,b], Abdul ROUDSARI[a,c]

[a]*Centre for Heath Informatics, City University, London, UK*
[b]*King Abdulaziz Medical City, National Guard Health Affairs, Riyadh, Saudi Arabia*
[c]*School of Health Information Science, University of Victoria, Canada*

Abstract. This paper briefly examines some major cultural/social factors influencing the quality of healthcare services in Saudi Arabia, then offers a telecare model used to provide the National Guard diabetic patients at King Abdulaziz Medical City in Riyadh with an alternative method of receiving healthcare services, to improve services and cope with healthcare, social, and cultural obstacles.

Keywords. Saudi Arabia, telecare, model, diabetes, methodology, soft systems

Introduction

The quality of services in primary care in many nations is suffering and under enormous pressure due to the increasing demand for access to care and the limited resources available. This is no different to the situation being faced by the healthcare industry in Saudi Arabia. Conservative social and cultural factors add to the problem. This paper proposes using telecare solutions as an alternative method of delivering quality healthcare services to overcome religious, cultural, and traditional aspects of a society. It introduces a telecare solution, selects a methodology to implement it, and then integrates it into the healthcare system at the National Guard Health Affairs to be used at the clinic by the diabetic educators (DEs), physicians, and diabetic patients at King Abdulaziz Medical City (KAMC) in Riyadh, taking into account the different influencing factors. It concludes by devising a model which illustrates how a telecare solution can be applied and integrated into existing systems.

1. Review of Current Saudi Telecare Services

1.1. National Guard Health Affairs (NGHA)

For the past decade, the NGHA management has worked vigorously to improve the quality of the healthcare services offered through the realization of how the investment in health informatics can assist in facing the growing obstacles in the healthcare industry. To begin with, they implemented a state-of-the-art network infrastructure which incorporates its sites kingdom-wide. From here, IT projects were launched and focus was on examining alternative methods of providing quality healthcare services.

Attempts started as early as 2000, during the live broadcast of the Siamese Twins Separation Surgery over the Internet. NGHA also offered free medical consultancy for one week, over a live video-conferencing link, to patients in a rural area. Since then, NGHA has taken huge steps to invest in eHealth. The establishment of the College of Public Health & Health Informatics at King Abdulaziz bin Saud University for Health Sciences, an affiliate, being a bold move in this direction.

1.2. Other Healthcare Providers in Saudi

Although little information is available of institutes offering Telecare, King Faisal Specialist Hospital and Research Centre is considered a leader in eHealth offering outreach programs and medical services via teleconferencing. Also, the Ministry of Health is now focusing on eHealth directions and strategies [1] with a five-year plan.

2. Factors Influencing Design

2.1. NGHA Resources

NGHA has a stable network infrastructure connecting its sites kingdom-wide. It launched a number of health systems, such as the Clinical Information Management System and is now deploying the Electronic Medical Record and the Picture Archiving & Communications System. All systems comply with universal health standards.

2.2. Social Factors

It is fair to say that Saudi is unique in its culture. Let us identify some of the factors that truly make it a unique place, which requires acceptable solutions.

- Saudi law prohibits females from driving. In addition, no efficient public transportation is available.
- Due to cultural factors, many patients request same-sex physicians. This can be difficult to satisfy, especially in rural centers with limited resources.
- When faced with serious illnesses, Saudis prefer getting second opinions from medical centers abroad. This may not necessarily be the best option.

2.3. Technology Available

Telecare services can be delivered through simple mobile and internet technology, which are both spreading widely in Saudi, easy to use, and affordable. Currently, there are three mobile phone providers in Saudi; Saudi Telecom Company with 21.1m lines, Mobily at 1.1m lines, and Zain with under 1m lines, bringing the total to approximately 23m users indicating that 80% of Saudi residents own mobile phones. With regards to internet usage in Saudi, statistics by The World Bank organization in 2008, show that 31% of the population use this technology [2]. These statistics indicate that both mobile and internet technologies are practical tools to use in the proposed telecare model.

3. Design of Model

3.1. Methodology Selection and Justification

A number of methodologies were considered, two were found suitable: *Soft Systems Methodology*, and *Ontology*. The former was selected due to the following reasons:

- the 'messy situation' (i.e. obstacles faced by patient/physician interaction)
- the social aspects in Saudi which plays a major role in the success of implementing such solutions (i.e. cultural, religious, and traditional)
- 'subjective view of social world' of Soft School better suits this area

3.2. Applying Soft Systems Methodology (SSM)

After acknowledging the problem, stakeholders were identified and goals set. Unified efforts lead to results presented in the SSM stages as indicated by Flood and Carson [3].

3.2.1. Stages 1 and 2

Figure 1 is a Rich Picture Diagram representing the application of a telecare solution within the Saudi National Guard Health Affairs healthcare system, starting with remote data entry by patient, management of data by healthcare official, and data storage.

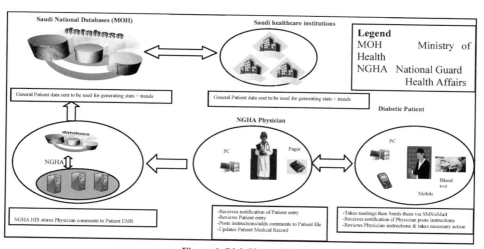

Figure 1. Rich Picture Diagram

3.2.2. Stages 3 and 4

A root definition is developed, and a CATWOE analysis is applied where C represents diabetic patients at KAMC, W represents the benefits gained by the Saudi government from controlling the spread of disease and providing healthcare services to more patients, and E represents the conservative Saudi society and illiteracy. This leads us to the development of the conceptual model (Figure 2), which is created from a number of statements used to describe the system, then assembled in a diagrammatic form.

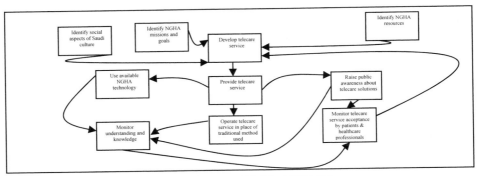

Figure 2. Conceptual Model – NGHA Telecare

3.2.3. Stage 5

A comparison between the conceptual model and the real world has been conducted. Findings show that eight out of the ten activities in our model have been achieved.

3.2.4. Stage 6 and 7

These stages focus on the changes to the structures, procedures, or attitudes that are socially feasible and applicable to the system at hand. As Checkland indicated [4], communication with 'Concerned actors' is essential when discussing changes.

Table 1. Desirable changes

Area of Change	Desirable Changes
Changes to System Structure	• Changing the way current NGHA healthcare services are being offered • The integration of required technology • Introducing new participants, teams and skills to the structure • Ownership of new system needs to be determined (Risks, Components, etc)
Changes to System Procedures	• The nature of the Patient-Physician relationship will change • Patients and physicians will need training on new procedures
Changes to Attitudes	• Patient acceptance of telecare services • Physician acceptance of healthcare policies and procedures • Raising public awareness of patients and their families

3.3. Model Selection and Justification

The Soft Systems Methodology (SSM) was selected since we are dealing with a complex human and organizational problem situation. The model will be developed using results gathered from the implementation of SSM, and also using the Soft System Diagram (SSD) approach. However, we have adopted the modified version of this Model, proposed by Checkland using sentences broken down into phases [5].

The justification is: our attempt to reflect social factors impacting on a system, our research area can be viewed as that involving 'purposeful human activity', and the area of research can be categorized as a 'messy situation'. Furthermore SSDs deal with messy situations consisting of 'purposeful human activity', and DFDs are used to represent a situation where 'problem solving' activities are applied and when an 'end' is known. Our 'end' is our set of objectives.

3.4. Model Development

First we identify the model components and their relationships: patient, physician, hospital and national information systems, telecare application, and the Diabetic Educators (DEs) at the clinic who are the first line of communication with patients.

Patients can use internet or SMS to electronically send their blood sugar readings. In addition, a dedicated landline handled by DEs is included, in order to capture more information from the patient. The DE then uses the telecare application to determine the next course of action. Figure 3 presents the model developed.

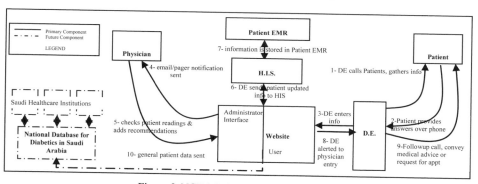

Figure 3. NGHA Telecare Model for diabetes clinic

4. Conclusion

The healthcare system in Saudi Arabia is finding it difficult to cope with the rapidly growing number of diabetics. Due to a number of factors, both cultural and systematic, we find that telecare solutions can assist in overcoming these obstacles. This model has been discussed with 'Concerned actors' at NGHA to determine its effectiveness and accuracy. Accordingly, corrections have been made. As of now, the model has been evaluated and implemented. An application has been developed, integrated into the current system, and launched for a limited trial period. Almost 80 patients have joined, managing their diabetes remotely via the application.

References

[1]   http://www.moh.gov.sa/ehealth/
[2]   http://www.stc.com.sa/cws/content/en//stc/files/Financial-Statements/annual-report2009.pdf , 31.
[3]   R. L. Flood, R. Ewart, Carson, *Dealing with Complexity*, 1993, 109.
[4]   P. B. Checkland, *Systems Thinking, Systems Practice,* 1981.
[5]   P. B. Checkland, Techniques in 'Soft' Systems Practice: Part 1. Systems diagrams-Some tentative guidelines. *J App Sys Anal*, **6** (1979), 33.

On-Line Communities

International Perspectives in Health Informatics
E.M. Borycki et al. (Eds.)
IOS Press, 2011
© 2011 ITCH 2011 Steering Committee and IOS Press. All rights reserved.
doi:10.3233/978-1-60750-709-3-251

Getting Better Together? Opportunities and Limitations for Technology-Facilitated Social Support in Cardiac Rehabilitation

Julie MAITLAND [a,1]

[a] People-Centered Technologies Group, National Research Council of Canada

Abstract. Social support has long been positively correlated with cardiac outcomes. However, sources of tension surrounding peer-involvement in the period following acute cardiac events are well documented. Informed by a previous study of patient perspectives of peer-involvement in cardiac rehabilitation, this paper draws from the cardiac and computing literature to provide actionable insights into how technology could be designed to promote appropriate peer-involvement and the challenges that may be faced when designing technologies to support the unsupported.

Keywords. social support, cardiac rehabilitation, computer-mediated communication.

Introduction

Social support is positively correlated with cardiac outcomes including recovery from myocardial infarction (MI) [1], participation in cardiac rehabilitation programs [2], and health-related behavioral change [3]. It can be so strongly linked that the lack of a social support network (social isolation) has been deemed to be a risk factor for both the development of coronary heart disease (CHD) and prognosis of established CHD [4,5] equivalent to "classic" risk factors, such as high cholesterol and smoking [6]. While there are social support structures (both health professional- and peer-based) in traditional cardiac rehabilitation programs in hospital and community settings, the primary focus remains on physiological recovery through cardiovascular exercise, rather than psychosocial interventions. However, patient-based support groups appear to be promising venues for non-traditional support provision [5,7].

Reflecting the focus of traditional cardiac rehabilitation, technological innovations and research in this area are grouped around web-based delivery of rehabilitation programs and physiological monitoring. Here, we are concerned with examining the potential role for technology in promoting social support for cardiac rehabilitation participants. As such, informed by the cardiac and computing literature, this paper draws on the insights gained into patients' perspectives of peer-involvement during a qualitative study of cardiac rehabilitation participants [8,9] to identify avenues of opportunity and constraint for technological interventions in this area. Before that, we

---

[1] Corresponding author: Julie Maitland, National Research Council of Canada, 46 Dineen Drive, E3A 4J1, Fredericton, Canada; email: julie.maitland@nrc-cnrc.gc.ca

commence with a brief overview of the study, the methodological and analytical approach employed, and the findings. For further details, we refer the reader to [9].

1. Method

Participants were recruited at the end of a ten-week cardiac rehabilitation program. Nineteen cardiac rehabilitation participants were recruited for the study. The majority of participants were male (n=14). Of the five female participants, three were widowed, one was married and the other was living with her common-law husband. All but one of the male participants was married or living with their common-law wife, the other lived alone but had a long-term partner. One of the married male participants also lived alone. Apart from the gender bias, the participants represented a broad demographic: participants were aged between 43 and 78 (average age= 63.1; s.d. = 10.8) and occupations (and pre-retirement occupations) spanned the manual-professional continuum, including janitor, domestic, policeman, nurse, engineer and laborer.

The interviews were performed at the participants' homes, and were structured around topics such as their cardiac event and rehabilitation, health-related behaviours and change, peer-involvement, and technology use. Each interview lasted between 45-90 minutes. All interviews were audio recorded and transcribed. Employing inductive analytic methods advocated by Lofland et al. [10], transcripts were initially subjected to open coding, whereby each sentence was analyzed in a process of sensitisation. The emergent codes were then subject to more focused coding, whereby similar codes were grouped together to form categories of phenomena. Similarities and differences were compared and contrasted, and the data was repeatedly revisited. Themes emerged that were then used to structure the data presented in [8,9], the latter of which we draw from here.

2. Results

Although experienced to a degree by members of an individual's family, a heart attack happens to the individual and it is the individual who needs to physically recover. We observed two broad categories of social network members found in this study: the inner core group and others. Inner core members were typically immediate family and provided the bulk of support. The distinction within an individual's social network between their inner group and others resonates with the notion of support cliques and sympathy groups discussed by Dunbar et al. [11]. Peer-involvement typically took the form of practical assistance, behavioral guidance or emotional support. The degree to which family members were involved in an individual's recovery and rehabilitation depended on many things including perceived need for support, desire for independence and social proximity (geographic and emotional). In particular, the findings highlighted two aspects of peer-involvement, namely tension between an individual and their peers, and the challenges of providing social support to those who have none. Here we reflect on the study's findings and consider the implications for research and design in the area of technology to promote social support within cardiac rehabilitation.

We found that following the event, both the individual and his/her family members undergo a period of uncertainty regarding what is physically safe for the individual to do and what will be possible for the future. In the cardiac literature, this is referred to as the period of adjustment. The supervision and encouragement of the rehabilitation staff, combined with the physical progress that the individuals can see and feel over the course of the rehabilitation program, serve to increase the individual's confidence with respect to what is physically possible. Family members, however, do not see what the individuals do during the exercise classes and so have to gain confidence by proxy: through verbal reassurance from the individual. Much of the cardiac literature calls for a greater involvement of spouses in the cardiac rehabilitation program [12-15]. However, for participants such as those who viewed the rehabilitation as their private battle, the prospect of further involving peers in the process is likely to be frowned upon.

Only three participants voiced dissatisfaction with the level of support that they had received from their families. Not wanting to be a burden, none of the participants had discussed these issues with their family. In each case, the issues did not seem to be exclusive to the cardiac condition but rather to stem from the nature of the existing relationships.

3. Discussion

Instead of proposing ways in which technology can assist peers in becoming more involved in an individual's rehabilitation, as we had first imagined, we suggest that technology be designed in such as way so as to build confidence by proxy. We propose and discuss three design strategies to promote peer confidence by proxy (see Table 1).

Pervasive monitoring technologies of could be utilized during rehabilitation classes to convey objective measures of progress to their peers, in an effort to build peers' confidence, and potentially alleviate unnecessary mollycoddling. Rather than automatically broadcasting progress to the inner core we would suggest that the individual should control information disclosure, as is currently practiced. Although the retention of information was cited as a source of frustration for peers elsewhere [15], controlled and selective disclosure is intrinsic to the maintenance of privacy. It is also especially important when considering the importance of the act of enquiry itself. Alongside interactions elsewhere viewed as controlling and potentially harmful, such as verbal instructions and emotional blackmail [3], enquiries were considered to be a caring gesture; a meaningful expression of concern. If information were automatically broadcast about a person to immediate family, this would reduce the need for him or her to ask how the individual is feeling that day. In other medical situations, such as when a family member is in intensive care the automatic broadcasting of updates may ease the burden of responding to enquiries [16], but here we suggest that it may reduce interactions that contribute to an individual's sense of support. Furthermore, the automatic broadcasting of information may be seen as demanding attention from the family members, something actively avoided by many participants.

Table 1. Designing to promote peer confidence by proxy.

Utilise pervasive monitoring to convey objective measures of progress to their peers
The individual should control information disclosure
Deliver peer-specific rehabilitation programs that run separately to the individual's program

As well as the difficulty in finding a balance between acceptable dependency and being a burden, finding a balance between peer involvement and interference is another well-documented source of tension [3,15,17,20]. In contrast to previous work, for the most part we found that individuals were tolerant and even appreciative of potentially intrusive involvement of their family because of an implicit understanding of the underlying motivation behind the family members' actions: caring concern. However, our study was concerned with establishing the response of the individual to peer involvement and we did not measure behavioural outcomes. Given the findings in the cardiac literature that suggest spousal control contributes to negative health outcomes, perhaps technology could contribute to reducing this area of tension. In addition to the earlier suggestion of a system to provide confidence by proxy, technology could also be used to deliver peer-specific rehabilitation programs that run separately to the individual's program. In this way peers could benefit from a cardiac rehabilitation program while the individual retains ownership of their program.

Similarly, participants appreciated offers of help and assistance even if they did not need to or want to call on those offers. The evident importance of anticipated support supports findings from gerontology that suggests anticipated support is more valuable to elders than practical support [19]. It is easy to envisage a computer-mediated anticipated support system by which friends and relatives leave virtual post-it notes containing good wishes and offers of assistance, a virtual get well card. However, particularly in view of this population's attitude towards technology (an overall reluctance to use technology "for technology's sake" [8]), the question that must be asked is what value would such a system add? The vast majority of our participants were happy with their existing levels of support, which, when from people who weren't co-located, came in the form of personal visits, phone calls and emails.

Here we find the crux of the problem when considering the design of peer-based technologies for cardiac rehabilitation. The people who feel that they are well supported do not necessarily need technology to mediate or augment the support processes and structures that they have in place, and clinically there is little to be gained from further enhancing moderate or strong support [1]. For those with weak support structures, it is naive to think that technology can improve what is essentially the nature of their relationships with their peers. Peer-based systems that forge new social ties such as forums may offer some purchase on this problem, but there are limitations in addition to the relative technical and literate expertise required to access and participate in traditional forums. Firstly, when considering the experiences of this study's participants, much of the value of the offers of support and good wishes was in the underlying emotions that they conveyed which are unlikely to be replicated in newly established social ties. One strategy to overcome the limitations of online support would be for portals to point to local community resources as well as relevant online communities.

Lastly, and perhaps more importantly, those who are not used to seeking support may not feel able or willing to proactively search for it. Note that two of the participants with the weakest support structures were the only ones not to engage in discussions with the other rehabilitation participants in their class. Technology can play a limited role in that anonymous and asynchronous communication seems like possible technical strategies to promote the establishment of social ties. However, it is likely that in cases where individuals are unaccustomed to seeking or receiving social support, such skills may need to be developed independently of any technological intervention.

Indeed, Arthur [1] similarly suggests: "A pre-requisite for benefit from peer support groups is the availability, and prior use, of social support networks in other aspects of life." Before technologists can realistically contribute to increasing the provision of support to those who currently have none, more research is required to understand the nature of support seeking practices of individuals with poor support structures.

4. Conclusion

In highlighting and discussing the problems of peer tension and supporting the unsupported, the original study deconstructed the somewhat abstract notion of social support. The further analysis and discussion presented in this paper now provides actionable insights into how technology could contribute and the challenges that may be faced.

References

[1] H.M. Arthur. Depression, isolation, social support, and cardiovascular disease in older adults, *J Cardiovasc Nurs*. 2006; 21(55): 52-57.
[2] B.J. Shen, H.F. Myers, C.P. McCreary, Psychosocial predictors of cardiac rehabilitation quality-of-life outcomes, *J Psychosom Res*. 2006; 60(1): 3-11.
[3] M.M. Franks, M.A.P. Stephens, K.S. Rook, B.A. Franklin, S.J. Keteyian, N.T. Artinia, Spouses' provision of health-related support and control to patients participating in cardiac rehabilitation, *J Fam Psychol*. 2006; 20(2): 311-318.
[4] S.J. Bunker, D.M. Colquohoun, D.E. Murray, Stress and coronary heart disease-psychosocial risk factors: National Heart Foundation of Australia Position Statement Update, *Med J Aus*. 2003; 178: 272-276.
[5] G.B. Sullivan, M.J. Sullivan, Promoting wellness in cardiac rehabilitation: exploring the role of altruism. *J Cardiovasc Nurs*. 1997; 11(3): 43-52.
[6] F. Mookadam, H.M. Arthur, Social support and its relationship to morbidity and mortality after acute myocardial infarction: systemic overview, *Arch Int Med*. 2004; 164(14): 1514-1518.
[7] H.M. Arthur, D.M. Wright, K.M. Smith, Women and heart disease: the treatment may end but the suffering continues, *Canadian Journal of Nursing Research*. 2002; 33(3): 17-29.
[8] J. Maitland, M. Chalmers, Self-Monitoring, Self-Awareness, and Self-Determination in Cardiac Rehabilitation. In: *Proceedings of the 28th international conference on Human factors in computing systems*. New York, NY: ACM; 2010: 1213-1222.
[9] J. Maitland, Patient Perspectives of Peer-Involvement in Cardiac Rehabilitation. *In Submission*.
[10] J. Lofland, D.A. Snow, L. Anderson, L.H. Lofland, *Analyzing Social Settings: A Guide to Qualitative Observation and Analysis*. Georgia: Wadsworth Publishing; 2005. 304p.
[11] R. Dunbar, M. Spoors, Social Networks, support cliques and kinship, *Human Nature*. 1995; 6: 273-290.
[12] S.S. Dickerson. Cardiac spouses' help-seeking experiences. *Clin Nurs Res*. 1998; 7(1): 6-24.
[13] T.B Hong, M.M. Franks, R. Gonzalez, S.J. Keteyian, B.A. Franklin, N.T. Artinian, A dyadic investigation of exercise support between cardiac patients and their spouses, *Health Psychology*. 2005; 4: 430-434.
[14] A, Karner, M.A. Dahlgren, B. Bergdahl, Coronary heart disease: causes and drug treatment- spouses' conceptions, *J Clin Nurs*. 2004; 13: 167-176.
[15] S. McLean, F. Timmins, An exploration of the information needs of spouse/partner following acute myocardial infarction using focus group methodology, *Nurs Crit Care*. 2007; 12(3): 141-150.
[16] W. Moncur, J. Masthoff, E. Reiter, What Do You Want to Know? Investigating the Information Requirements of Patient Supporters, In: *Proceedings of the 21st IEEE International Symposium on Computer-Based Medical Systems*. Washington, DC: IEEE Computer Society; 2008: 443-448.
[17] J. Wingham, H.M. Dalal, K.G. Sweeney, P.H. Evans, Listening to patients: choice in cardiac rehabilitation, *Eur J Cardiovasc Nurs*. 2006; 5(4): 289-294.
[18] C. Condon, G. McCarthy. Lifestyle changes following acute myocardial infarction: Patients perspectives, *Eur J Cardiovasc Nurs*. 2006; 5: 37-44.N. Krause, Longitudinal study of social support and meaning in life, *Psychol Aging*. 2007; 22(3): 456-469.

International Perspectives in Health Informatics
E.M. Borycki et al. (Eds.)
IOS Press, 2011
© 2011 ITCH 2011 Steering Committee and IOS Press. All rights reserved.
doi:10.3233/978-1-60750-709-3-256

The Role of User-Centred Design Within Online Community Development

Erin ROEHRER[a1], Elizabeth CUMMINGS[a], Leonie ELLIS[a], Paul TURNER[a]

[a]*eHealth Services Research Group, School of Computing & Information Systems, University of Tasmania, Australia*

Abstract. Research has evidenced the benefits of using information and communications technology (ICT) in chronic disease management including improving information availability, communication methods and raising individual patient's self-awareness of their own conditions. Extending ICT use to support patients in the community through online services draws attention to the complex task of how to meaningfully acquire input from all potential users of such systems and to balance their competing interests. This paper explores these issues across system analysis, specification and design for a community based patient support system. The paper highlights user-centred design challenges in a situation where the patient-users were not able to be included during the planning stage and explores how this impacted on the subsequent development

Keywords. user centred design, online communities, patient-centred systems

Introduction

The use of information and communication technology (ICT) in health service provision over the last two decades is fast becoming commonplace and applicable to a broader range of situations [1, 2]. This paper will use a community based patient support system project to demonstrate and explore the issues relating to system analysis, specification and design when patients are not included in the planning.

In Tasmania a team of clinicians, researchers and information technology developers is currently exploring methods to provide a means of overcoming geographical and medical barriers to communication, mentoring and health service delivery in the cystic fibrosis (CF) community. Tasmania has a high incidence of CF and many of the people with CF are geographically dispersed and isolated within this island state. This can create logistical challenges in accessing specialised services for some families. This can lead to decreased attendance at regular clinical appointments and the adoption of a reactive approach to care, rather than a proactive, preventative approach [3]. More specifically, there are commonly a number of virulent and resistant respiratory bacterial associated with CF. The possibility of cross contamination with one or more of these bacterium has led to the increased separation of patients when in hospital or attending outpatients clinics. The flow-on effect of this is further isolation

---

[1] Corresponding Author: Erin Roehrer, School of Computing & Information Systems, University of Tasmania, Private Bag 87, 7001, Hobart, Tasmania.;E-mail: Erin,Roehrer@utas.edu.au

of the people with CF and their families particularly in relation to any regular contact between people with CF that may provide a base for a supportive network [4].

Research has shown the potential of using information and communications technology (ICT) to improve the information available, the communication methods and the individual's self-awareness of their own conditions within the chronic disease domain [5]. The role that ICTs can play within enabling and fostering self-management behaviours has been encouraging, but not conclusive. Some research has demonstrated that individuals not only increase their own knowledge and levels of self-efficacy for self-management but additionally have improvements in some clinical outcomes and enjoy greater levels of social support [1, 2].

Building upon previous research [6-8] in the use of ICT and self-management, the research team from the University of Tasmania and the Department of Health and Human Services decided that expansion of the original research may be advisable. The revised project included web and mobile based education, self-monitoring and mentoring resources, specific for the CF community. The intention is to create an online community for individuals and families living with CF, allowing for the sharing of experiences and ultimately the improvement of self-management abilities.

1. The Challenge

Norman and Draper (1986) first developed the concept of user-centred systems design, stressing the importance of ensuring that systems development occurred through a high level of understanding of the user's situation and requirements. This understanding however did not necessarily need the active involvement of the users themselves [9]. Through their own exploration of user-centred system design literature and processes, Gulliksen et al [9] indentified the following 12 principles of user centred design (UCD) developed in order to improve upon the varying existing definitions of the concept [9].

Table 1. Table adapted from Gulliksen et al [9]. p409.

1. User Focus	The goals of the activity, the context of use, end-users requirements should guide initial development.
2. Active User Involvement	Representative of user groups should be actively involved throughout the entire Systems Development lifecycle.
3. Evolutionary systems development	Systems Development approach should be iterative and incremental.
4. Simple design representations	Design must be represented so that all stakeholders have easy understanding.
5. Prototyping	Prototypes should be used as early as possible in order to allow for the visualisation of ideas and designs and to enable users to interact with them.
6. Evaluate use in context	Baseline usability goals and design criteria should control the development.
7. Explicit & conscious design activities	Development process should contain dedicated design activities.
8. A professional attitude	Multidisciplinary teams should be involved in the development process.
9. Usability Champion	Usability experts should have early and continuous involvement through the Systems Development lifecycle.
10. Holistic Design	All aspects that influence the future use situation should be developed in parallel.
11. Processes customisation	The user-centred systems design process must be specified, adapted and/or implemented in each organisation.
12. A user-centred attitude	This should always be established from the commencement of any systems design process.

In the field of health informatics (HI) emphasis on principles 1, 2, 4, 6, 9 and 10 may ensure the design process captures all stakeholders within the project, particularly when the end-users involve both the health service professionals and health service recipients. This emphasis provides an avenue to include all apparent and non-apparent orientations to the systems development.

The challenge for HI is that many 'user-centred' approaches don't involve all of the stakeholder groups until the final phase of the systems development lifecycle. This is particularly apparent within those system developments that include patients as a beneficiary or end user of the enhanced or altered service. In these cases initial development phases are reliant upon representation and conceptualisation of 'the typical patient' as provided by health care professionals. This creates assumptions about the requirements of the end-users, the usage behaviours that will be present and inherent prejudices each individual will have towards the final product.

The late use of user-centred system design within the systems development lifecycle can then translate a potential holistic project into one of a narrowed focus. The communication between the design and project team may become frustrated as assumptions and agenda's cloud the representations of the health service recipient end users. The communication processes may also become cyclic in nature, encountering similar problems with the design but without the potential solution the included involvement of all stakeholders can bring.

The experiences of the ICT development team within this research project have been that the clinical team has a close relationship with their patient population and tend to protect them from outsiders. Attempts at early involvement of patients in the development of the system have experienced many barriers. The clinical team insisted upon having a polished, operational system before the patients were included. Thus the patients become final testers of the system rather than involved in the conceptualisation, design and development.

2. Several Orientations – One ICT Platform

Health care providers require objective evidence of not only the effectiveness, but the safety of ICT platform design [10]. This evidence is to be collected whilst removing any burden to patient safety and confidentiality, essentially excluding the majority of patients from a user design process. This, in turn, may create difficulties within the creation of a service platform for varying user needs when the overall needs analysis has taken place through a single user cohort on behalf of all users. In the example of the CF project, the health service providers have presented a conceptualisation of a 'typical patient' and encompassed those anticipated needs and behaviours into the requirements of the ICT platform.

The potential for a 'needs gaps' to arise once the participants finally have the opportunity to use the platform increases through this approach. One of the dilemma's encountered within the project's website design and development was trying to find a balance between functionality and form. Functionality allows the participants and health care providers to use the site according to the design stipulations and ensures information security. The form of the site is concerned with the overall layout and style. How the users can access information, how task intensive that process is and how the users interact and perceive the site will assist them in achieving the highest level of functionality. As visual creatures, different users also find different layouts aesthetically pleasing. Through the design and development phase the ICT team were concerned with this balance. The underlying nature of such a site is that the functionality is of paramount importance; the site must be able to achieve what the research team had envisioned. However, all user groups must be drawn to the site and want to interact with it. Thus functionality and form are linked essentials.

Kushniruk et al [11] suggest the analysis of Human Computer Interaction issues can allow the inclusion of user groups in the design stage, and be continuously cycled through the implementation stages. Usability engineering can provide varying methods of analysis that allow for the study of how the end users interact with the platform [11]. These methods can provide the end users perspective within the development stages, allowing for cost effective, safe and practical platforms to be developed.

Consistent with changes in the health care system, health information systems as a discipline, has been undergoing a transformation in regard to the conceptualisation of 'the patient' in the overarching research and development process. Traditionally health information systems were designed primarily to meet the health care providers needs and requirements, in order to deliver patient care [12]. This is now evolving to the involvement of patients within the system, creating further avenues for health service interaction and information [12]. The additional involvement of the patient within the system indicates the need for increased involvement in the design processes to allow a more congruent method of ensuring the system fulfills the major requirements of both patient and health care provider. Broader user involvement in the design of the ICT platform can allow previously unidentified requirements to be worked into the system [10, 13]. Powell and Armstrong [14] promote the use of "health consumers" in the varying stages of HI research, noting that focus groups, workshops and intervention pre-tests are of particular value when the extra dimension of input is created. This involvement has the potential to shape future research projects to be truly multi-focused and increased the range of usability across the varying health care orientations.

HI projects frequently evolve due to a perceived need's gap identified by those involved in the provision of health care services or researcher within the area. The projects have ranging diversities and stakeholders can be limited to inter-professionals within a particular health service, a single unit within an organisation to those involving improving service and communication gaps for health care recipients.

3. Conclusion

To assist in remaining clear to the aims of HI, the involvement of users need to take place within the very first phase of the systems development lifecycle, incorporating the user-centred systems design principles most relevant to HI developments. Barriers to access and usability concepts can then be dealt with when presented by all project stakeholders, as first hand representations. Through this interaction, and the involvement of a user-centred systems design, the need to implement ICT may prove to be of greater harm than good, or the role of the ICT may be that of service complimentary, rather than a true service provision platform.

With the initial conceptualisation of the revised project, the ICT team had the intentions of providing the health care recipients access to the development and design of the ICT platform, anticipating the formulation of the online community would stem from a user-centred design process. The clinical team found it difficult to facilitate this involvement in the design process and insisted that they only be involved once the platform was developed to a fully functional level. These differing views have led the project to difficult situation of continuous development that cannot be resolved easily until the involvement of all end-users becomes possible. This is not an unusual situation within health information systems development.

4. References

[1]   E. Murray, J. Burns, S. See Tai, R. Lai, I. Nazareth. Interactive Health Communication Applications for people with chronic disease (review). *Cochrane Database of Systematic Reviews* 2005.

[2]   M.R. Solomon. Information Technology to Support Self-Management in Chronic Care. *Disease Management and Health Outcomes* **16** (2008), 391.

[3]   E.H. Wagner, B.T Austin, C. Davis, M. Hindmarsh, J. Schaefer, A. Bonomi. Improving Chronic Illness Care: Translating Evidence Into Action. *Health Affairs* **20** (2001), 64.

[4]   R. Bradbury, A. Champion, D. Reid. Poor clincial outcomes associated with a multi-drug resistant clonal strain of Pseudomonas aeruginosa in the Tasmanian cystic fibrosis population. *Resp* **13** (2008), 886.

[5]   G. Paré, M. Jaana, C. Sicotte. Systematic Review of Home Telemonitoring for Chronic Diseases: The Evidence Base. *JAMIA* **14** (2007), 269.

[6]   H. Cameron-Tucker, M. Jessup, E. Cummings, J. Busch, P. Turner, L. Joseph, H. Saddington, C. Wainwright, D. Reid. Mentoring for people with cystic fibrosis: evaluation of the preperation & process. *Euro Cystic Fibrosis Conf.* Brest, France, 2009.

[7]   H. Cameron-Tucker, L. Joseph, E. Cummings, J. Busch, P. Fitzpatrick, P. Turner, E.H Walters, D. Reid. Health-Mentor Training of Health Professionals to Facilitate Self-Management for People with Cystic Fibrosis. *Intl Cong Chronic Disease Self-Management.* Melbourne, Australia, 2008.

[8]   M. Jessup, J. Busch, P. Fitzpatrick, P. Turner, H. Cameron-Tucker, L. Joseph, E. Cummings, E.H Walters, D. Reid. Pathways Home Project: A Pilot Study of Chronic Disease Self Management in Cystic Fibrosis (CF). *7th Australasian Cystic Fibrosis Conference.* Sydney, Australia, 2007.

[9]   J. Gulliksen, B. Goransson, I. Boivie, S. Blomkvist, J. Persson, A. Cajander. Key Principles for user-centred systems design. *Behav Inf Tech* **22** (2003), 397.

[10] P. Sanderson. Designing and Evaluating Healthcare ICT Innovation: A Cognitive Engineering View. In: J.I Westbrook, E.W Coiera, J.L. Callen, J. Aarts, editors. *Information Technology in Health Care 2007.* Sydney, Australia: IOS Press, 2007. p.3.

[11] A.W Kushniruk, E.M Borycki, S. Kuwata, F. Ho. Emerging Approaches to Evaluating the Usability of Health Information Systems. In: A.W Kushniruk, E.M. Borycki, editors. *Human, Social, and Organizational Aspects of Health Information Systems.* Hershey, New York: Medical Information Science Reference, 2008.

[12] J. Dawson, B. Tulu, T.A. Horan. Towards Patient-Centered Care: The Role of E-Health in Enabling Patient Access to Health Information. In: E.V. Wilson, editor. *Patient-Centered E-Health.* Hershey, New York: Information Science Reference, 2009. p.1.

[13] A. Mauro, F. Gonzalez Bernaldo de Quiros. Patient-Centered E-Health Design. In: E.V. Wilson, editor. *Patient-Centered E-Health.* Hershey, New York: Information Science Reference, 2009.

[14] J. Powell, N. Armstrong. Involving Patients and the Public in E-Health Research. In: E.V. Wilson, editor. *Patient Centered E-Health.* Hershey, New York: Information Science Reference, 2009.

International Perspectives in Health Informatics
E.M. Borycki et al. (Eds.)
IOS Press, 2011
doi:10.3233/978-1-60750-709-3-261

A Requirements Engineering Approach for Improving the Quality of Diabetes Education Websites

Omid SHABESTARI[a,1], Abdul ROUDSARI[a,b]

[a] *Centre for Heath Informatics, City University, London, UK*
[b] *School of Health Information Science, University of Victoria,*
British Columbia, Canada

Abstract. Diabetes Mellitus is a major chronic disease with multi-organ involvement and high-cost complications. Although it has been proved that structured education can control the risk of developing these complications, there is big room for improvement in the educational services for these patients. e-learning can be a good solution to fill this gap. Most of the current e-learning solutions for diabetes were designed by computer experts and healthcare professionals but the patients, as end-users of these systems, haven't been deeply involved in the design process. Considering the expectations of the patients, this article investigates a requirement engineering process comparing the level of importance given to different attributes of the e-learning by patients and healthcare professionals. The results of this comparison can be used for improving the currently developed online diabetes education systems.

Keywords. Web 2.0, diabetes mellitus, patient education as topic, eLearning; requirement engineering, healthcare professionals, adolescent, young

Introduction

Diabetes mellitus is one of the major chronic diseases. The characteristic sign of this disease is high blood glucose level (hyperglycemia). Diabetes has two main types based on the pathogenic process which causes the hyperglycaemia. Type 1 is caused by complete or near total deficiency of insulin, whereas type 2 can be caused by a different set of factors like variable degrees of insulin resistance, impaired insulin secretion, and increased glucose production.

Diabetes is considered to be one of the most important chronic diseases for several different reasons. Not only it has a relatively high prevalence in the UK (4.95% in 2010), it also has a high incidence rate of 0.33% which can be explained both by new cases and better methods of case detection and monitoring used in the recent year which helps to identify undiagnosed cases. Another reason is its chronic multi-organ complications. These complications can involve eyes, nerves, cardio-vascular system, gastrointestinal system, genitourinary system and the skin. These complications are mostly irreversible and once the patient starts developing such complications, it will

---

[1] Corresponding Author: Dr. Omid Shabestari, Centre for Health Informatics, City University, Northampton Square, London, EC1V 0HB, UK   Email: omid.shabestari.1@soi.city.ac.uk

cause a very high impact on the health system with a total cost of approximately a tenth of NHS budget each year. The shift of the type 2 of diabetes toward younger people has increased the risk of longer life with complications of this disease causing considerable increase in the costs [1] .

Two main research projects on type 1 and type 2 of diabetes have shown that intensive management of diabetes can reduce the risk of these complications. These studies were Diabetes Control and Complications Trial (DCCT) [2] on type 1 and UK Prospective Diabetes Study (UKPDS) [3] in type 2 . Most routine diabetes care processes such as carbohydrate intake control, blood glucose metering, and insulin injection in type 1 and diet control and weight-watching in type 2 are done by patients themselves. Also control of certain complications such as foot problems can be performed by the patients, in addition to scheduled visits to clinics. Providing the patients with enough knowledge about these tasks can play a crucial part in diabetes care. This goal can be achieved by patient education. The statistics show that the coverage of education for the people living with diabetes is unsatisfactory [4]. There are several limitations that do not allow face-to-face education to expand within current capacities such as the limitation of time among the educatees and the limitation of the human resources among the educators. So there is a need for other methods of communication to deliver this education.

E-learning is defined as the use of electronic technologies for the purpose of education. It has been widely used in other sectors like schools and universities and it is a method that most of the computer native generation are quite familiar with. Several trials have been conducted to measure the feasibility and the impact of this method of education in the diabetes. Although many of these studies has demonstrated a positive impact in this method, they mostly used this channel of communication as an alternative method for delivering the topics that has been used in face-to-face education without empowering their training with the special features of this new medium. Introduction of social networks and Web 2.0 technologies has enabled this channel of communication to be more collaborative by increasing the role of the patients in these systems.

Although the examples of diabetes education which were previously mentioned were designed for the patients, they have not been involved in the design of the system from the beginning. There are some patient-centred projects, but they were mostly designed by computer experts according to the requirements provided by healthcare professionals [5-10]. Bull et al studied the user friendliness, accessibility, interactivity and support level of the existing diabetes education web sites and reported that the sites fall short of their potential to help consumers [11].

In this paper the expectations of the patients as the end-users of the system and the healthcare professionals are compared using value theory and the parameters from End-User Computing Satisfaction (EUCS) model [12]. This model is selected because it includes the participation concept behind collaborative networks. This comparison can highlight the difference between the opinions from those two groups and can be used as a requirement engineering model to change the currently developed systems to something more acceptable by its end-users.

1. Methods

An online survey was designed for this research. Invitation to this study was emailed to the healthcare professionals working in diabetes clinics of collaborating hospitals and also was posted to the patients aged from 10 to 30 registered in those clinics. For the purpose of simplicity the healthcare professionals will be addressed as professionals in the rest of this article.

The characteristics of the online diabetes education were classified in four main groups. According to King and Epstein a rating scale which can be as reliable as a ranking scale [13] was used in this study. Based on the recommendation from Kahle and Kennedy [14], a zero to six rating model was chosen for this value survey. A special user-defined component was developed for collecting the answer to each question based on the Likert-type scaling [15] and slider tools in dot net technology. This tool was designed to highlight the chosen response of the user with both annotation and colours using traffic light model. The research was conducted as a multi-centre study in the three educational hospitals in London including Barnet, chase Farm and Mayday hospitals. Each of the participants had a unique user-name and password and they only had access to their own answers to ensure the confidentiality of the system. Only the principal investigator had access to the responses of all participants.

2. Results

39 patients and 13 professionals completed the online questionnaire. The professionals participating in this study were a good combination of the different professions involved in the diabetes care including 6 doctors, 5 diabetes specialist nurses and 2 dieticians responding to this survey. A data preparation procedure was followed to ensure the cleanness of the data for final analysis. No missing data was identified as the response to the questions was mandatory in the interface.

Although this questionnaire was validated in the information science the collected data was checked for multicollinearity and any bias caused by data items. No highly correlated items pointing to similar concept were identified. In the next step the collected data was controlled for outlier responses using three methods of Residual Statistics, Mahalanobis Distance and Cook's Distance. Five outlier responses were identified in the patients group. They were closely examined and serial response pattern was identified in them. Those responses were excluded from the final analysis.

In the next step the reliability of the responses were measured to ensure the extendibility of the results in this study. In the patients group the Cronbach's alpha test was equal to 0.942 and in the healthcare professionals it was equal to 0.925 which shows a very high level of reliability. After ensuring the reliability of the data, the normality of the distributions was checked. This test was used to select the proper statistical method for comparing the responses from the patients and the professionals. Shapiro-Wilks test showed not normally distributed data in all of the e-learning attributes, so non-parametric tests was used to compare the two groups.

Table 1. Significant differences in values of online diabetes education between the patients and professionals

Attributes significantly higher among the patients	P-Value
System security	0.03
Learning flexibility	0.043
Attribute significantly higher among the professionals	**P-Value**
Different system tools	0.024

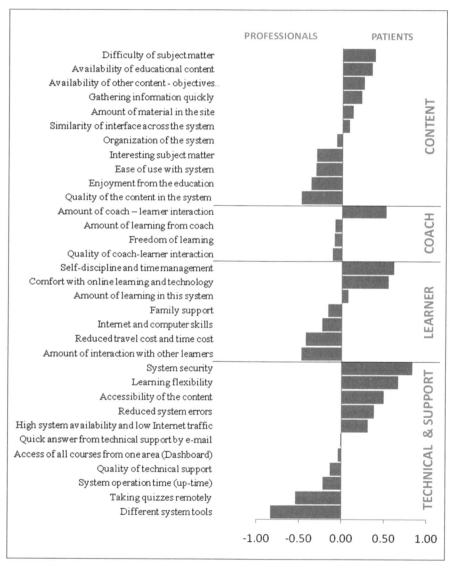

Figure 1. Comparison of the values between the patients and the healthcare professionals

There was no significant difference between the mean values of all online diabetes education attributes in the two groups (P=0.953) using Mann-Whitney, but comparison of the individual items showed the significant difference listed in table 1. Also the mean value of the rating for each attribute was calculated and summarized in Figure 1.

3. Discussion

Although the two groups had no significant difference on the overall picture about this method of learning, their view had considerable differences about the detailed attributes of it.

In terms of the system content, the patients gave more value to the difficulty of the subject matter and availability of the content. These are the items that need more investment in the current systems. On the other hand, enjoyment from the education and quality of the content had less importance comparing the patients with professionals and increased investment in them will have less value.

Among the coaching-related attributes only amount of coach-learner interaction had a higher values voted by the patients and the others received less relative value than the rating from the professionals. For the learning values the patients were more concerned about self-discipline and comfort with online learning and their concern was less than professionals regarding family support. This shows good evidence for their interest in independence. Also it emphasizes that organizers of these systems should ensure that their users have the required level of computer knowledge to utilize their service properly. The other interesting evidence in the learner-related attributes is that patients gave much less value to the interaction with other users. It shows that the professionals are more interested in increasing the collaboration among the patients but patients consider these systems as a method to expand their direct channels of communication with their care team. High level of ratings for learning from the coach is more evidence for this result. In technical and support related attributes, the patients have much higher expectation on system security and learning flexibility. Their perceived level of importance was much lower than professionals on taking quizzes remotely and different system tools. These ratings show that the patients see such systems more as a secure extension for their communication with their care team than a complete educational package.

Their low rating about the system tools was investigated in series of secondary interviews. This follow-up showed that some patients did not have the insight into the possibility of integration between their clinical data and personalized education, or they believed that the technology for automated transfer of clinical data from their gluco-meters to the centralized server available to their care team was not feasible. Also they believed that even if such services could be provided, their care team would not have enough time to monitor all of them on a regular basis. The professionals gave a high value to such communication but agreed that it needed additional human resources.

4. Conclusion

The considerable difference between the patients and the professionals in this study shows that implementing them can help to improve the currently existing online diabetes education systems and make them more acceptable for their end-users. This research was limited to the adolescent and young people living with diabetes because of being more familiar with computing and online education. An extended research is required to confirm these results in elder people living with diabetes.

Acknowledgement

The data used in this study was collected as part of the formative evaluation of a study on using Web 2.0 technologies for diabetes education of adolescent and young patients (CareNet). The CareNet study was conducted for fulfilment of PhD degree in Health Informatics by the first author of the paper. None of the authors have financial interest in this project. The authors of this paper like to extend their gratitude to the healthcare professionals in the collaborating hospitals for their valuable support in this study.

References

[1]   F. R. Kaufman. Type 2 Diabetes in Children and Young Adults: A "New Epidemic". *Clinical Diabetes* October **20**(4) (2002), 217-8.

[2]   D. J. Chrisholm. The Diabetes Control and Complications Trial (DCCT). A milestone in diabetes management. *Med J Aust* Dec 6-20, **159**(11-12) (1993), 721-3.

[3]   C. E. Nasr, B. J. Hoogwerf, C. Faiman, S. S. Reddy. United Kingdom Prospective Diabetes Study (UKPDS). Effects of glucose and blood pressure control on complications of type 2 diabetes mellitus. *Cleve Clin J Med* Apr **66**(4) 1999, 247-53.

[4]   Healthcare watchdog survey of people with diabetes suggests NHS is meeting Government standards on diabetes check-ups. 2007 [cited20/05/2008];Available from: http://www.healthcarecommission.org.uk/newsandevents/pressreleases.cfm?cit_id=5356

[5]   S. Shea, J. Starren, R. S. Weinstock et al. Columbia University's Informatics for Diabetes Education and Telemedicine (IDEATel) Project: rationale and design. *JAMIA* Jan-Feb **9**(1) (2002), 49-62.

[6]   G. Viklund, E. Ortqvist, K. Wikblad. Assessment of an empowerment education programme. A randomized study in teenagers with diabetes. *Diabetic Medicine* **24**(5) 2007, 550-6.

[7]   J. M. Wiecha, V. K. Chetty, T. Pollard, P. F. Shaw. Web-based versus face-to-face learning of diabetes management: the results of a comparative trial of educational methods. *Fam Med JT* 9 ed, 2006, 647-52.

[8]   T-I Lee, Y-T Yeh, C-T Liu, P-L Chen. Development and evaluation of a patient-oriented education system for diabetes management. *Int J Med Inf* **76**(9) (2007), 655-63.

[9]   Glasgow RE, Boles SM, McKay HG, Feil EG, Barrera M. The D-Net diabetes self-management program: Long-term implementation, outcomes, and generalization results. *Prev Med* **36**(4) (2003), 410-9.

[10] H. G. McKay, R. E. Glasgow, E. G. Feil, S. M. Boles, M. Barrera. Internet-based diabetes self-management and support: Initial outcomes from the diabetes network project. *Rehab Psych* **47**(1) (2002), 31-48.

[11] S. S. Bull, B. Gaglio, H. G. McKay, R. E. Glasgow. Harnessing the potential of the internet to promote chronic illness self-management: diabetes as an example of how well we are doing. *Chron Illn* Jun;1(2) (2005),143-55.

[12] W. Doll, G. Torkzadeh. The measurement of end-user computing satisfaction. *MIS Quart* **15**(1) (1988) 5-9.

[13] W. R. King, B. J. Epstein. Assessing information system value: An experimental study. Dec Sci **13**(4) (1982), 34-45.

[14] L. R. Kahle, P. Kennedy. Using the list of values (LOV) to undeerstand consumers. J Serv Market **2**(4) (1988),49-56.

[15] R. Likert. A technique for the measurement of attitudes. *Arch Psych* **140**(5) 1932,1-55.

Methods

International Perspectives in Health Informatics
E.M. Borycki et al. (Eds.)
IOS Press, 2011
doi:10.3233/978-1-60750-709-3-269

Application of a Non-Linear Autoassociator to Breast Cancer Diagnosis

Joel A. FERSTAY[a,1], Kimberly D. VOLL[b]

[a,b] *Department of Computer Science, University of British Columbia, Vancouver, British Columbia, Canada*

Abstract. Fast and accurate, non-linear autoassociators perform well in the face of unbalanced data sets, where few to no positive examples are present. In cancer diagnosis, for example, this can be convenient if only benign data is available, or if only a very small proportion of malignant data is available. As proof of concept, we apply a non-linear autoassociator to breast tumor data to predict the presence of cancer using only benign examples to train the autoassociator. Our results indicate that the non-linear autoassociator approach to automated breast cancer diagnosis is convenient and yields accurate results with minimal overhead.

Keywords. breast cancer, autoassociator, diagnosis, classification, connectionism.

Introduction

A challenging task that requires consideration of many variables, automated diagnosis of breast cancer can increase accuracy, reducing patient stress and the potential litigation of misdiagnosis, as well as saving medical practitioners time. Connectionist networks such as multi-layer perceptron (MLP) networks have had past success in breast cancer diagnosis [1,2,3,4]. Such approaches for medical diagnosis, however, have been limited by the requirement for training corpora consisting of both positive and negative examples of data in relatively equal numbers [5,6,9]. As a consequence, obtaining corpora in sufficient size for effective training is often difficult, limited by the harder-to-obtain class of examples [5,6,9]. To avoid this difficulty, we propose the use of a non-linear autoassociator (NLA) network. NLAs can be trained on data sets that contain only one class of sample (e.g. only benign samples) [5,6,9]. We use the Breast Cancer Wisconsin (BCW) corpus to demonstrate that NLAs achieve competitive classification results on an established, benchmarking dataset, while only requiring negative (benign) instances of the diagnostic class for training [7,8]. This paper is organized as follows: first, a brief introduction to NLAs is given, second, the experimental methods and analysis are described, and third, the results and future directions are discussed.

---

[1] Corresponding Author: Joel A. Ferstay, Department of Computer Science, University of British Columbia, 201-2366 Main Mall, Vancouver, B.C. V6T 1Z4, Canada; E-mail: joel.ferstay@gmail.com

1. Background on Non-linear Autoassociators

Connectionist models inspired by the neuronal substrate of the brain, MLP networks consist of a collection of nodes arranged in layers with all but the input and output layers hidden from observation and direct manipulation. The nodes are linked between layers via weighted connections; each node in the input layer is connected to every node in the hidden layer, and each node in the hidden layer is connected to every node in the output layer. On training, data is provided to the network by activating the input layer nodes, whose activations are then propagated through the network to the nodes at the output layer, whose activations are then interpreted. Based upon comparison to the expected output, the weights within the network are adjusted through continual testing until the network settles into a stable configuration that produces the correct output for a given input.

NLAs are MLP networks with two caveats: first, they have fewer hidden nodes than input and output nodes, and second, they are trained to reconstruct their input on their output nodes – this aspect is described in more detail below [9]. An example of the structure of an NLA is given in Figure 1.

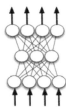

Figure 1. The structure of a non-linear autoassociator. Nodes are shown as circles, and weighted connections are shown as lines between nodes. Arrows indicate the input and output layers. NLAs are trained to reconstruct the given input on their output nodes.

As with MLP networks, NLAs can be trained via modifying the weights of the internal network connections. We will apply the standard error-backpropagation to train our network. Backpropagation adjusts network weights on the basis of a differential analysis of the actual output versus the desired output, and incrementally propagates weight changes backwards through the network [10].

NLAs further differ from other classifiers in that they are not trained to explicitly output the class to which a given input belongs, but instead reconstruct the input pattern on the output nodes [9]. In order to train an NLA to discriminate one class from another we train on only instances of one particular class. After training, exposure to subsequent examples of that same class should result in a low "input reconstruction error", while negative examples of the class should result in high input reconstruction error. Input reconstruction error is calculated using the mean-squared error between the NLA input and its output. The actual discrimination between classes is determined on the basis of an error threshold– anything with error less than or equal to a predetermined threshold[2] is a positive instance, and anything greater is negative.

---

[2] An appropriate threshold can be established using a variety of techniques [6,9]. In this experiment we determined the threshold using Japkowicz et al.'s method [6].

2. Diagnosis of Breast Cancer using Non-linear Autoassociators

2.1. Description of the Breast Cancer Dataset

To assess performance of the NLA on breast cancer diagnosis we used the Breast Cancer Wisconsin (BCW) dataset, originally formed by Wolberg and Mangasarian [7]. This dataset has 683[3] samples, each with nine features, including clump thickness, uniformity of cell size, uniformity of cell shape, marginal adhesion, single epithelial cell size, bare nuclei, bland chromatin, normal nuclei, and mitosis. Each feature is assigned a discrete integer score, from 0-10. A sample is assigned to one of two classes, malignant and benign; there are 444 benign samples and 239 malignant samples.

The BCW dataset was chosen because of the inherent difficulty in breast cancer diagnosis, the availability of positive and negative data for comparative analysis, and its availability on the World Wide Web [1,2,3,4,7,8].

2.2. Experimental Methods

As only one class of examples from the breast cancer corpus is needed in training we selected the largest class, thus creating a separate, benign-only dataset. To get a better estimate of the NLA's performance on more varied data, we applied k-fold cross-validation during our training. A k value of 10 was chosen to give an estimate that is statistically likely to be accurate [10]. The 444 benign samples were consequently split into 10 subsets (9 sets of 44 and 1 set of 48). From these subsets 10 different training sets were formed, each training set omitting a different one of the 10 subsets for variation. For evaluation purposes, 10 test sets were formed using one of the 10 subsets from above combined with all of the malignant samples. Ten NLAs were constructed, each with weights and biases initialized based upon a random sampling[4]. The network consisted of 9 input nodes, 4 hidden nodes, and 9 output nodes, based on performance testing and the methods of Japkowicz et al. [6, 9]. Each of the 10 NLAs was tested on one of the 10 training sets. The number of training epochs was determined experimentally to be 800 iterations, based on good classification performance [6, 9]. After training, each of the 10 networks was tested on the one of the 10 test sets that corresponded to its omitted benign dataset.

2.3. Results and Analysis

After performing 10-fold cross validation the classification accuracy averaged over all 10 test sets was calculated to be 96.90% for the BCW corpus. Sensitivity was on average 97.07% over the 10 folds, while the specificity was on average 96.17 % over the 10 folds. The F-measure (Eq. 1), a measure of the test's accuracy using the harmonic mean of sensitivity and specificity, was 96.62%. See Table 1 for a summary of the NLA network's performance.

---

[3] As with previous experiments using the BCW dataset, the sixteen samples with missing values are removed leaving the dataset with a total of 683 samples.

[4] These weights were determined experimentally based on good classification performance.

$$F - Measure = \frac{2 \times (Sensitivity \times Specificity\ )}{(Sensitivity\ + Specificity\ )} \tag{1}$$

Table 1. Performance of the NLA on the WBC dataset.

Classification accuracy (%)	Sensitivity (%)	Specificity (%)	F-Measure (%)
96.90	97.07	96.17	96.62

Further analysis of the NLA classifier's performance is done through calculating the true positive (TP) rate and false positive (FP) rate of the benign and malignant classes. The *F*-measure (Eq. 2), as a measure over the class accuracy, was also calculated for both benign and malignant classes. The TP and FP rates, along with the *F*-Measures are given in Table 2.

$$F - Measure = \frac{2 \times TP}{2 \times TP + FP + FN} \tag{2}$$

Table 2. Detailed accuracy by classes: TP = True Positive, FP = False Positive, and F-Measure = Frequency over Class Accuracy.

Classes	TP Rate	FP Rate	F-Measure
Benign	0.96	0.03	0.91
Malignant	0.97	0.04	0.98

Comparing these results to the top previous attempts at classification of the BCW corpus, Verma and Hassan were able to obtain a 97.90% classification accuracy on the breast cancer data set, and Marcano-Cedeno et al. were able to obtain a classification accuracy of 98.91% using modified MLP (non NLA) networks trained on both positive and negative examples [1, 2]. Verma and Hassan report an F-measure of 0.97 for their malignant class, and 0.96 for their benign class [1]. Marcano-Cedeno et al. did not report F-measures [2].

All results were generated using NLAs implemented in Python, and run on a 2GHz Intel Core 2 Duo iMac with 1GB of SDRAM, running Mac OS X version 10.5.8. The NLA network takes 1243.64 seconds, or 20.73 minutes, to perform 800 iterations of training over 400 samples from the WBC dataset, and 4.11×10^{-4} seconds to classify a single sample.

3. Discussion and Future Work

The NLA approach motivated here is able to perform at levels comparable to more traditional network classifiers, but with the added benefit of requiring only one class of samples; this is particularly advantageous in health informatics as benign or negative data tends to be present in higher numbers than positive samples. This opens up further domains to testing that were not considered formerly due to a lack of data.

We are currently investigating further data sets, including a broken-ankle dataset that includes a large percentage of negative examples, as well as the application of our techniques to challenges associated with wound assessment, especially in telemedical applications. Furthermore, NLAs may also find use in areas such as lung cancer diagnosis, which is currently the leading cause of death in the Western world. Often, patients are only diagnosed once they are experiencing advanced symptoms, meaning there is often more malignant lung cancer data than benign data, or early, pre-cancer data [11]. An NLA system may improve early diagnosis in light of such unbalanced datasets. Work is also underway to improve the overall accuracy of the system. Obtaining a larger training corpus may be necessary given that not all examples are used (i.e. the malignant samples are discarded), and may explain why our results are slightly lower than other researchers classification systems on the BCW corpus. In addition, study of the network parameters and learning algorithms is ongoing.

4. Conclusion

Non-linear autoassociators (NLAs) are a viable system for medical classification and diagnosis, requiring only one class of examples for training. As a result such networks are ideally suited to areas of medical classification for which it is hard to obtain corpora of relatively equally represented classes of examples, such as some cancer datasets that contain mostly benign samples but few to no malignant samples. By way of proof of concept, we have demonstrated that our NLA performs comparably to some of the best performing classification techniques on the Breast Cancer Wisconsin corpus, an established and well-used dataset, and we are expanding our study to include further such corpora.

References

[1]   A. Marcano-Cedeno, F. S. Buendia-Buendia, D. Andina, in *Bioinspired Applications in Artificial and Natural Computation*, J. Mira, J.M. Ferrandez, J.R. Alvarez, F. de la Paz, F.J. Toledo, Springer, Heidelberg **5602** (2009), 48-54.
[2]   B. Verma, S. Z. Hassan, Hybrid ensemble approach for classification, *Applied Intelligence* (2009) Available from: http://www.springerlink.com/content/f624146358627704/
[3]   C. E. Floyd CE, Lo JY, Yun AJ, Sullivan DC, Kornguth, PJ, Prediction of breast cancer malignancy using an artificial neural network, *Cancer* **74** (1994), 2944–2998.
[4]   D. B. Fogel, E. C. Wasson, E. M. Broughton, Evolving neural networks for detecting breast cancer, *Cancer Letters* **96**(1) (1995), 49-53.
[5]   N. Japkowicz, Concept-learning in the absence of counter-examples: an autoassociation-based approach to classification, PhD thesis, New Brunswick Rutgers, The State University of New Jersey, 1999.
[6]   N. Japkowicz, C. Myers, M. Gluck, A novelty detection approach to classification, *in the proceedings of the Fourteenth Int Joint Conf on Artificial Intel* (1995), 518-523.
[7]   W. H. Wolberg, O. L. Mangasarian, Multisurface method of pattern separation for medical diagnosis applied to breast cytology, *Proceedings of the Nat Acad Sci* **87**(990), 9193-9196.
[8]   C. L. Blake, C. J. Merz, UCI repository of machine learning databases, http://www.ics.uci.edu/~mlrepository.html. *University of California, Irvine, Dept. of Information and Computer Sciences*, 1998.
[9]   N. Japkowicz, S. J. Hanson, M. A. Gluck, Nonlinear autoassociation is not equivalent to PCA, *Neural Comp* **12**(3) (2000), 531-545.
[10] S. Russell, P. Norvig, *Artificial Intelligence: A Modern Approach,* Pearson, Upper Saddle River, New Jersey, 2010.
[11] S. S. Birring, M. D. Peake MD, Symptoms and early diagnosis of lung cancer, *Thorax* **60** (2005), 268-269.

International Perspectives in Health Informatics
E.M. Borycki et al. (Eds.)
IOS Press, 2011
© *2011 ITCH 2011 Steering Committee and IOS Press. All rights reserved.*
doi:10.3233/978-1-60750-709-3-274

From Complexity Theory to a Generalized Governance Model: A Practical Architectural Pattern for Health Care and Wellness Economies

Bogdan Motoc[a,1]
a Allied Bionics Inc., Cochrane, Alberta, Canada

Abstract. Using tools from the domain of Complexity Theory, the present paper offers a simple and intriguing modeling methodology for organizations and organizational ecosystems within the wellness and health care economy. The model is used to deliver a high usability cross-domain analysis tool, the driver for integrated social, business and technology architecture. The outcome of the proposed methodology consists of practical steps towards implementing evidence based governance within the given context of operation. Improved and multi-domain governance leads to higher efficiency and better integration of organization domains (culture, business and technology).

Keywords. complexity theory, autopoiesis, social systems, analysis, general systems theory, decomposition, integration, sustainability, kpi, governance, integration, models.

Introduction

Is the world today essentially different from what our forefathers used to live in? According to the Complexity Theory, the only difference resides in our ability to model the reality at its increasing rate of change. In complex self-producing systems, the rate of change has an exponential growth based on the two engines of evolutionary transformation – efficiency and functional agility.

Through time, the winning answer to the pressure of evolution has been a growth in complexity through specialization and integration. Within the domain of human culture, including scientific theories and products of technology, while specialization has benefitted of clear metrics of improvement, integration has lagged in progress due to its inherent need for cross-boundary expertise and validation, the need for somehow contradictory abilities to generalize while still having a good grasp of the detail.

Within the field of integration of specialized agencies, technology had most advances. Service Orientation is an architectural pattern that offers both specialization and ease of integration. Service Orientation brings a good grasp on governance. The domain of business follows, with more and more businesses using outsourcing, mergers, acquisitions and corporate splitting. The area that needs attention is culture.

---

[1] Bogdan Motoc, bogdanm@allied-bionics.com

We "do" culture for quite a while (1 million years or so) but we never had to integrate it with such aggressively changing domains like business and technology. While theories exist, there is no current accepted methodology to capture and model cultural aspects of a social group as part of an architectural effort to optimize an organization as a whole (social consistency, business effectiveness with optimal technological support in a dynamic, perpetual transformation).

This paper proposes a modeling technique for such complex systems that enables both simple and powerful analysis, modeling and integration of otherwise complex multi-dimensional aspects (cultural, business and technology) of an organization. As an exemplification, the paper brings practical examples from the wellness and health economies. The author puts together elements of Autopoiesis, Generalized Theory of Evolution, Constructal Theory, Living Systems Theory, Social Systems Theory, Viable System Model and Systems Control Theory aggregated to offer a method of identification of core relations and supporting infrastructure within an organization and its operating environment.

The proposed analysis, modeling and synthesis methodology is recursively applied to social agencies at increasing levels of social complexity (individual specialists, teams, departments, organizations, economies). It is the author's hope that the presented modeling approach will raise the interest of other researchers and practitioners to further explore and develop competing or symbiogenetic methods of analysis, decomposition and integration leading to the integrated improvement of culture, business and technology aspects within the domains of Wellness and Health Care (WHC), in support for a healthier society.

1. Methods and Supporting Theories

We will have a brief look at some of the core contributors of the methodology brought together in this paper.

1.1. Autopoiesis: The Pattern of Life

Coined as a term in the mid 1970's by Francisco Varela and Umberto Maturana, the term of autopoiesis identifies the main architectural pattern for living systems. Through its generality, novel perspective and implications, it has been and is instrumental to a series of offspring theories and hypotheses in biology, physiology, medical sciences, cognitive sciences, psychology, philosophy, business, social sciences, general systems theory to name just a few. The theory states that, for a system to be considered alive, it needs to fulfill the following conditions:

- To consist of a network of relations (chemical, biochemical or of an other nature)
- The relations shall be self-producing (the maintenance of the network is done by the network activity)
- The network should be distinguishable form the background (the network architecture should provide its identity)

While initially strictly limited to the biological domain, the generic definition for life has opened the use of the model in many non-biological domains of knowledge. For the purpose of this presentation, the domain of interest is social networks of organizations in the domain of wellness and health care.

Figure 1. An Iconic Representation Proposed by the Author for the Autopoietic Pattern.

In Figure 1, the ring symbolizes the recurrent pattern of self-production while the wiggly arrow suggests a generic flow through an open thermodynamic system.

1.2. Generalized Theory of Evolution: The Pseudo-purpose of Life

As presented so eloquently by Prof Dr. Richard Dawkins, the pressure of change in our ecosystem or, in lack of a better term, the "purpose" of life, consists of two goals: survival and growth.

It is these two goals that, through the webbing of specialization and integration, have led to the vast complexity of form and behavior that surrounds us. This aggregation of simple in complex is even more visible in the social activity for health preservation, where both social and health are compounding complex processes.

1.3. Constructal Theory: An Universal Pattern of Change

The core concept of the Constructal theory introduced by Prof. Dr. Adrian Bejan states: "for a finite-size flow system to persist in time (to live) it must evolve such that it provides greater and greater access to the currents that flow through it".

This theory, arguably competing for the IVth principle of Thermodynamics, points to a direction, a vector of change for all systems, biological and non-biological. Its use, in our context, is related to providing a metric of fitness, a vectorial kpi, of a composite agency in an ecosystem, or more specific, a basis for performance measurement of agencies, be they human, non-human or hybrid (ex: humans integrated with IT tools), within a given socio-economic context.

1.4. Living Systems Theory: The Universal Decomposition of Living Systems

Dr. James Grier Miller, an MD, as an outcome of his passionate work on General Systems Theory, proposed in 1978 a universal decomposition of living systems, biological or non-biological. His model provides a good pattern for an initial approach to decomposition of an organization. The model lists a set of 20 functional patterns identifiable in all living systems, with a higher or lesser contribution to the autopoiesis of the host.

A list of his functional components grouped in classes, includes:

- input/output components like boundary, ingestor, extruder, input and output transducers
- transport/distribution components like motor, distributor and channel with network
- processing components like producer, convertor, supporter, decoder/encoder and matter/energy storage
- coordination components like associator, memory, decider, timer, reproducer and internal transducer

1.5. Social Systems Theory: A Bio-mimetic Model for Organizations.

Working on the systemic path of thought, the general systems theory, the German sociologist, Nicklas Luhmann, identified social agencies, organizations, as obeying the autopoietic pattern of self-production. While his initial work pre-dates the publication of Autopoiesis, later refinements have brought the two theories to consistency.

Modern tools of relation analysis and visualization (Social Network Analysis – see Figure 2) 30+ years later, have illustrated the validity of his bio-mimetic model for Social Systems.

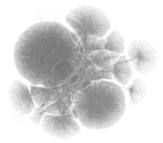

Figure 2. SNA Visualization of Inter-Employee Communication in an Organization.

2. Applying the Model

The specific of these complexity theory tools is their metaphoric character. By applying the models listed above to the domain of wellness and health care, analysts and architects can decompose, evaluate solutions and integrate **better** systems, with consistency and objectivity, avoiding the mudding impact of high detail in the early stages of analysis. The "better" qualifier is a multi-modal attribute spanning through cultural comfort, business sustainability and technological performance.

This author firmly believes that only such a multi-domain effort of analysis, modeling, architecture and evaluation can optimally lead to a sustainable transformation process, with measurable benefits, towards more efficient and agile organizations, with an effective societal role.

The specifics of wellness and health care economies multiply the complexity of social agencies (social activity within a business context) by the complexity of the inner biological functionality of our specie (as opposed to a machine repair shop).

The very simplified block diagram of the model, shown in Figure 3, represents an organization in continuous transformation, with two interdependent loops. One loop has fast iterations and is intended at defining the patterns and change in patters specific to the organization's internal components. The second loop deals with governance adjustments at the organization level for a sustainable relation with the ecosystem the organization is part of. Both loops have to obey the Nyquist systemic requirement for control.

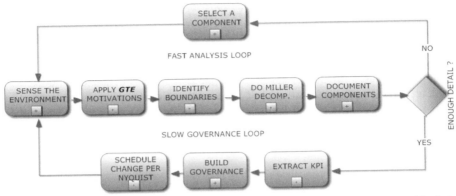

Figure 3. High level workflow diagram of the proposed method.

In a wellness and health care (WHC) organization context, these components can materialize as departments (cardiology, neurology, obstetrics/gynecology and so on), teams, individuals or even procedures (short lived patterns of social collaboration). Due to space limitations, out of the 20 Miller components, the author touches just the boundary related components as follows:

- Boundary – the component that delimits the network defining the agency from a certain point of view; WHC context – the scope of a hospital or practice, physical or virtual, that includes patients, specialists, technology, buildings and so on.
- Interface Transducers - sensorial components that trigger internal processes; WHC context – R&D, needs for health care assistance, wellness program opportunities
- Ingestor - component mediating incoming flow through boundary; WHC example is the Admission procedure.
- Extruder - component mediating outgoing flow through boundary; WHC example would be Discharge and Transfer procedures
- Actuator- component enabling migration of living agency to better survival environments; WHC functions of strategy planning, marketing, public awareness programs, anything that changes the boundary of the organization.

This decomposition is applied to an ecosystem containing the following wellness and health care agencies:

- Consumer/patient (the consumer of wellness and health services including its public interfaces as caregivers and/or legal guardians)
- medical specialty agency (includes all health and wellness specialists, other health management related technologies including IT, research and education)
- societal agency (all activities leading to maximization of societal value of the WHC service)
- business agency (all activities securing sustainability of wellness and health care activities, supporting technologies, investment motivation and financial risk mitigation)
- pharmaceutical agency (pharmaceutical products, clinical trials)
- biotechnology (diagnostic, visualization and devices)

For each of these components, the presentation proposes a method of discovery of KPIs relevant to the sustainability of the organization (efficiency and transformational agility) expanding through the domains of culture, business and technology, in support of evidence based governance.

The accent on governance improvement in this presentation is anchored in the belief of the author that, at present time, the maturity of the specialization in the WHC industry is higher than the maturity of the integration process. This unbalance can be addressed by a systemic, evidence based, cross-domain, governance approach.

3. Conclusions

The analysis, modeling and architecture (synthesis) of Wellness and Health Care organizations is a complex endeavor. Modern tools brought to the community by the Complexity Theory enable novel, better adapted approaches. Current paper proposes such an integrated model in support for a systemic decomposition, analysis and integration (synthesis) of a sustainable organization. Future steps include complete models with identification of attributes vital to sustainability, in support for an evidence based organizational architecture and governance process.

References

[1] H. Maturana, F. Varela. *Autopoiesis and Cognition: the Realization of the Living*, D. Reidel Publishing Co., Dordrecht, 1978

[2] L. von Bertalanffy, An outline of General Systems Theory, *British Journal for the Philosophy of Science*, 1950, 134–165.

[3] J. G. Miller, *Living systems*, McGraw-Hill, New York, 1978

[4] N. Luhmann, *Social Systems*, Stanford University Press, Palo Alto ,1995

[5] R. Dawkins, *The Selfish Gene*, Oxford University Press, Oxford, 1976

[6] S. Beer, *Cybernetic and Management*, English Universities Press, London, 1959

[7] S. Beer, *Brain of the Firm*, The Penguin Press, London, 1972

[8] K. Stephenson, *The Quantum Theory of Trust: Power, Networks and the Secret Life of Organisations*, New York Times Press, Manhattan, 1996

[9] A. Bejan, *Constructal Theory of Social Dynamics*, Springer Publishing Co., New York, 1996

[10] M. Csikszentmihalyi, *Good Business: Leadership, Flow, and the Making of Meaning*, Penguin Publishing, London, 2003

[11] F. Varela, *The Embodied Mind: Cognitive Science and Human Experience*, MIT Press, Cambridge, 1993.

International Perspectives in Health Informatics
E.M. Borycki et al. (Eds.)
IOS Press, 2011
© 2011 ITCH 2011 Steering Committee and IOS Press. All rights reserved.
doi:10.3233/978-1-60750-709-3-280

Who's Users? Participation and Empowerment in Socio-Technical Approaches to Health IT Developments

Andre W. KUSHNIRUK[a], Paul TURNER[b]

[a]School of Health Information Science, University of Victoria, Victoria, Canada

[b]eHealth Services Research Group(eHSRG), CIS, University of Tasmania, Australia

Abstract. Health informatics researchers advocating socio-technical approaches to the design, implementation and evaluation of health information technology (HIT) consistently promote the important role of users. Aside from conventional ethical and legal considerations around their involvement, there are a number of philosophical and methodological issues that have received less attention because of the tendency for researchers to assume the term 'user' is well defined and understood. It is however, evident that there are significant differences amongst users, and differences in how researchers engage, involve and interact with them during health IT developments. Failure to acknowledge these differences and their impact on Health IT developments makes comparisons across different studies problematic and raises fundamental questions about participation and empowerment of end-users in our developments. This paper re-examines the term user in the context of socio-technical approaches to HIT and presents a preliminary approach to differentiating between types of users and our changing expectations of their roles in enhancing different HIT projects across design, implementation and evaluation.

Keywords. socio-technical design, user-centered design, system design and evaluation.

Introduction: Bridging the Knowledge Gap

Acceptance within academic and business circles that approaches involving users are valuable for informing the design, development and implementation of health information systems highlights the maturation of user-centred approaches. These approaches have been shown to enhance technology adoption and use by influencing developments in ways that increase users' satisfaction, trust and ease of use with particular applications/technologies/systems. Beyond these successes however, there remains some concern about the process of translation from the user insights generated through socio-technical analysis to the health information systems that are finally produced and implemented. How users are defined, engaged and their participation mediated by health information technology (HIT) projects may relegate the rich insights advocated to simply adjuncts of conventional usability testing. Without care in analysis, opportunities to open up genuine dialogue on innovative ways of thinking, designing and empowering may be marginalised [1]. These 'failures in translation' are partly because many HIT developments are too often uncritically framed as problems with technological solutions. It is also evident that while 'lip-service' to user- and/or patient-centred approaches are common, business/career imperatives strongly encourage and/or reward developers for feature and functional complexity whether users require it or not. More prosaically, there is always the risk that in the name of technical, financial or other factors research insights end-up being used to subvert, marginalise or even obscure the very 'user' issues they identify [2].

In the health care domain, socio-technical approaches have been strongly advocated in the development of health information systems. Following Berg et al. these approaches argue for the importance of users and share a number of common starting points including that: '(i) health care work is seen as a social, 'real life' phenomenon guided by a practical rationality that can only be overlooked at a high price (i.e. failed systems), (ii) technological innovation is a social process, in which organizations are deeply affected, (iii) in-depth, formative evaluation, of these approaches can help improve system design and implementation.' [3].

Involving users in HIT research and development is clearly complex and difficult. In order to make the rich insights that can be obtained from socio-technical analysis applicable and useful in the lifecycle of health information systems, we argue that greater consideration of who the user is and how the user is involved and their inputs mediated needs to be further articulated [4]. To address these issues it is useful to try to be more precise about who the users are, when and where they are engaged, what expectations we have about our users and why.

This paper re-examines the term user in the context of socio-technical approaches to Health IT to draw out the complex and dynamic interplay between social, cultural, political and technical factors available for observation and analysis. This work is part of a larger research program aimed at helping to provide aid and assistance to developers and designers of systems when contemplating the selection and role of users in complex healthcare information systems projects. Towards this end, we have developed an initial framework for considering the user in socio-technical design.

1. Towards a Framework for Considering the "User" in HIT

There are several dimensions in our framework for considering users in socio-technical design described below. The first dimension is consideration of the important question of exactly "who is the user"?

1.1. Who is the User?

Socio-technical approaches and in particular participatory design have rightly taken into account the important role of the potential users of a system in the design process itself [5]. However, this has also lead to complexity and blurring of the distinction between design and evaluation when considering and envisaging who the user of the system will be and how to recruit representative users (who will also serve in the design process itself).

In contrast to more strictly prescribed subject identification approaches used in some methodologies (such as usability testing) [6], where detailed target user profiles are created to delineate classes of potential users who will be "sampled" during such system testing), in socio-technical design a restricted number of users (restricted due to issues of practicality) may be engaged to serve both as representatives of the end user community, and participate in the design process itself. This complicates important decisions regarding exactly which classes of users will participate in the design and which users will be the target for the completed system and its evaluation.

This is particularly true in the case of healthcare IT where the range and distinctions among possible user types are potentially greater than in other organizational domains. In addition to wide possible variance in demographics (e.g. age, sex, computer literacy) healthcare brings in variance due to specialty, nature of healthcare (e.g. chronic versus acute) and considerable local, regional, and national practice variation [7].

We also need to consider who the user is in terms of motivation, (i.e. whether they are altruistic (volunteers), self-selecting participants (leading to a range of possible biases), mandated users by their employers and/or whether they receive remuneration for use [8]. Each of these distinctions has important implications for the meaning of the results obtained from the participation of the users regarding how generalizable the results from any one set of subjects will be.

1.2. What Expectations are There in Relation to Users?

The role of potential users and what researchers expect from them during the design and evaluation process of the systems development cycle is also an implicit assumption that is often left unexplored by those advocating socio-technical approaches to the development of HIT. Given the importance that is associated with the "user" it would seem to be critical for the success of our studies and development work that there is an explicit articulation of researcher expectation. Unfortunately, this poses its own problems, including how, and to what extent researcher communications about his/her expectations of users, impacts on the outcomes. Clearly the role of the user will also depend to a great extent on the software development methodology employed as there are marked differences in the involvement required between, for example, extreme programming and agile methodologies as compared to more conventional system development methods.

Beyond this it would also seem sensible to consider in detail the motivations and expectations held by users. As Heaven et al. have argued in the context of health trials 'participants bring their own coherent models of understanding about trial participation' [9]. It seems likely that this is also the case for users involved in the health IT developments and that this has an impact on the results and outcomes from our studies that requires further consideration. This is particularly the case given that the result of most IT developments involves a change of behaviour that goes beyond participation and into engagement, similar in some ways to that expected of patients who participate in health behaviour modification trials [10].

1.3. When do We Engage the User?

The complex issue of when to bring in different types of users to the design, development and evaluation processes can be considered in our framework within the context of the basic activities common to all system development lifecycles, whether they adopt a traditional approach, a socio-technical approach or whether a more flexible iterative agile approach is utilised.

We therefore consider the question of when to engage users in the activity of early design and system envisagement, requirements gathering and modeling, design and testing of early and late prototypes, and testing of early releases of a new healthcare system/application/service. The intent of each of these different activities has important implications for who we select as users, what we expect of them, and when they appear during the overall design, development, testing and evaluation processes. Some approaches to system development, for example extreme programming, have very specific recommendations regarding when and for how long to engage users [13]. In contrast socio-technical approaches are less explicit about this and its potential impact on the results of the user studies are often less well-defined.

One perspective for considering when to engage different types of users involves consideration of the stages that healthcare IT projects go through as this will have important implications for choosing the type, number and role of users to be engaged in system design and development. One potentially useful approach here is to consider these decisions along the continuum of the System Development Life Cycle (SDLC) [11]. When considered within the context of the SDLC, we can develop a more explicit analysis of the type of users we may need to engage and their potential role [12]. For example, in the early system planning and envisagement stages, criteria for selection of type of users (and also consideration of the number of users) that are needed to aid in design processes may differ from later in the SDLC, e.g. during the detailed design process, or later yet, during beta-testing and through to final system release. Both socio-technical and user-centered design processes and activities need to keep this consideration in mind when "engaging the user", as for complex healthcare system design, this may involve engaging multiple classes of users, at multiple stages in system development, and for multiple purposes. These considerations further highlight the complexity of 'user-studies' and their roles in HIT developments.

It is also evident that rarely do our studies recognize and/or respond to the impact on users of extended participation in our approaches. Co-design, user-engagement and iterative feedback are potentially useful processes for obtaining important insights. They do however run the risk of a kind of 'Hawthorn Effect' or in extreme cases a 'Stockholm Syndrome' whereby our users become overly willing to reflect back to us our own biases and expectations. The key question here is not whether this happens but rather how should we remain sensitive to it when it occurs and how should we accommodate it in our analyses.

1.4. Where do We Engage Users?

Consideration of where we engage users obviously depends on the design methodology chosen but there are a number of emerging trends, including the move towards examination of user goals, understanding and complex workflow (particularly in HIT) in-situ within the rich social and cultural milieu of the workplace. Traditional approaches to evaluation of user needs and requirements within artificial settings, fixed usability laboratories and meeting room locations (for holding participatory design focus groups) has lead to a move towards interviewing and interacting with users within rich cognitive and social settings, including use of more realistic simulations and within the actual healthcare environment itself. Consideration of the impact of naturalistic recording however also requires careful understanding of when users' behaviours are truly natural and users are not responding to the "lens".

Recent work has argued for implementing highly unobtrusive recording devices and the running of extended baseline recording periods prior to analyzing data collected using such ethnographic techniques [12]. In addition, the level and extent of intrusion introduced in the environment by the analysis varies from extremes of direct participant observation to use of highly unobtrusive and "invisible" recording methods (not covert surveillance). This may lead to requirements for formal opt-in and op-out agreements with users as the move to unobtrusive naturalistic analysis continues.

1.5. Why Engage Users?

Ultimately we must ask what our intentions are in engaging users in design and development at each stage in the process of envisaging, designing, implementing and deploying healthcare IT systems. Furthermore, the reason for working with users will vary along each of the dimensions described above. This may lead to the need to consider involving a greater variety, number and range of users to participate throughout the life-cycle of the system development. However, it is likely that this will actually involve the identification of users most appropriate to different development activities when considered along the entire timeline from early project planning through to deployment, beta testing and full-scale release. This in-turn potentially increases the research burden for those engaging in user- or patient-centred systems developments.

2. Conclusions

Health informatics researchers deploying socio-technical and related approaches to the design, implementation and evaluation of health IT need to ensure that in promoting the importance of users in their work, they ensure that the who, what, where, when and why of those involved is articulated explicitly. Significant differences amongst users, and differences in how researchers engage, involve and interact with them during health IT developments makes comparisons across different studies problematic and raises fundamental questions about participation and empowerment of end-users our IT developments. Issues related to identification of the role of users at different stages of system development warrant careful consideration. Engagement of a limited number of users through participatory design (i.e. due to practical constraints related to optimal size of design teams [13]) needs to be considered in the context of the generalizability of the design decisions made through their engagement. On the other hand, user involvement in user-centered evaluation processes, where the role of the user is more circumscribed, need to be better integrated with participatory design processes.

This paper has presented our thoughts towards an initial framework for considering the user in healthcare system design. It is anticipated that the considerations described in this paper will assist researchers to more accurately distinguish among types of users in their work and to be more explicit about researcher expectations of their roles in enhancing different health IT projects across design, implementation and evaluation.

We would argue that such consideration will ultimately be necessary for more effective engagement and empowerment of Health IT users.

References

[1]   S. Gasson, Human-centered vs. user-centered approaches to information systems design. *J Inf Tech Theory App* **5**(2) (2003), 29-46.

[2]   S. Kujala, User Involvement: A review of the benefits and challenges. *Behav Inform Tech* **22**(1) (2003), 1-16.

[3]   M. Berg, J. Aarts, J. Van der Lei, ICT in health care: Sociotechnical approaches, *Meth Inf Med* **42**(4) (2003), 297-301.

[4]   J. A. Kelder, P. Turner, People, places and things: Leveraging insights from distributed cognition theory to enhance the user-centered design of meteorological information systems. *JITTA* **7**(1) (2005), 77-92.

[5]   E.B.N. Sanders, From user-centered to participatory design approaches, In *Design and the Social Sciences*. J.Frascara (Ed.), Taylor & Francis Books Limited, 2002.

[6]   D. Hinderer, Challenges in participant recruiting for usability testing, *Annual Conference of the IEEE Professional Communication Society*, IPCC98' Proceedings, 1998.

[7]   A. Maynard (ed). *The public-private mix for health: Plus ça change! Plus ca meme chose!* Nuffield Trust, London, 2004.

[8]   W. W. Cotterman, K. Kumar, User cube: A taxonomy of end-users, *Comm ACM* **32**(11) (1989), 1313-20.

[9]   B. Heaven, M. Murtagh, T. Rapley, C. May, R. Graham, E. Kaner et al, Patients or research subjects? A qualitative study of participation in a randomised controlled trial of a complex intervention. *Patient Educ Counsel,* **62** (2006), 1485-1494.

[10]   U. Felt, M. D. Bister, M. Strassnig, U. Wagner, Refusing the information paradigm: informed consent, medical research, and patient participation. *Health: An Interdisc J* **13** (2009), 87-106.

[11]   A. W. Kushniruk, Evaluation in the design of health information systems: Applications of approaches emerging from systems engineering. *Comp Bio Med* **32**(3) (2002), 141-149.

[12]   A. W. Kushniruk, V. L. Patel, Cognitive and usability engineering approaches to the evaluation of clinical information systems. *J Biomed Inf* **37**(1) (2004), 56-57.

[13]   S. McConnell, *Rapid development: Taming wild software schedules.* Redmond Washington: Microsoft Press, 1996.

International Perspectives in Health Informatics
E.M. Borycki et al. (Eds.)
IOS Press, 2011
© *2011 ITCH 2011 Steering Committee and IOS Press. All rights reserved.*
doi:10.3233/978-1-60750-709-3-286

Grounded Theory Evolution and Its Application in Health Informatics

Elizabeth CUMMINGS [a,1], Elizabeth M. BORYCKI [b]

[a] *eHealth Services Research Group, CIS, University of Tasmania, Hobart, Australia*
[b] *School of Health Information Science, University of Victoria,*
Victoria, British Columbia, Canada

Abstract. The value of utilising qualitative research approaches to identify, describe and evaluate the impact of health information systems upon healthcare processes is becoming increasingly clear. The use of grounded theory has increased over the past decade within the health informatics discipline. However, for researchers new to the approach, the theory and conduct of grounded theory can be both confusing and daunting. This paper begins to dispel some misconceptions about the use of grounded theory and aims to assist researchers starting out using grounded theory in health informatics research. It also discusses the past and potential future application of grounded theory in health informatics.

Keywords. grounded theory, evaluation, methodologies

Introduction

In health informatics there exist a number of qualitative methods that can be used to identify, describe and evaluate the impact of health information systems (HIS) upon healthcare processes. Qualitative approaches that are frequently employed by health informatics researchers include ethnography, grounded theory and case study research. Grounded theory, as a qualitative approach, has been found to be especially effective in identifying and describing the impact of HIS upon health care processes especially in cases where the impacts of HIS and their associated devices (e.g. palm devices) are as yet un-discovered or are not easily described by quantitative approaches [1]. Methodologically, grounded theory's use in health informatics has evolved since its introduction to this field of research in the early 1990's [e.g. 2]. In this paper the researchers will: review the historic and theoretical origins of grounded theory; discuss the evolution of grounded theory and theory generation; reflect upon the challenges and processes involved in using grounded theory; and discuss the evolution of grounded theory use in information systems research and health informatics.

---

[1] Corresponding Author; Elizabeth Cummings, eHealth Services Research Group, School of Computing and Information Systems, University of Tasmania, Private Bag 87, Hobart, Tasmania, Australia 7001. Email: Elizabeth.Cummings@utas.edu.au.

1. Historic and Theoretical Origins of Grounded Theory

Grounded theory was developed as a methodology by sociologists. Its theoretical origins can be traced back to the literature on symbolic interactionism and the work of Mead [2]. Symbolic interactionism espouses the view that individuals develop a sense of self through their interactions with others [2]. In 1969 extensions to symbolic interactionism (see Blumer [3]) proposed that the meanings individuals and groups ascribe to things influence how they react to these objects in their environment. Individuals and groups who ascribe meanings to these objects also do so through their interactions with others. These interactions, in turn, shape and alter an individual's or group's interpretation of objects, events or situations. Therefore, grounded theory attempts to: (a) determine how individuals derive meaning (i.e. meaning from experienced objects, events and situations), (b) describe those objects, events and situations, and (c) describe how these meanings guide individual and/or group behaviours, actions and their experiences of the consequences of these actions. Grounded theory can therefore be described as a methodology that aims to understand how individuals and groups interact, act and engage in response to phenomena (i.e. objects, events and situations) they experience or encounter in their everyday lives. It is within this context that theory is developed that describes these underlying social processes and researchers conduct this work to better understand these processes [4].

2. Evolution of Grounded Theory and Theory Generation

Over the past several decades grounded theory as a methodology has evolved since its initial inception in the general sociology literature. In the early 1960's grounded theory was initially associated with a positivist epistemology using quantitative data [5]. However, researchers observed that grounded theory provided "a logically consistent set of data collection and analysis procedures aimed to develop theory" [6:245]. Therefore, the approaches to coding that underlie grounded theory methods developed as key processes that researchers could undertake to systematically reduce and categorize data. Coding in grounded theory provided a link between the raw empirical data gathered by researchers and theoretical concepts that emerged from the data [7]. It is through the process of researcher identification of patterns in the data and analysis of these patterns empirically that theory can be developed [8,9]. In order for a researcher to be able to create theory the chain of evidence used in the analysis needs to be described precisely. This means the researcher must show how classification, theme identification and the linking of key properties occurs.

Since this work there has emerged a debate regarding the conflicting assumptions of the inherent positivist or interpretivist philosophical position of grounded theory (see [10, 11]) and this has affected how researchers conduct data analysis in grounded theory. Glaser suggested Strauss and Corbin's [4] coding and analytical method (as described above) forced issues or problems to emerge. The precise process of coding has been a point of contention between Glaser and Strauss. Both Glaser [12] and Strauss and Corbin [4] describe coding as an essential aspect of transforming raw data into theoretical constructions of social processes [13]. However, Glaser [12] distinguishes between two types of coding, substantive (open) and theoretical, whereas Strauss and Corbin [4] define three levels, open, axial and selective coding. Essentially open and substantive coding, and theoretical and selective coding are considered similar, making axial coding the point at which the two approaches diverge [13]. Many researchers have entered into this debate. For example, Parker and Roffey [14] suggested that Strauss and Corbin's approach provided a structured approach to data analysis, whereas Glaser's approach is often considered more difficult to operationalise. Strauss and Corbin seemed to offer more procedural advice than Glaser [14].

There has also emerged as a debate as to whether prior theoretical ideas should be set aside prior to coding the data. Some methodologists such as Creswell [15] and Dey [16] espouse the view that grounded theory aims to generate or discover a theory. In their work both Creswell and Dey suggested there is a need to set aside other theoretical ideas to allow for a substantive theory to emerge from the data. The theory generated through this method usually focuses on how individuals interact with the phenomenon under investigation and attempts to expose plausible relationships between concepts and sets of concepts that emerge from the data. In this view of grounded theory a range of data is acquired by the researcher through the conduct of fieldwork including, but not restricted to, interviews, observations and documents. Subsequent data analysis is systematic, iterative and commences as soon as data are available. Concepts are developed and refined through the analysis and constant comparison of new and old data. Alternatively, other researchers have suggested prior theoretical knowledge may be brought to bear in the process of coding.

3. The Challenges to Using Grounded Theory

As a result, there are a number of challenges associated with using grounded theory. Firstly, there appears to be an internal conflict with the process of "setting aside theoretical ideas". However, this does not mean that the researcher can separate from previous theoretical knowledge but that they should not be restricted by their previous knowledge and so fail to question their existing assumptions or impose preconceived ideas on the data. This process can particularly be at odds with the academic world where some researchers consider it to be a less rigorous method. The truth is that "grounded theory is by definition a rigorous approach" requiring significant time, a chain of analysis, and the relating of findings back to other theories [17]. Secondly, one characteristic of research employing grounded theory is that often there is only a problem area identified at the commencement of the research. This can be confusing for researchers new to the approach. This is the reason why grounded theory is so well suited to the examination of processes rather than commencing with fixed research questions. Here, the research questions are developed and iteratively refined as an outcome of the open coding process. Glaser [12:25] notes that 'out of open coding.., theoretical sampling and analyzing by constant comparison emerge a focus for the research'. This process can be in conflict with the "scientific" requirements within the health informatics research community. The third challenge is confusion over the philosophical basis of grounded theory. In grounded theory, segments or slices of data are examined thereby providing researchers with expanded opportunities for data gathering. This includes the opportunity to employ different data types, data collection techniques, and to analyse the data to explore "different views or vantage points from which to understand a category and to develop its properties" [8:65]. This is not supported by the facts [18]. Consistent with Klein and Meyers [19] and Olson [20] qualitative methods can be used in any underlying epistemology and so grounded theory can be influenced by researchers from any epistemological stance [21]. Glaser [22] provided the following assertion: "Let me be clear. Grounded theory is a general method. It can be used on any data or combination of data." So the authors assert that irrespective of the research paradigm they are using health informatics researchers can safely use grounded theory approaches to analyse research data using any philosophical stance as long as they are systematic and clear about the method undertaken and the assumptions underpinning them.

4. Evolution of Grounded Theory in Information Systems Research

It is interesting and worthy to note, information systems researchers have suggested that the procedures outlined in grounded theory should be thought of as rules of thumb, rather than hard or fixed rules - and has advised researchers to study these rules of thumb, use them, and *modify* them in accordance with the requirements of the research. Thus, increasingly grounded theory is being used more flexibly and treated as a set of guidelines rather than a structured methodology in the field of information systems research [18,23]. Increasingly information systems researchers are using a hybrid of both Strauss and Corbin's and Glaser's coding approaches. These researchers have adopted a hybrid approach to assist with data reduction and organisation. To illustrate Strauss and Corbin's three phase approach of open, axial and selective coding, is acknowledged by information systems researchers as a useful technique for breaking down and organising the data. However, some researchers have exercised caution when imposing the 'coding paradigm' advocated by Strauss and Corbin [4] rather than allowing theory to emerge [18]. So information system researchers have combined these approaches with the original concepts of constant comparison to provide a balance. The three-stage coding process has evolved as a result into the following commonly adopted steps:

1. **Open Coding** - reducing the voluminous data into more manageable chunks though the assignment of codes to passages within the data;
2. **Axial Coding** - comparing the open codes and identifying relationships between the codes so that categories emerge. This process facilitates building connections within categories; and
3. **Selective Coding** - the process of selecting and identifying the core category and systematically relating it to other categories. It involves validating the relationships, filling in, and refining and developing those categories. At this point, the researcher synthesizes or makes sense of the findings, and this forms the basis of theory discovery from data, as argued by Glaser and Strauss [8].

When employing a grounded theory approach a vital step in the development of theory from the data is using theoretical (or analytical) memos and integrative diagrams [4,12,24,25]. Through the use of these tools, whenever a researcher has an idea during coding, they write a memo to develop the ideas. "Memos are the theorizing write-up of ideas about codes and relationships as they strike the analyst while coding" [25:83]. They are recorded throughout the coding process as a way of fixing impressions of what was going on, and are written at the same time as, or as close as possible to, data collection and analysis in order to retain a fresh impression.

5. Grounded Theory in Health Informatics

Qualitative researchers were the first to have employed grounded theory in health informatics. These studies were conducted by researchers who wanted to obtain a better understanding of the underlying reasons for HIS successes and failures as quantitative studies were unable to do so [26]. Grounded theory, as a methodology, was therefore able to illuminate some of the factors that affect HIS success or failure. For example, in a series of studies Ash and colleagues [27, 28] documented the issues and factors that affect the diffusion of innovations such as physician order entry in hospital settings. Grounded theory has been used to identify key themes associated with the diffusion of innovations and the findings from these studies have been interpreted within the context of existing frameworks such as classical Diffusion of Innovations Theory [e.g. 27]. Such work has been essential to informing the field of health informatics about the success factors associated with some types of information systems [28] and has been used to inform system implementers about factors they must consider when implementing such systems in healthcare organizations [27,28]. In other works grounded theory has been used in an attempt to better understand how health professionals (e.g. physicians and nurses) derive meaning from their interactions with HIS and devices in health care settings. Here, researchers have attempted to understand and develop models that describe the interactions between the health professional and the social system within the context of the organization where they conduct work. More specifically, they have documented how these interactions influenced health professional perceptions of the technology, their subsequent interactions with the technology (including their decisions to adopt the health information system). For example, Peute et al. [29] investigated the human, social and organizational issues involved in implementing physician order entry. In this work the researchers not only identified lessons learned and recommendations on how to manage these issues but they outlined their work within a conceptual model that could be used to understand the impacts of physician order entry involving a laboratory system upon aspects of health professional work (e.g. workflow) [29]. In these studies researchers have developed or used theoretical frameworks to describe how health information systems are adopted [26] and the factors that influence their adoption from a human, social and organizational perspective [26,27,28,29]. Having demonstrated the ability of grounded theory to provide a greater understanding of the factors that affect the implementation process as well as the implementation process itself these researchers have used grounded theory to develop models and frameworks that can be used to guide practitioners in the real-world [27,28,29]. In the process these health informatics researchers have widened the use of this methodology in health informatics.

In health informatics one of the most powerful and emergent uses of grounded theory as a methodology has been its application to the development of frameworks, models and theories that form the basis for ontologies and models for HIS design [30, 31]. The application of grounded theory by Kuziemsky and colleagues has proven to be a useful and significant area of work [30,31]. The researcher has successfully developed ontologies that were later implemented during the development of HIS. Evaluations of the HIS developed using these ontologies have been positive among the user community (e.g. physician and nurses) [30, 31]. Health informatics as a research discipline has been informed by both the social sciences and information systems research where grounded theory is concerned. In the social science grounded theory has traditionally been used in a very structured manner. More recently, information systems and health informatics researchers have begun to use the method more flexibly (see for example [11,18]). This has encouraged the use of grounded theory methods for broader applications within the discipline. The use of grounded theory methods can positively contribute to improving not only the evaluation phases of implementations but can be used for specification identification and development. To illustrate, research by Cummings and Turner [32] demonstrated that grounded theory could be used to not only learn about the experiences of users of a new HIS, but could be used to determine the potential outcomes of implementing such systems. Here, such information could be used to inform future systems development as well as modifications to existing systems to improve software quality.

Grounded Theory, as a methodology, has led to significant changes in the way HIS are designed, developed, implemented and evaluated in the health informatics community. Initially, grounded theory challenged the accepted primacy of the use of randomised control trials and other quantitative methods as the primary approach to evaluating HIS, demonstrating its value and ability to undercover the underlying factors that influence HIS success or failure. Today grounded theory is emerging as a methodology that can be used to gather requirements, develop ontologies, and develop systems (in addition to) being used as an evaluation approach. Further to this, grounded theory has allowed researchers to develop empirically based models and frameworks that can be used to guide systems design and implementation. Therefore, grounded theory is coming of age as a research methodology and tool to be used by health informatics professionals.

6. Conclusions

Researchers and health informatics professionals are increasingly using grounded theory. However, there is a need to further encourage the increased and appropriate use of grounded theory as it is emerging as a powerful methodology to be used in the design, development, implementation and evaluation of HIS. This paper has presented: a review of the historic and theoretical origins of grounded theory; discussed the evolution of grounded theory and theory generation; reflected upon the emergence of grounded theory as a powerful methodology; and discussed the evolution of grounded theory use in information systems research and health informatics. This is not an exhaustive review of the method or a full explanation of the processes involved in grounded theory but it offers some exploration of the current uses of grounded theory. The authors remain convinced that what is required is an easy navigation tool for students and new researchers in the processes involved in qualitative research using grounded theory. The authors offer a final word of caution, using grounded theory for data analysis is very time consuming. The researcher needs to be prepared to spend many months immersed in their data.

References

[1] B. Kaplan, P.F. Brennan, A. F. Dowling, C. P. Friedman, V. Peel, Towards an informatics research agenda. Key people and organizational issues. *JAMIA* **8**(3) (2001), 235-241.
[2] G. H. Mead, *Mind, self, and society*. Chicago: The University of Chicago Press, 1934.

[3] H. Blumer, *Symbolic Interactions.* Englewood Cliffs, California, 1969.

[4] A. L. Strauss, J, Corbin. *Basics of qualitative research: Grounded theory procedures and techniques.* Thousand Oaks, California: Sage Publications, 1990.

[5] B. G. Glaser. *Organizational Scientists: Their professional careers.* Indianapolis: The Bobbs-Merrill Company Inc, 1964.

[6] K. Charmaz. In: N.K. Denzin, Y.S. Lincoln editors. *The American Tradition in Qualitative Research, Vol. II.* London: Sage Publications, 2001.

[7] J. Seidel, U. Kelle. Different functions of coding in the analysis of textual data. In: U. Kelle editor. *Computer-aided Qualitative Data Analysis: Theory, Methods, and Practice.* Thousand Oaks, CA: Sage Publications, 1995.

[8] B. G. Glaser, A. Strauss. *The Discovery of Grounded Theory: Strategies for Qualitative Research.* Chicago, IL: Aldine Publishing Co, 1967.

[9] P.Y. Martin, B. A. Turner, *J Applied Behav Sci* **22** (1986), 141-157.

[10] A. Bryant, Re-grounding Grounded Theory. *J Inform Tech Theory Applic* **4**(1) (2002), 25-42.

[11] C. Urquhart, Regrounding Grounded Theory - Or Reinforcing Old Prejudices? A Brief Reply to Bryant. *J Inform Tech Theory Applic* **4**(3) (2002), 43-54.

[12] B. G. Glaser. *Basics of Grounded Theory Analysis: Emergence vs. Forcing.* Mill Valley, CA: Sociology Press, 1992.

[13] J. Kendall, Axial coding and the grounded theory controversy. *W J Nurs Res* **21**(6) (1999), 743–757.

[14] L. Parker, B. Roffey. Methodological themes back to the drawing board: revisiting grounded theory and the everyday accountant's and manager's reality. *Acc Aud Acc* **10**(2) (1997), 212-247.

[15] Cresswell JW. *Qualitative Inquiry and Research Design: Choosing Among Five Traditions.* London: Sage Publications, 1998.

[16] I. Dey. *Grounding Grounded Theory.* CA: Academic Press, 1999.

[17] C. Urquhart. In: E.M. Trauth, editor. *Qualitative Research in IS: Issues and Trends.* Hershey, PA: Idea Group Publishing, 2001.

[18] C. Urquhart, W. Fernandez. *Grounded Theory Method: The Researcher as Blank Slate and Other Myths.* ICIS 2006 Proceedings, Paper 3, 2006.

[19] H. K. Klein, M. D. Myers, A set of principles for conducting and evaluating interpretive field studies in information systems. *MIS Quart, Spec Issue Inten Res* **23**(1), (1999).

[20] H. Olson. Qualitative "versus" quantitative research: the wrong question. *CAIS/ACSI 95, Annual Conference of the Canadian Association for Information Science, Connectedness: Information, Systems, People, Organizations*, Edmonton, Alberta, 7-10 June 1995.

[21] K. Charmaz, *Constructing Grounded Theory: A Practical Guide Through Qualitative Analysis.* Thousand Oaks, CA: Sage Publications, 2006.

[22] B. G. Glaser. *The Future of Grounded Theory. Qual H Res* **9**(1) (1999), 836–845.

[23] C. Urqhart, R. A. Currell, P. J. Wainwright, Evidence-based policy making in health informatics: indications from systematic reviews of nursing record systems and telemedicine. *H Inf J*, **6**(4) (2000), 204-211.

[24] A. Strauss, *Qualitative Analysis for Social Scientists.* Cambridge: Cambridge University Press, 1987.

[25] B. G. Glaser, *Theoretical Sensitivity: Advances in the Methodology of Grounded Theory.* Mill Valley, CA: Sociology Press, 1978.

[26] B. Kaplan, N.T. Shaw, Future directions in evaluation research: People, organizational and social issues. *Meth Inf Med* 43(3) (2004), 215-231.

[27] J.S. Ash, L. Lyman, J. Carpenter, L. Fournier. A diffusion of innovations model of physician order entry. *Proceedings of the Am Med Infor Assoc Symp* (2001), pp. 22-6.

[28] Ash JS, Chin HL, Sittig DF, Dykstra DF. Ambulatory computerized physician order entry implementation. *Proceedings of the Am Med Inf Assoc Symp* (2005), pp. 11-5.

[29] L. W. Peute, J. Aarts, P. J. Bakker, M. W. Jaspers. Anatomy of a failure: A sociotechnical evaluation of a laboratory physician order entry system implementation. *Int J Med Inf* **79**(4), e58-70.

[30] C. E. Kuziemsky, F. Lau. A four stage approach for ontology-based health information system design. *Art Intel Med* (2010).

[31] C. E. Kuziemsky, J. H. Weber-Jahnke, F. Lau, G. F. Downing, An interdisciplinary computer-based information tool for palliative severe pain management. *JAMIA* **15**(3) (2008), 374-82.

[32] E. Cummings, P. Turner. Patient self-management and chronic illness: Evaluating outcomes and impact of information technology. *Stud Health Tech Inform* **143** (2009), 229-34.

International Perspectives in Health Informatics
E.M. Borycki et al. (Eds.)
IOS Press, 2011
doi:10.3233/978-1-60750-709-3-293

Use of Qualitative Methods Across the Software Development Lifecycle in Health Informatics

Elizabeth M. BORYCKI[a,1], Mowafa HOUSEH[c],
Andre W. KUSHNIRUK[a], Craig KUZIEMSKY[b]

[a] School of Health Information Science, University of Victoria,
Victoria, British Columbia, Canada
[b] Telfer School of Management, University of Ottawa, Ottawa, Ontario, Canada
[c] College of Public Health and Health Informatics,
King Saud Bin Abdulaziz University for Health Science, Riyadh, Saudi Arabia

Abstract. In this paper the authors review and discuss four different qualitative approaches as they are used to evaluate health information systems: (1) grounded theory, (2) ethnography, (3) verbal protocol analysis/usability engineering and (4) action research. The authors describe the historical origins, current uses, strengths and weakness of the three qualitative methodologies that are frequently used in health informatics and they discuss an emerging approach: action research. More importantly, they identify how each of the approaches can be used across the SDLC to inform planning, analysis, design, implementation and support of health information systems.

Keywords. grounded theory, ethnography, usability engineering, verbal protocol analysis, action research, qualitative methods, software development lifecycle, evaluation

Introduction

In health informatics (HI) evaluation can take place throughout the software development lifecycle (SDLC): from the beginning of a project in its initial project planning stages through to its implementation and maintenance [1]. Some researchers have suggested the SDLC offers key points where health informaticians can evaluate health information systems (HIS) and they have suggested such formative evaluation can improve the quality of the software and its adoption by health professionals [2]. Over the past several years, there have emerged many differing types of methodological approaches that can be used to evaluate health HIS. Initially, researchers employed quantitative approaches. These approaches were successful (in some cases) in determining the effects of a HIS upon patient and organizational outcomes (e.g. 3,4). In other cases these studies identified that there were no improvements in either patient or organizational outcomes. Therefore, the results from these quantitative studies were mixed, leading some researchers to conclude that

---

[1] Corresponding Author: Elizabeth Borycki, School of Health Information Science; Email: emb@uvic.ca

quantitative approaches alone are ineffective in determining the reason(s) for a system's success or failure (i.e. in terms of improving patient or organizational health outcomes) [5].

In the early 1990's we saw the introduction and initial application of qualitative approaches to the evaluation of HIS [5]. Researchers found that qualitative approaches could be used effectively to determine the underlying reasons for a HIS's success or failure. Qualitative approaches can employed across the SDLC to evaluate a HIS [5]. Over the years we have seen the use of several differing types of qualitative approaches in HI in the evaluation of systems, among them: grounded theory, ethnography, protocol analysis, and action research. Each of these approaches has both strengths and weaknesses associated with their use. The purpose of this paper will be to review and discuss the four different approaches that are currently used to evaluate HIS, namely: (1) grounded theory, (2) ethnography, (3) verbal protocol analysis/usability engineering and (4) action research and how they can be used within the context of the SDLC. To the best of our knowledge, this work represents the first attempt to use the SDLC as a framework that can be used to select a qualitative method for use in evaluating HIS within the context of the SDLC. We begin this paper by first reviewing the underpinnings of the SDLC.

1. Software Development Lifecycle

A range of software models have been developed in the general and healthcare software engineering industry. These models guide the planning, design, development, implementation and maintenance of HIS (e.g. electronic medical records, electronic patient records). More recently, a number of software engineering models have been developed that support information systems evaluation throughout the SDLC. This work has led some researchers to identify evaluation methods that can be used to inform software developers across the SDLC. In HI qualitative approaches, were introduced and tested by researchers, to determine their ability to evaluate HIS [1]. The conventional SDLC as outlined by researchers [6] is comprised of five stages: planning, analysis, design, implementation and support (see Figure 1). In each of these five stages, differing qualitative approaches can be used to provide significant insights into the quality (e.g. usability), future and actual use (e.g. ability of the health professionals to adopt) of HIS in real world settings. In the next section of this paper the authors will discuss the use of these four qualitative approaches and discuss their application within the context of the SDLC.

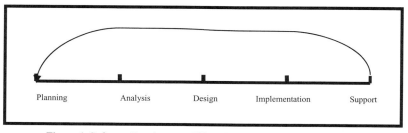

Figure 1. Software Development Lifecycle. Adapted from Kushniruk [1]

1.1. Grounded Theory

Grounded theory (GT) was developed by researchers as a method that could be used to study of social phenomenon using a symbolic interactionist perspective (i.e. the study of the construction, maintenance and change of social institutions) [7]. GT emerged in the 1960's and challenged the view that qualitative research only produced descriptive case studies and could not be applied to theory development [8]. GT is a general methodology that is used to develop theory. GT is grounded in data that has been systematically gathered and analyzed by researchers. The hallmark of GT is its three coding cycles: open coding, axial coding and selective coding [8]. In open coding raw data are coded according to concepts and categories. In axial coding these concepts and categories are refined and interconnected. Lastly, selective coding establishes the final concepts and categories. The strength of GT is in its ability to develop theory from the data. These theories have been used in various stages of the SDLC including requirements engineering [9], systems design [10] and the evaluation of HISs [3]. GT is especially valuable for providing an empirical basis for the development of conceptual models (e.g. ontologies) [11]. The systematic coding methodology that forms the basis of GT is rigorous and provides a way to analyze and understand data such that models are empirically tied to the data (and not based on assumptions or preconceptions). The challenge to using GT is time as it is a time consuming method.

1.2. Ethnography

Ethnography's historical roots can be traced back to the 19th century. Anthropologists used ethnography to study cultural traditions and traditional societies. Since then, ethnography has been used by other disciplines (e.g. medicine, nursing and HI) [5,6]. In HI, ethnography has been used to describe what people do in response to a HIS (e.g. their actions and interactions with the HIS and its artifacts such as computer workstations) [6]. Specific ethnographic data collection methods employed by health informaticians include observation, focus groups and interviewing [6,12]. In terms of the SDLC, ethnography has been used to inform the planning, analysis, implementation and support of HIS. Ethnography has helped health informaticians to better understand the work of HIS project planning teams during implementation [15]. Health informaticians have used these data collection methods to gather requirements for software designers [16], develop an understanding of the intended and unintended consequences of HIS [16], and evaluate the quality of health professionals/patients interactions with a HIS. One of the strengths of ethnography as a methodology is its ability to collect data about the actions and interactions that arise from introducing HIS. Such knowledge can be used to inform those working in the field. One of the weaknesses of ethnography is the limited generalizability of the findings of these evaluations to other settings.

1.3. Verbal Protocol Analysis/Usability Engineering

The use of verbal protocol analysis was first pioneered in psychological research and involves the principled analysis of the verbalized thoughts of human subjects as they carry out tasks in complex domains (e.g. chess, physics, and medicine) [17]. The resultant verbalizations are typically transcribed, coded and analyzed to identify the cognitive processes involved in decision making and reasoning in the domain being studied [17]. The approach has since found considerable use in HIS especially when used in conjunction with methods emerging from usability engineering (the foremost of these methods being usability testing). Usability testing involves observing representative users of information systems while they carry out representative tasks with the system under study. A variety of studies [18] have applied the approach at various stages of the SDLC, ranging from usability testing of completed systems to testing earlier in the SDLC emerging prototypes and design models in an iterative cycle of design and evaluation. The value added by using these methods has ranged from identification of usability problems, user information needs as well as application in the testing of systems to ensure their ultimate safety prior to final release [18].

1.4. Action Research

Action research was first used in the social sciences to understand "social illnesses" that transpired following World War II [13]. The method evolved as a result of collaborative research efforts between scientists and clinicians to understand the reasons behind various social issues impacting society [13]. Within the field of HI, action research has been identified as a method that can link "theory with practice through an iterative process of problem diagnosis, action intervention, and reflective learning" [14]. While working collaboratively with stakeholders, action researchers collect various subjective and objective data (e.g. documents, interview data, meeting notes, survey data, discussion group data, log data, and computer usage reports). These various data sources help to understand the problem, take action, and reflect on the learning process. The use of action research within HI is increasing (i.e. calls have been made for its use in developing and evaluating patient-centered electronic health records) [4]. In terms of the SDLC, action research can help inform planning, analysis, design, implementation, and support as it involves researchers, administrators, clinicians, and other stakeholders who would be involved in the SDLC. In action research, researchers and stakeholders work collaboratively to identify issues, solve them, and reflecting on the process in each of the SDLC phases. Action research would then lead to a more user centered approaches to design. A major disadvantage of action research is the bias that may arise from researchers working too closely with stakeholders or from user resistance associated with participating in research.

2. Discussion and Conclusions

As described above, qualitative approaches have been used to evaluate HIS across the SDLC [1]. Differing qualitative approaches (i.e. grounded theory, ethnography, verbal protocol analysis and action research) have strengths and weaknesses in evaluating HIS across the SDLC. The authors of this paper have described the use of these varying methodologies within the context of the SDLC taking into consideration their strengths and weaknesses. Each of these approaches can be compared and contrasted in terms of effectiveness and usefulness in addressing the practical issues of evaluation throughout the SDLC (i.e. from software planning through to implementation and maintenance). The SDLC was used as a guiding framework for this discussion. In this context grounded theory has been used in a variety of studies early in the SDLC to obtain requirements, inform systems design and later in the SDLC to evaluate HIS [3,9,10,11]. In contrast, verbal protocol analysis in conjunction with usability testing has been applied more extensively later in the SDLC, particularly during the design, implementation and support phases, when a prototype or system has been implemented and is available for such testing [17,18]. Ethnographic approaches have found utility at various stages in the SDLC, as both preliminary to system design and later in the SDLC to assess the impact and safety of completed systems [15,16,17]. Action research is emerging as an approach and is finding application across the SDLC informing researchers and stakeholders such as administrators and software developers involved in HIS implementation and support [4,13,14]. In conclusion, the concept of the SDLC can provide a valuable framework for comparing and contrasting differing qualitative methods that can be applied from the planning to implementation and deployment to support of HIS. Selection and application of qualitative methods should be considered in the context of the SDLC in order to maximize their usefulness in improving software design, implementation and support.

References

[1]   A. W. Kushniruk, Evaluation in the design of health information systems: Application of approaches emerging from usability engineering. *Comp Biol Med* **32** (2002), 141-9.
[2]   E. M. Borycki, A. S. Kushniruk, Towards an integrative cognitive-socio-technical approach in health informatics: Analyzing technology-induced error involving health information systems. *Open Med Inf* **4** (2010), 181-187.
[3]   E. M. Campbell, D. F. Sittig, J. S. Ash, K. P. Guappone, R. H. Dykstra, Types of unintended consequences related to computerized provider order entry. *JAMIA* **13** (2006), 547–56.
[4]   W. J. Winkelman, K. J. Leonard. Overcoming structural constraints to patient utilization of electronic medical records: a critical review and proposal for an evaluation framework. *JAMIA* **11**(2) (2003), 151-61.
[5]   W. Jackson, N. Verberg, *Methods: Doing Social Research* 4th ed. Toronto, Canada, 2007.
[6]   J. G. Anderson, C. E. Aydin. *Evaluating the Organizational Impact of Healthcare Information Systems* 2nd ed. United States of America: Springer, 2005.
[7]   B. G. Glaser, A. Strauss. *The Discovery of Grounded Theory: Strategies for Qualitative Research.* Chicago, IL: Aldine Publishing Co, 1967.
[8]   A. Strauss, J. Corbin. "Grounded Theory Methodology: An Overview" In *Handbook of Qualitative Research*, 1994, N.K. Denzin and Y.S. Lincoln (eds.), Thousand Oaks: Sage, pp. 273-285
[9]   S. Garde, P. Knaup. Requirements engineering in health care: The example of chemotherapy planning in paediatric oncology. *Req Eng* **11** (2006), 265–278
[10]   C. E. Kuziemsky, J.H. Weber-Jahnke, F. Lau, G. M. Downing, An interdisciplinary computer based information tool for palliative severe pain management. *JAMIA* **15** (3) (2008), 374-382.
[11]   C. E. Kuziemsky, F. Lau, A four stage approach for ontology-based health information system design. *Art Int Med*, 2010, in press.
[12]   M. Angrosino, *Doing Ethnographic and Observational Research*. Los Angeles: Sage, 2007.
[13]   R. Baskerville, M. D. Myers. *Special Issue on Action Research in Information Systems: Making IS Research Relevant to Practice*: Foreword (pp. 329-335) Stable URL: http://www.jstor.org/stable/25148642.
[14]   F. Lau, R. Hayward. Building a virtual network in a community health research training program. *JAMIA*. Jul-Aug **7**(4) (2000), 361-77.
[15]   D. Martin, J. Mariani, M. Rouncefield. Implementing a HIS project: Everyday features and practicalities of NHS project work. *Health Inf J* **10**(4) (2004), 303-313.
[16]   W. Ventres, S. Kooienga, N. Vuckovic, R. Marlin, P. Nygren, V. Stewart. Physicians, patients and the electronic health record: An ethnographic analysis. *Ann of Fam Med,* **4**(2) (2006), 124-131.
[17]   K. A. Ericsson, H. A Simon. *Protocol analysis*. Cambridge MA: MIT Press, 1993.
[18]   A. W. Kushniruk, V. Patel. Cognitive and usability engineering methods for the evaluation of clinical information systems. *J Biomed Inf* **37** (2004), 56-76.

International Perspectives in Health Informatics
E.M. Borycki et al. (Eds.)
IOS Press, 2011
doi:10.3233/978-1-60750-709-3-298

Health Information System Access Control Redesign – Rationale and Method

Kenneth A. MOSELLE[a]

[a] *Vancouver Island Health Authority, Victoria, British Columbia, Canada*

Abstract. This paper addresses the question of why a health service system might find it necessary to re-engineer the access control model that mediates the interaction of clinicians with health information systems. Factors that lead to increasingly complexity of the access control models are delineated, and consequences of that complexity are identified. Strategies are presented to address these factors, and a stepwise procedure is suggested to structure the access control model re-engineering process.

Keywords. access control model, role based access control, organization based access control, privacy, principle of least privilege, need-to-know

Introduction – Drivers Behind Access Control Redesign

Within the healthcare arena, an access control model describes a set of permissions and constraints that manage the interaction of users with an array of information systems. An effective model must reconcile the twin task demands of privacy protection (*via* controls on access and use) with the service provider's need for information to support standards of care. In an ideal case, as new technologies, clinical services and users enter into the mix, and as new legislation is passed, new components would be added to the model in an incremental fashion without requiring extensive changes to the entire model. However, several factors can converge to create a need to re-engineer the information access control model for a health service system.

Complexity of the model – from a purely fiscal perspective, the model has become too complex when the organization cannot manage the administrative burden (and cost) associated with changes to the model as new categories of users are added and as new functions are deployed within the technology base. From a functional perspective, the model has become too complex when end users are no longer able to understand the model, which impacts on their capacity to appropriately self-regulate their interactions with the information systems.

When users do not understand the access control model and the principles on which it is based, they are at risk for breaching access control policies. To compensate, proactive controls (restrictions placed on use) may need to drill down even more deeply into the data sets and processes that constitute the information system, in which case the model becomes more complex, which compounds the problem. As well, as the logic that governs access becomes more granular and local role/context specific, more generic auditing functions lose their capacity to discriminate appropriate from inappropriate uses of information (auditing sensitivity and specificity decreases).

Access control interoperability challenges – horizontal integration of peer point-of-service systems, or vertical integration of such systems with the interoperable electronic health record (EHR), will create the necessity for harmonized access control policies. The standards foundation for such interoperability (e.g., policies; role taxonomies; permissions/constraints catalogues) is under construction. One consequence is that implementations that predate emerging access control standards will conflict at the level of access control policies, or similar policies may implemented in different ways across systems. The process of reconciling these differences across systems or jurisdictions may be difficult, even if the technology were capable of supporting complex access control policy brokering.

History – different components of enterprise electronic health record solutions are likely to be implemented in phases, to different programs and professional roles. It is impossible to anticipate all information access control challenges at the point of initial deployment, if for no other reason than the mix of clinical services and roles changes over time, service delivery standards change, and technologies change. Decisions made early on in a deployment may become increasingly difficult to reconcile with later information access requirements. As a result, the model either becomes increasingly inconsistent and complex, or legacy access control decisions (that may not be fully compatible with current standards of care) may be imposed on new situations.

For all of these reasons, as electronic health record technologies and standards mature, and as the deployment of these solutions matures within a given health region and across the entire health service system, the need to re-engineer the information access control model may emerge.

1. Challenges to Building an Access Control Model that Supports Best-possible Standards of Clinical Practice while Protecting Privacy.

The challenges around configuring effective access control models in enterprise health information systems reflects the convergence of several factors:

Complexity is inescapable – Within health information systems, this complexity is driven by a host of factors, including: (a) heterogeneous clinical populations served by the system; (b) the range of clinical activities undertaken by the service system as a whole; (c) large numbers of site and function-specific service delivery workflows; (d) broad range of different professions and functionally-based roles in the service system; (e) functionality of the health information system(s); (f) data structures in the systems; (g) access control services provided (and often not provided) by the technology; (h) diversity of point-of-service and interoperable EHR technologies; and (h) legislation and organizational policies and procedures.

Principle of least privilege – Application of this principle is linked to the proliferation of roles in role-based access control (RBAC) models: this principle asserts that users should be allowed access only to the *minimal* amount of information or resources in the information system that are required for them to do their work. It is tied conceptually to the "need-to-know" principle in access control, which asserts that users should only have access to information they require to do their work. In practice, this means that if there are two service providers who are distinguishable on the basis of required access to a specified system resource or type of information, they *should* be distinguished as two separate roles in the model, in order to uphold the position that the access control model is architected around the principle of least privilege.

Classification challenges – if access to information and information system services (e.g., order entry) is governed by the need-to-know principle, and if need for information is going to be specified in an explicit manner, then the access control model would require the following factors to be classified: (a) client conditions (clinical/functional/behavioural characteristics); (b) interventions that can be 'applied' to clients; (c) data that users can access and activities that users can perform within the health information systems (c) provider professional roles and job functions; and (d) service settings or locations. Furthermore, even if all of these classification systems existed, an access control model is a description of the *mappings* between these factors, so all relevant linkages would need to be fully articulated, e.g., when a client presents with a specified set of conditions in a specified setting, a provider of a particular professional designation functioning in a particular role would need to have access to a defined and bounded set of data and would be permitted to perform a set of activities in the electronic health record.

In an ideal client-centred access control model, where access is driven by client need for services, all of these classifications and mappings would be specified *a priori*, and then permissions could be derived through an four-stage procedure: (1) specify a clinical sub-population and a set of care contexts; (2) look up a set of clinical functions that would be required for those clients in context; (3) look up a set of information requirements associated with those functions; and (4) assign permissions to users based on steps 1-3. However, in practice, the requisite classification systems are incomplete, and the required mappings between them have not been specified in a comprehensive, technology-and-service-system-agnostic manner.

The fall-back strategy is to rely upon *post hoc* role-engineering methods, e.g., to investigate the need-to-know information requirements for new roles and bodies of information as they emerge over time, and to build the new roles and associated permissions in a way that is responsive to these immediate requirements. The challenge is to carry out such a *post hoc* strategy in a way that does not result in a complex, possibly inconsistent model that is difficult to administer and communicate out to users.

Dynamic need-to-know vs static permissions - the underlying basis for need-to-know access is the client's condition, which changes as the underlying health condition changes (due to intrinsic factors and/or the impact of treatment). However, unless the access control model has been built around an event-driven architecture, the access control model will be implemented as a static set of permissions that are assigned to roles. As a result, when the model is being constructed, and permissions are mapped to roles, there is no other option than to try to anticipate all of the possible information requirements for a given user, i.e., "need-to-know-based access" gives way to "might-need-to-know-based access". The result of this shift is an opening up of access, with the attendant risks to privacy. This is an inevitable side-effect of the intersection of dynamically unfolding need for information and statically assigned permissions.

2. Strategies for Addressing Challenges to the Construction of Access Control Models that Reconcile Privacy Protection with the Clinician's Need to Access Pertinent Health Information.

While there are no perfect solutions to address these challenges, there are strategies that can enhance privacy protection while supporting access to needed information:

Organization-based access control - if an access control model is going to function to protect privacy, it must incorporate some means for delimiting bodies of information and controlling who has access to those bodies of information. Rather than tackling the challenges of delimiting bodies of information by classifying client clinical/diagnostic profiles and mapping onto a classification of clinical interventions, information can be indexed by an organizational entity that is relatively homogeneous with respect to client-type, intervention-type, possibly sensitivity of information, and associated information use. For example, treat all information that is generated by users within an organized body of addictions services as an entity, and assign/deny users access to information associated with that organization. This would constitute an organization-based access control model [1].

The organization-based access control model can be integrated with RBAC – users within roles are assigned access to distinct bodies of information that are indexed by organization. For example, emergency room nurses may be assigned access to all acute care organizations, all ambulatory organizations, including mental health and addictions organizations. Nurses working in a sub-acute rehabilitation unit may be granted access to medical acute care organizations but may be denied access to the mental health and addictions organization (unless some exception-handling procedure is activated, e.g, "break-the-glass" functionality within the EHR). This hybrid structure is characteristic of the more current iterations of the RBAC model, referred to in the literature as "role and organization-based access control", or "ROBAC" [2].

Enterprise risk management – when the principle of least privilege is called into play, it results in a net total reduction in the amount of information flowing out to users, which in theory will reduce the risks to privacy. However, this may also increase the risk to quality of care, and it will result in additional complexity in the model, which is a risk to effective privacy protection. From an enterprise risk management perspective, if the model can be simplified by collapsing two roles together, without increasing risks to privacy or to quality of care, then those roles should be collapsed down to one, even if one role is granted access to some information that may not be required to perform role-based job functions.

Standardize post hoc methods for creating new roles – *post hoc* methods for adapting an access control model to new roles or technologies do not necessarily have to devolve into *ad hoc* methods. The scenario-based functional role-engineering process developed by Neumann and Strembeck [3], which has been adopted by the Veterans Health Administration in the United States[4], has been granted the status of a *de facto* standard by virtue of its uptake by standards organizations such as HL7[5]. This procedure has the advantage of being very explicit about the tasks that are assigned to roles, and the information that is attached to tasks.

3. Context for Access Control Redesign Within VIHA

The Vancouver Island Health Authority (VIHA) is one of six health authorities in British Columbia. VIHA addresses the needs of approximately 750,000 individuals, providing a full spectrum of services that includes acute care, hospital and community-based emergency response, outpatient clinics, case management services, and residential care. Various enterprise-standard point-of-service applications are in place, along with access to interoperable EHR functionality (e.g, PharmaNet, which is the province-wide network that links all BC pharmacies to a central set of data systems) .

The Cerner® health information system was deployed in phases in VIHA, beginning in 2001. Rollout was initiated in medical acute care settings, and in a host of hospital and community-based mental health/addictions services operated by the health authority. The original deployment was limited to the approximately half of the services and clients living in the greater Victoria part of Vancouver Island. Over time, the scope of the Cerner® deployment extended across the entire health authority, new functionality was implemented, and new roles and clinical functions were incorporated. The principle of least privilege has been employed consistently throughout the deployment. The result is an access control model that has become quite complex and difficult to administer. As well, the model has become increasingly difficult to communicate out to users, who fill the void with their own understandings or concerns around the way that access is managed.

In the case of the Cerner® access control model in VIHA, the problem is also key to the solution: the set of roles and associated permissions within Cerner® constitutes a catalogue of almost every access control issue the organization has encountered since the launch of Cerner®. As such, a re-engineered access control model that is responsive to the issues addressed in the Cerner® model is likely to anticipate many future situations, even if the redesign process does not tackle what is probably the impossible challenge of positioning the model on a 'pure' *a priori* classification foundation. The re-engineering process in VIHA is organized around steps: *Step 1:* Review legislated and organizational policy-based requirements related to privacy and security. This scan should include authoritative documents that have been developed by organizations representing professional disciplines, e.g., the *BC Physician Privacy Toolkit* [6]. *Step 2:* Review access control architectures and develop a technology-agnostic ideal model that provides the greatest degree of control over access to information and systems functionality. *Step 3:* Evaluate functionality of existing technologies against the ideal model. Identify essential functions in this idea model that are not present in the existing technology base, and evaluate risks to information access or privacy that are inherent in the functions that *are* available. Develop a compromise architecture that leverages as much as possible off of the existing technologies. *Step 4:* Identify 'problem' roles within existing access control models in key enterprise technologies in VIHA, and abstract the rules and principles that have been applied to set permissions for the roles. These problem roles are typically those roles where the permissions are not clearly tied to a person's professional designation, so the basis for setting permissions is not always clear. *Step 5:* Identify 'problem' service delivery contexts, where it is not clear what information from which organizations/locations should be made available to persons working in different roles. Abstract the rules and permissions involved in attaching organizations (and associated information) to roles.

Step 6: Alignment, standardization – identify points of convergence/divergence with emerging standards, taxonomies and nomenclatures, including: (1) roles identified as part of the BC Provincial eHealth initiatives, e.g., the Provincial Laboratory Information System [7]; and (2) various front-runners for standards in the work undertaken by the US Veterans Health Administration on role and organization based access control [8-11]. *Step 7:* Risk assessment – evaluate the protection of privacy versus quality of care costs and benefits associated with the application of identified rules and principles. Determine a set of principles and generate clarity around application of rules in a way that does not incur unacceptable risk with regard to quality of care. *Step 8:* Risk management – proactive controls that do not compromise quality of care cannot reduce risks to privacy down to a level that obviates the need for auditing, particularly if the model has been simplified and permissions are not tailored to every job function in every setting. To mitigate these risks, auditing must be strengthened, and breach management policies and procedures must be enforced. *Step 9:* Once rules and principles have been clarified, and requirements around enhanced auditing have been determined – re-engineer the problematic roles using the scenario-based functional role engineering process. *Step 10:* Validate new roles and permissions against the legacy model through consultation with senior clinical and administrative leadership. Adjust the revised principles and rules (Step 7) accordingly, and revise the new role permissions. *Step 11:* Repeat Step 10 until the new permission build for problem roles and settings is validated. Revise the remaining portion of the model on the basis of the revised and validated principles and rules. *Step 12:* Reconfigure auditing procedures to reflect the new principles and rules, and to address as effectively as possible the limitations that are inherent in the access control services supplied by the transactional systems.

4. Evaluation

Success of the access control redesign efforts will be gauged against:
- The extent to which the roles and associated permissions incorporated in the re-engineered model can be mapped to the roles and permissions included in the BC Provincial eHealth initiatives, and the structural roles identified in the work of the Veterans Health Administration. This supports the goal of vertical access-control interoperability with the interoperable EHR.
- Reduction in the total number of roles included in the model, while preserving distinctions among roles that enhance privacy protections or uphold service standards and professional practice scope.
- Stakeholder acceptance of changes to permissions associated with roles.
- Adoption of a standardized scenario-based role-engineering process on a go-forward basis, to resolve issues around access control as they arise, and to enable the model to keep pace with changes in technology, service delivery processes, and workforce composition and scope of practice.

5. Conclusion – Beyond Technology Solutions to Access Control Issues.

Organizations mature in their understanding of access control issues. Initial efforts to manage access may rely heavily on access control services built into the transactional systems. However, as health information systems become a critical component of service delivery processes, and when clinicians become increasingly invested both in accessing required information and in safeguarding the privacy of clients, they become aware of issues in the access control model and will drive their concerns forward in the organization. As well, as data from multiple systems start to stream into data warehouses, and as service system evaluators and evidence-based planners and policy makers become users of new sources of information that originate in a variety of source systems, issues around secondary use will come to the fore. As the enterprise EHR implementation matures, it becomes increasingly apparent that access controls anchored in the underlying information systems technology cannot cover off all of the issues that arise. Information governance policies must be developed, organizational processes must be launched to operationalize those policies, and information stewardship roles and responsibilities must be clarified. As well, users must be educated to enhance their capacity to self-regulate their use of systems in a manner that is aligned with access control policies. Finally, access control protocols legislate the flow of information across professional and program boundaries. Decisions on how and where this flow can occur should not entail a process of unilateral decision-making on the part of business owners of the processes that gave rise to information in the first place – the information ultimately belongs to the client receiving services, and information flows should be determined by the need that emanates from their health-related concerns, which span program and professional boundaries. There must exist some mechanism for senior administrative and clinical leaders to come together, in order to adjudicate on different views regarding information flow, and to ensure that a single strong organizational voice is heard when it comes to information management issues that affect *both* quality of care and the protection of privacy.

References

[1] F. Cuppens, A. Miege. Modeling Contexts in the Or-BAC Model, *Proceedings of the 18th Annual Computer Security Applications Conference*, 2003.

[2] Z. Zhang, X. Zhang, R. Sandhu, ROBAC: Scalable Role and Organization Based Access Control Models, *International Conference on Collaborative Computing: Networking, Applications and Worksharing*, 2006.

[3] G. Neumann, M. Strembeck. A Scenario-drive Role Engineering Process for Functional RBAC Roles, *SACMAT '02*, Monterey California, June 3-4, 2002.

[4] Veterans Health Administration (VHA). *Implementing Role Based Access Control (RBAC) in Healthcare – Draft Standard for Trial Use, Adoption and Interoperability between Standards Organizations*, May 2, 2007

[5] *HL7 Role-based Access Control (RBAC) Role Engineering Process, Version 1.1*, November 2005

[6] BC Medical Association, College of Physicians and Surgeons of BC, Office of the Information and Privacy Commissioner of BC, Physician Privacy Toolkit, 2nd edition, June 15, 2009.

[7] Province of British Columbia. *Provincial Laboratory Information Solution (PLIS) and Interoperable Electronic Health Record (iEHR) - Project Summary*, August 2007

[8] Veterans Health Administration (VHA). *Health Information Systems Privilege Management Infrastructure – VHA Structural Roles Catalog, Version 8.0*, June 2007.

[9] Veterans Health Administration (VHA). *VHA Functional Roles, Version 8.0*, June 2007.

[10] Veterans Health Administration (VHA). *VHA Role Based Access Control (RBAC) Healthcare Permission Catalog, Version 2.7*, May 1, 2007

[11] Veterans Health Administration (VHA). *VHA Role Based Access Control (RBAC) Security and Privacy Constraint Catalog, Version 1.36*, May 9, 2008

International Perspectives in Health Informatics
E.M. Borycki et al. (Eds.)
IOS Press, 2011

305

doi:10.3233/978-1-60750-709-3-305

National Patient Flow Framework: An Ontological Patient-Oriented Redesign

Fragoulis PAPAGIANNIS [a, b], Abdul ROUDSARI [b, c], Konstantinos DANAS [d]

[a] *American College of Thessaloniki, Greece,*
[b] *Centre for Health Informatics, City University, UK,*
[c] *School of Health Information Science, University of Victoria, Victoria, British Columbia, Canada,*
[d] *School of Computing, IS and Mathematics, Kingston University, UK*

Abstract. This study introduces the necessary ontological redesign regarding patient-oriented frameworks. Different national healthcare frameworks around the world as well as semantic gaps have been discovered and demonstrate the need for a new healthcare management framework. This study's Patient-Oriented Management and Reporting framework (POMR framework) will introduce and measure the concept of value-added, patient-oriented flow. The ontological introduction of leading patient-oriented measures is also considered as a novel approach to solving problems. These measures are included in this POMR framework which introduces a unique ontological model redesign (POMR model) and its patient-oriented supporting information system (POMRS) adding value to the concept's implementation in CLIPS technology.

Keywords. patient-oriented, ontology, framework, measures, redesign

Introduction

Most of the contemporary studies focus on the redesign and optimisation of the patient flow without consideration of this study's conceptual framework. This study focuses on specific patient flow transactions and measures that should be encompassed within the patient flow framework that is designed. The contemporary healthcare at the national level would thus be redesigned around patient needs. This study will focus on the Greek patients as they are paying the most out of their pockets [1]. Greece's single payer system's aim should be equally available for everyone delivering effectiveness and efficient performance [2]. Other relevant research provides, as well, sufficient evidence of the need for an alternative patient oriented flow in the country [3]. Based on enterprise ontology this study will redesign the core patient flow processes. Simultaneous introduction of a patient-oriented model and its supporting information system will conceptualise and implement this ontological framework aiming towards the quantity and quality flow redesign and basic information exchange. This study also aims at fulfilling the NHS objectives, if in existence, with regard to patient-centred care.

1. Method

This research problem is defined as: "The contemporary lack of patient-oriented external parameters and internal transactions that guide and measure the quality service of the patient flow primarily within the healthcare premises that currently lead to lack of patient satisfaction, treatment and high hospitalisation costs." The solution to that problem concerns an intervention in the problematic areas of the patient flow process as far as patient value-added is concerned, based on a proposed Object System (OS) or rather POMR framework. The terms OS and POMR framework might be considered for the purpose of this study almost identical to the degree that framework is considered as a re-usable measurable design for this study's proposed OS [3]. Proactive transactions in healthcare could develop the Using System (US) to deliver patient satisfaction outcomes for the healthcare organisations to study in order to remain competitive [4]. The DEMO redesign methodology is selected since based on enterprise multilayer structure, it develops a framework that bridges mostly semantic gaps between technical and social issues which are very important according to the literature review for the nature of this study. So, developing an OS is to define, at the ontological level, the prototype model (POMR) and next its supporting information system (POMRS) to this model of a world that assists the framework's concept at info-logical and data-logical level.

2. Analysis

Based on Dietz's ontology [5] this redesign study follows these methodology steps:
1. Requirement analysis for the US with the White Box model (WB model)
2. Structural decomposition of the US with the WB model
3. Identification of the Black Box model's redesigning requirements (BB model input)
4. Redesigning of the specifications of the results and measures function (BB output)
5. Devising specification of the OS with the WB model
6. Redesigning and implementation of the OS with CLIPS technology

Step 1: Requirements Analysis for the US with the WB Model

The framework figure produced next should encompass the POMRS, its infrastructure and POMR model for the implementation of a patient-oriented flow concept:

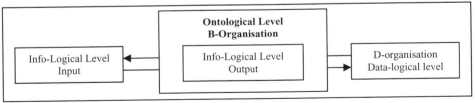

Figure 1. Framework Infrastructure of the OS

Step2: Structural Decomposition of the US with the WB Model

The process of the patient flow based on the WB devising processes and research findings is having four core US sub-processes: P01: Patient appointment to GP, P02:

Patient referral process, P03: The contemporary treatment process, P04: The discharge process. These sub-processes need to be redesigned. The US of the P02 ontological diagram (Figure 2) is produced in enterprise ontology software design package: Xemod 2008.

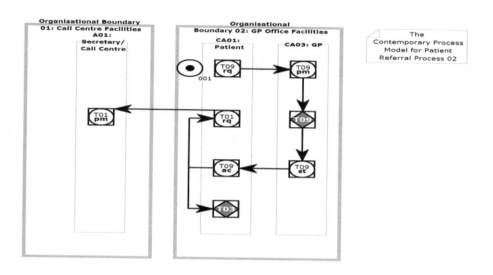

Figure 2. The US Process 02 Model of the Contemporary Situation

Step 3: Identification of the Black Box Model's Redesigning Requirements (BB Model Input)

Based on Figure 2, the US process from the examination results acceptance of the patient (T10 acceptance) is haphazard as there are multiple choices due to lack of policies and procedures from all the previous systems gaps presented in this section. Thus a measurable transaction structure that focuses on the patient relation rather than patient transaction should be redesigned. All other transactions to be followed in the patient's flow, at primary level, are based on the doctor's decision-making process which is taking place solely on doctor's tacit knowledge. Thus the US process 02 (Figure 2) requires the abolishment of the current series of multiple appointments and time spent by the patient before the process completion. That is why the Figure 2 ends with the initiation of a loop for the first contemporary process (P01). Thus, it is imperative that patient's choice to be supported by value-added information, as patients should pay for results and not for procedures.

Step 4: Redesigning of the Specifications of the Results and Measures Function

The following transactions are being redesigned, as Table 1 indicates, providing relative measurable results. These results are produced in a unique primary, secondary and tertiary level hierarchy, and should be introduced to support these ontological transactions at all levels. These core patient flow transactions' results to specific process steps delivered through the construction and organisational synthesis.

Transaction Type	Transaction Result
T1 Healthcare appointment management	R1 Initiation of a patient relationship management
T2 E P R analysis	R2 Complete patient record
T3 Doctor's referral for further treatment	R3 Patient treatment proposal based on POMR2
T4 Hospital inflow	R4 Patient-oriented hospital registration And room allocation
T5 Hospital discharge and/or rehabilitation treatment initiation	R5 Patient treatment and/or outpatient hospital rehabilitation procedures report program
T6 Patient relationship monitoring	R6 Verification of rehabilitation procedures and delivery of POMR1, POMR4
T7 Patient record management	R7 Storage, indexing, retrieval of patient records
T8 Information retrieval from NHS bill of examination database	R8 Interpret information based on expertise
T9 Patient Examination	R9 Diagnosis of the patient's problem
T10 Patient-oriented measurements analysis for patient condition	R10 Treatment proposal based on relevant POMR3
T11 Initiation of patient's treatment circle	R11 Patient POMR based counselling
T12 Electronic study management treatment	R12 Electronic verification of treatment process and medical operations
T13 Proactive treatment continuation	R13 Prevention plan.
T14 Doctor's expert opinion	R14 Patient quality communication
T15 Laboratory tests	R15 Safe laboratory results
T16 Clinical tests	R16 Safe clinical results
T17 Electronically recorded treatment performance	R17 Patient's awareness of medical performance
T18 Electronically recorded narration of treatment methodology	R18 Patient's awareness of the full treatment circle

Table 1. The TRT of the Proposed Patient Flow

Step 5: Division of the Specifications of the OS with the WB Model

The first of these sets of measures will focus on equal patient access via accessibility function of the healthcare system. The next two sets of measures will focus on efficiency via the safety function and structural operation function. The last set focuses on effectiveness via the outcome function. So, several measures are included in such coded reports as Figure 3 exhibits, at info-logical level for the supporting POMRS. Next, at data-logical level, object model coding is in order. An indicated report coded as Patient-Oriented Measurement Report number one (POMR1), is exhibited:

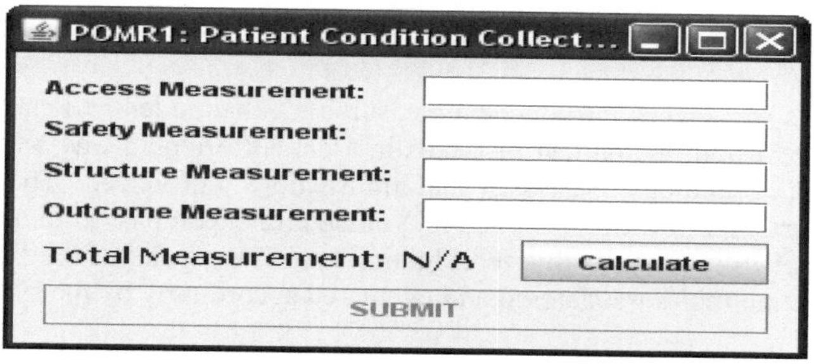

POMR1: Patient Condition Collect... ▭ ▭ ✕

Access Measurement: [_____]

Safety Measurement: [_____]

Structure Measurement: [_____]

Outcome Measurement: [_____]

Total Measurement: N/A   [Calculate]

[SUBMIT]

Figure 3. "POMR1: Patient Condition Collection Measure" Screen

Step 6: Redesigning and Implementation of the OS with CLIPS Technology

The 0S P02 process follows the OS P01 process. As the GP's assistance prepares for the appointment, the patient has a good chance to proceed efficiently for further treatment. Any other referrals that are not relevant to extraordinary ad hoc patient conditions are considered evidence towards ineffective P01 according to the following measure which is included in the POMR1 report (Figure 3):

$$\text{Referral measure (n)} = S(n)\,T03\,/\,S(n)\,T04 \qquad \text{Eq. (1)}$$

Where n equals number of instances in integer numbers (example: "patient condition"). Upon successful loading of the ontological model's processes knowledge base on CLIPS the rule base is launched and implementation occurs.

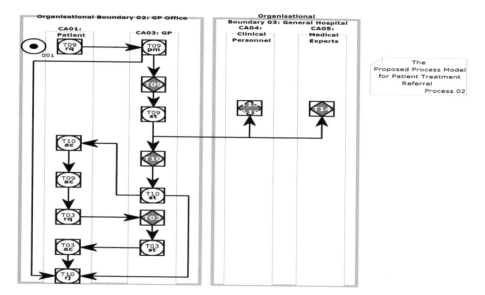

Figure 4. The OS Process 02 Model of the Proposed Situation

3. Conclusions

This study's framework introduced a measurable value-added patient flow. According to this novel redesign, the patient proceeds in a patient-oriented way which is specified by the enterprise ontology processes and transactions introduced. The ontological rules which govern this flow are designed in Xemod and encompassed in a CLIPS knowledge base in order to implement this redesigned flow. The results of the flow of each patient entity are being monitored, stored and evaluated accordingly by the system's actors.

References

[1] OECD, Measuring up: improving health system performance in OECD system performance
     in OECD countries, Ottawa, Paris November 2001, Conference Proceedings Section A-4, 2002, 5-7.
[2] Y, Tountas, N, Economou N.,Health services and health systems Evaluation, *Arch Hellenic Medicine*, **24**
     (2007), 7-21.
[3] V. Papanikolaou, S. Ntani, Addressing the Paradoxes of Satisfaction with Hospital
     Care, *Int J Health Care Quality Assu*, **21** (6), (2008), 548-561.
[4] G. Steinke, C. Nickolette, (2003), Business rules as the basis of an organisations information systems,
     Indus Manage Data Systems, **103** (1) (2008), 52-63.
[5] J.L.G. Dietz, *Enterprise Ontology*, Springer-Verlag, Heidelberg, Germany, 2006.

International Perspectives in Health Informatics
E.M. Borycki et al. (Eds.)
IOS Press, 2011

doi:10.3233/978-1-60750-709-3-311

A Model For Representing Formal, Informal and Hybrid Communication in the Clinical Communication Space

Craig E. KUZIEMSKY[a,1]

[a] *Telfer School of Management, University of Ottawa, Ottawa, ON, Canada*

Abstract. The clinical communication space refers to the activities that take place in the context of clinical communication. Communication is an important part of healthcare delivery yet the communication space has been described a source of medical errors and other communication issues such as interruptions. Information and communication technologies (ICTs) can enhance the clinical communication space but before we can design ICTs we need to describe the space. In particular we need to understand the role that informal communication plays. This paper reports on an exploratory study of the clinical communication space. It uses an ontology to illustrate the range of processes, modalities and contexts within the communication space and the role of formal, informal and hybrid communication.

Keywords. communication space, ontology, health information systems design

Introduction

Communication is a key part of healthcare delivery. The clinical communication space refers to the activities that take place in the context of clinical communication and consists of the communicator, media, and the information that is exchanged in a communication act [1]. Although it comprises a large part of healthcare information flow the communication space has been described a source of medical errors and other communication issues such as interruptions [1,2]. Information and communication technologies (ICTs) can help overcome these issues and enhance activities within the communication space, but before we can design ICTs we need to describe and model the communication space [3].

There are several limitations to existing research on the communication space. First, existing models of the space tend to represent only certain parts of it such as communication errors [1]. There is no research that presents a systematic approach for modeling the communication space. Second, ICT design requires standardization of exchanged data and most research on communication standardization has focused on formal or structured types of communication. For example Garde et al. have proposed openEHR Archetypes as a means of facilitating interoperability during clinical processes such as communication [4]. Although ad-hoc communication can be

---

[1]Corresponding Author: Dr. Craig Kuziemsky, Telfer School of Management, University of Ottawa, 55 Laurier Avenue East,Ottawa, ON K1N 6N5, e-mail: Kuziemsky@telfer.uottawa.ca

supported if it is within the archetypes, we suggest that could be problematic. Informal communication is very common in healthcare and the complexity and variation of healthcare delivery will certainly require communication outside the archetypes. Therefore we need to understand the role of informal communication in the communication space. Third, communication is influenced by contextual factors such as the type of clinical unit where communication takes place and the providers involved in a communication act [2]. To effectively design ICTs to support communication we need to understand the entire communication space including the clinical processes and communication channels that exist within it both formal and informal. We also need to understand the contexts that influence communication activities. This paper reports on a study of team communication in three units of a pediatric hospital. We studied the clinical communication processes and designed an ontology of the communication space. The ontology models the clinical communication space so we can understand and analyze the formal, informal and hybrid communication activities that take place within it as well as the contexts that influence communication. The ontology provides starting point for the design of ICTs to support clinical communication.

1. Study Design

We studied clinical communication on three units of a pediatric hospital in Eastern Ontario. The current communication system of all three units is a hybrid of paper and electronic systems. The hospital is implementing a new electronic charting system that will replace many of the paper charts and provide a common charting document. The purpose of this study was to obtain a model of the clinical communication space prior to the implementation of the new system. We wanted to develop an understanding of the current communication space to proactively identify were implementation issues may arise with the new system.

1.1. Data Sources

We observed patient cases through the trajectory of care as they entered the intensive care unit (ICU) and then moved to one of two standard inpatient units. 71 hours of observations and 10 patient cases were observed from July to December 2009. We also conducted semi-structured interviews with 15 care providers (3 residents/fellows, 4 RNs, 2 Physicians, 1 social worker, 1 respiratory therapist, 1 pharmacist) and 3 patients/parents. Interview questions included questions about about communication and the different types of media (i.e paper, electronic) and channels (i.e. oral, written) that support it. Ethics approval was obtained for the study and consent obtained from all participants.

1.2. Methods

Ethnographic non-participant observation was used to collect the observation data on the clinical wards. A trained qualitative researcher collected the data. Grounded theory methodology [5] was used to analyze the data into concepts and categories.

2. Results

2.1. Ontology of the Clinical Communication Space

From our data analysis we developed an ontology of the clinical communication space (Fig. 1). The ontology has four main concepts: clinical processes, contexts, modalities and outcomes. Clinical processes are the high level concepts with each process having contexts, modalities and outcomes. Each concept of the ontology and how it is used to model the communication space is described in the sections below.

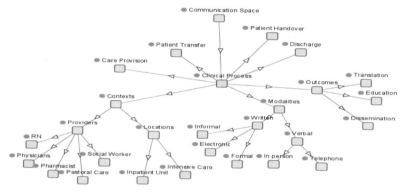

Figure 1. Ontology of the clinical communication space

2.2. Clinical Processes

Identification of clinical processes is the first task of modeling the communication space. To develop ICTs to support communication we first need to identify the specific communication processes that take place. In studying the communication space we realized that it is not a series of random events but rather there are specific and integrated processes. Four main clinical processes identified were identified: patient care provision, patient transfer, patient handover, and discharge. Patient care provision is a macro process comprised of several micro processes such as medication or treatment decisions, assessments, and viewing/accessing clinical data. It is essential that all the micro processes are identified. The clinical processes, particularly patient care provision, will vary in different settings, but there are two key things to look for in identifying clinical processes. First, it is important to identify processes that are communication 'impact points'. That means these processes have heavy communication flow and act as focal points for the flows. Second, clinical processes should act as integration points that use communication formats to connect the different processes. Patient care is not a series of random events but rather it follows an integrated flow. Communication is the thread that integrates the processes. In our study poor process integration was a common cause of communication issues. For example data from patient care provision needed to be effectively communicated to the patient transfer or handover processes in order for those processes to go smoothly. Although the four clinical processes existed in all three units in our study, the delivery of the processes and the communication that supported them was different. The remaining three ontology concepts: modalities, outcomes and contexts articulate these differences.

2.3. Modalities

All communication processes are not the same. The communication modalities concept refers to the different ways that communication is conducted in the four clinical processes. Two primary modalities were written and verbal. Verbal were synchronous activities either in person or by telephone. Written communication was formal (i.e. charting document) or informal (i.e. white board, sticky note) and could be either paper based or electronic. In our study informal communication was common. Written, informal communication documents were frequently created to customize formal documents. One of the challenges with clinical data is that it generic and intended for multiple providers. A common informal document for nurses and physicians were 'cheat sheets' to better fit the generic data with their clinical workflow. An example nursing 'cheat sheet' was the 'to do' list that included reminders, algorithms and other notes to personalize the charted data for nursing workflow. The 'to do' list was a common communication tool for patient handovers and transfers. Physicians, especially residents, used a patient summary 'cheat sheet' to ensure that all relevant clinical process concepts were communicated in patient rounds.

Modeling the different communication modalities also helped to quantify their frequencies of occurrence.   For example in the ICU we modeled 41 patient care micro processes of which 15 were written formal, 3 were written informal, 3 were written electronic, 4 were verbal telephone, 8 were verbal in person, 3 were a hybrid written formal/written informal, 2 were hybrid verbal in person/telephone/written formal, 2 were hybrid verbal in person/telephone, and 1 was hybrid written informal/verbal in person. Those numbers emphasize the variation in communication that exists and the extent of verbal, informal and hybrid forms of communication.

2.4. Outcomes

It is essential to understand the specific outcomes that communication is meant to provide. Although communication was used to support the clinical processes for day to day care delivery it was also used for education and the dissemination of policies and procedures.   The outcomes influenced the format and modalities of communication. Dissemination tended to be more general while education had to be tailored to specific providers.

2.5. Contexts

Different contexts of communication included the clinical unit and the number and/or type of provider involved in the communication acts. For example in the ICU there was a larger reliance on written communication as ICU patients had a careflow document that guided their care and the communication about care delivery. The chart for ICU patients also resided in the patient's room making it easily accessible. In contrast the standard inpatient units had more oral and less written communication. The charts in these units resided at the nursing station making them more mobile and often not available when needed. Oral communication was often used if the chart could not be located.   Different providers also had different communication practices. Providers involved in ongoing care delivery on a single unit (i.e nurses, attending physicians) had different communication patterns than providers who provided care across several units such as pastoral care, pharmacy, and social workers. Other contextual issues included environmental issues. During the H1N1 outbreak there was a large increase in oral and informal written communication because that was an unprecedented event. There were very few formal documents to support communication about that outbreak and so communication had to be adapted and was largely informal and by exception.

3. Discussion

This paper presented an ontology for modeling the clinical communication space. To date there is no comprehensive approach for modeling the space. The ontology also demonstrated the complexity of the communication space. It has been suggested that the communication space is simply part of the information space, which refers the processes by which information is exchanged between two or more people or ICTs [2]. We suggest communication is far more complex than that. As illustrated in this paper there are many factors beyond information exchange that need to be considered in the context of communication. Modalities of communication, the providers, clinical units, and the intended outcome of the communication act are all part of the communication space. Our ontology also highlighted the prevalence of informal, verbal and hybrid communication acts. Focusing solely on formal or structured communication will result in a poor model of the communication space. The ontology can also help us design ICTs to support communication. The variations in communication that exist mean there is no one size fits all ICT but rather ICT design will vary by provider, unit and intended outcome. Further, our ontology showed that communication processes are not disparate processes but rather they are integrated. Thus it is not practical to develop ICTs to support individual communication acts such as clinical rounds due to the integrated nature of the different clinical communication processes.

Shortcomings of this paper are that it presents preliminary findings of a study being conducted in three units of a pediatric clinical setting. Different representations of the ontology concepts will arise in other settings. However the ontology and method by which it was developed is a meta-model that provides a starting point for modeling and understanding the clinical communication space.

Acknowledgements

I acknowledge funding support from the Natural Sciences and Engineering Research Council of Canada.

References

[1] P.D. Stetson, L.K. McKnight, S.Bakken, C. Curran, T.T. Kubose, J.J. Cimino. Development of an ontology to model medical errors, information needs, and the clinical communication space. *JAMIA* 9(Nov-Dec suppl) (2002), S86–S91
[2] H. Pirnejad, Z. Niazkhani, M. Berg, R. Bal. Intra-organizational Communication in Healthcare. *Methods Inf Med* **47(4)** (2008),336-45
[3] E. Coiera. When Computation is better than Conversation. *JAMIA*. **7(3)** (2000), 277-286
[4] S. Garde, P. Knaup, E.J.S. Hovenga, S. Heard. Towards Semantic Interoperability for Electronic Health Records. *Methods Inf Med* **46** (2007), 332–343
[5] A. Strauss, J. Corbin J. Grounded Theory Methodology: An Overview In *Handbook of Qualitative Research*, N.K. Denzin and Y.S. Lincoln (eds.), Thousand Oaks: Sage, pp. 273-285, 1994

International Perspectives in Health Informatics
E.M. Borycki et al. (Eds.)
IOS Press, 2011
doi:10.3233/978-1-60750-709-3-316

The Action Case Method in Health Informatics Research

Mowafa HOUSEH[a][1]

[a] College of Public Health and Health Informatics
King Saud Bin Abdulaziz University For Health Science (KSAU-HS),
Riyadh, Saudi Arabia

Abstract. This paper introduces the action case as a research method that can be used in health informatics research. In general, this method has been used in information systems research but has been ignored within the field of health informatics. This paper defines the action case and provides suggestions for its use in the various stages of a research project.

Keywords. action case, research methods, health informatics

Introduction

Health informatics researchers generally use qualitative research methods such as grounded theory [1], action research [2], ethnography [3], and case studies [4]. An action case study examines a phenomenon in its natural setting, with the researcher acting as a participant in the research project [5]. This methodology has been primarily used in information systems research but is rarely, if ever, used by health informatics researchers. The purpose of this paper is to provide suggestions for the conduct of action case studies in health informatics.

This paper does not advocate that the action case be the sole research method used within the field. Each research strategy has advantages and disadvantages and no single strategy is more important than any other. Action case research is particularly appropriate for certain types of problems in which participants are not able to be directly involved in the research project and the researcher has a limited knowledge of the context and subject under study.

There are three reasons that action case research is a viable research method in health informatics. First, the researcher can study a particular system used by a group of people while maintaining minimal interaction with the participants. Second, the researcher can not only observe but also learn through participation in the research project. Third, it allows the researcher to actively learn and study a group of people or an organization in which few studies have been carried out and is therefore an appropriate method for doctoral students or new researchers seeking new topics within health informatics. In the rapidly changing field of health informatics, many new areas

---

[1] Corresponding Author: Dr. Mowafa Househ, King Saud Bin Abdul Aziz University for Health Sciences, College of Public Health and Health Informatics, Riyadh, Kingdom of Saudi Arabia; Email: househmo@ngha.med.sa

will emerge in the coming years; valuable insights may be gained from the use of the action case to investigate these topics.

1. Defining the Action Case

There is no standard textbook definition for the action case. For the purposes of this paper, the definition presented by Braa and Vidgen [5] will be used. An action case study examines a phenomenon in its natural setting with the researcher acting as a participant in the research project. It uses data collection and analysis methods similar to those used in qualitative case studies. The major difference between action case and case studies is the role of the researcher, who is a participant within the group in the action case. For perspective, it is useful to contrast this approach with other qualitative methods used by health informatics researchers, such as action research and case study research.

In health informatics, action research has been used in a number of settings. For example, in 2000, Lau and Hayward [2] published a paper on the use of action research to virtually train 25 health professionals in topics related to health policy, management, economics, research methods, data analysis, and computer technology. In that paper, the researchers introduced the intervention to the participants and worked collaboratively on the research project. As they note in their paper, action research "links theory with practice through an iterative process of problem diagnosis, action intervention, and reflective learning." In action research, the participants and the researcher work together through the processes of problem diagnosis, action intervention, and reflective learning.

Both hard (quantitative) and soft (qualitative) case studies have also been used in health informatics. Case studies have been primarily used to evaluate existing systems, groups, or organizations. Case studies differ from action research in that the researcher does not introduce any intervention to the group but rather acts as a non-participating observer studying the phenomenon at hand. For example, a quantitative case study conducted by Collins et al. [4] investigated the clinical information needs of clinicians at the point of care. They used generic question types and success rates for each of the clinicians included in the study. As another example, a qualitative case study by Nanji et al. [6] described the barriers and facilitators for the implementation of a pharmacy barcode scanning system and its ability to reduce medication dispensing errors. Pharmacy staff members were interviewed about their experiences with the system implementation. In both the quantitative and qualitative research cases, the researchers are non-participants within the groups.

The action case is a hybrid between action research and the case study method, as illustrated in Figures I A and B. Figures I A and B, adapted from Bra and Vidgen [5], present various methods (Figure I A) used in information system research and the research outcome for each method (Figure I B). In Figure I A (Methods), six methods are listed: action research, action case, soft case, hard case, field experiment, and quasi-experiment. In Figure I B (Research Outcome) each of these methods is mapped to a desired research outcome: change, understanding, or prediction. For example, action research is a qualitative research method that studies change as a result of an intervention. Soft case studies focus on understanding what happened in a specific study. Field experiments focus on outcome prediction and on relationships between variables within the study. Hard case studies take a quantitative approach to understanding what occurred within a specific study, aiming for both prediction and understanding. Quasi-experimental designs focus on understanding a change through the use of various quantitative methods; such designs therefore map somewhere between prediction and change. Finally, the action case focuses on understanding how an intervention took place within the study and maps somewhere between change and understanding.

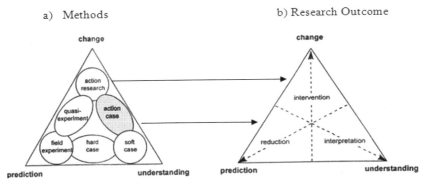

Figure 1. Adapted from Bra and Vidgen [5]

Others may argue that the action case is similar to the participant observation method used in sociology, psychology, and other fields. However, participant observation requires the researcher to immerse himself or herself in the participants' setting and become part of the social group, rather than sitting outside as an objective observer [7]. The action case does not require the researcher to become part of the social group; rather, the researcher plays an active role in supporting group activities but falls short of becoming a full-fledged group member.

2. Conducting Action Case Research

The researcher must determine whether the action case is an appropriate method to address a specific research question. The action case methodology is clearly useful in a natural setting in studies that are focused on a particular intervention that requires the participation of both the researchers and study volunteers. If there is no intervention to be studied or participation from the researchers or study volunteers is not required, then the action case is not an appropriate method. Similarly, the action case is not appropriate for projects that require a high level of researcher and participant involvement along with a major intervention within the group or organization.

The site of an action case study should be considered carefully and chosen based on the research topic. Studies can be carried out at the organizational, group, or technological level. For example, the site selection for a study of the impact of an electronic patient record on patient satisfaction within a hospital should be based on the characteristics of the hospital. These may include hospital size, public or private ownership, geographic location, and number of employees.

Today, potential research sites can be identified through the internet. Contact information for key people within organizations is readily available online. Masters and doctoral students should approach professors to talk to them about their research ideas and contacts within various healthcare organizations. Furthermore, it is important to obtain ethics approval that will provide confidentiality and/or anonymity for the organization being studied. This will develop an important sense of trust between the researcher and the organization or group being studied.

3. Action Case: Data Collection and Analysis

Multiple data collection methods can be employed in action case research. Ideally, there will be more than one source of information; sources may include interviews, observation notes, and meeting minutes. The goal is to collect a rich set of data that address the research question, describe the impact of the intervention, and illustrate the context in which the intervention took place. The researcher should keep a detailed record of observations. When relying on memory alone, the researcher may lose some important details that are (or become) relevant to the study. The record keeping should be detailed so that anyone is able to understand the project. Multiple data sources can enhance the validity of findings through the process of triangulation. Different methods of data analysis to address each type of data can be used in action case studies. These methods are similar to those found in qualitative analysis, such as grounded theory, thematic, or content analysis. Qualitative software systems such as NVIVO provide great tools for organizing the data analysis process.

4. Action Case Results

In the results section of an action case, it is most appropriate to reflect on the impact that the intervention has on the group or organization. The results section will show the reader the learning experiences derived from the intervention, as seen by the participants and analyzed by the research team. Linking the lessons learned in a particular case with previous literature on the subject is also important to show the contribution that the research has made to the field.

5. Conclusion

As described above, the action case is a research method that can be increasingly used in health informatics research projects where researchers are not able to be directly involved with other participant group members and the researcher has a limited knowledge of the domain area. The author believes that the action case can be a viable methodology in health informatics research because it requires a reduced amount of participation from the researcher and the participants of the research project. Future research should apply this research method in different health informatics settings. The use of this method will allow a better understanding more complete description of its advantages and disadvantages within the health informatics domain.

References

[1] C. Kuziemsky, J. Weber-Jahnke, F. Lau, M. Downing, An interdisciplinary computer-based information tool for palliative sever pain management. *JAMIA* **15**(3) (2008), 374-382.

[2] F. Lau, R. Hayward, Building a virtual network in a community health research training program. *JAMIA* **7** (2000), 361-377.

[3] E. Patterson, R. Cook, M. Render, Improving patient safety by identifying side effects from introducing bar coding in medication administration. *JAMIA* **9** (2002), 540-553

[4] S. Collins, L. Currie, S. Bakken, J. Cimino, Case report: Information needs, infobutton manager use, and satisfaction by clinician type: A case study. *JAMIA* **16** (2009), 140-142.

[5] K. Braa, R. Vidgen, Interpretation, intervention, and reduction in the organizational laboratory: A framework for in-context information systems research. *Acct Manage Inf Tech* **9**(1) (1999), 25-47.

[6] K. Nanji, J. Cina, N. Patel, Case report: Overcoming barriers to the implementation of a pharmacy bar code scanning system for medication dispensing: A case study. *JAMIA* **16** (2009), 645-650.

[7] W. M. Trochim, Research methods knowledge base: Types of data. [cited 2005 December 20]. Available from www.socialresearchmethods.net

[8] B. Berg, *Qualitative research methodology*. 3rd ed. Boston: Allyn & Bacon, 1989.

[9] N. Kondracki, N. Wellman, D. Amundson, Content analysis: review of methods and their applications in nutrition education. *J Nut Educ Behav* **34**(4) (2002), 224-230.

[10] W. J. Orlikowski, J.Yates, Genre repertoire: Norms and forms for work and interaction. *Center for Coordination Science Technical Report* #166. 1994.

[11] B. Jargen, H. Erling. Sensemaking in technology-use mediation: Adapting groupware technology in organizations. *Comp Supp Coop Work*, **15**(1) (2006), 55-91

Nursing Informatics

International Perspectives in Health Informatics
E.M. Borycki et al. (Eds.)
IOS Press, 2011
doi:10.3233/978-1-60750-709-3-323

Application of Language Processing Techniques to Capture the Use of Nursing Clinical Terms from Narrative Statements: Report of a Pilot Study

Noreen FRISCH [a], Larry FRISCH [b]

[a] School of Nursing, University of Victoria, Victoria, British Columbia, Canada
[b] School of Health Information Science, University of Victoria, Victoria, Bristish Columbia, Canada

Abstract. Objective: The authors piloted the use of the "General Architecture for Text Engineering" (GATE) program in an analysis of writings from the nursing literature to determine if this standard language processing technique could be used to capture the use of complex nursing terms. This work was undertaken as an initial step in evaluating if widely-available natural language processing methods could be applied to narrative nursing notes in a way that a nursing diagnosis could be identified and extracted from a narrative text. Methods: For purposes of the pilot study, the complex nursing term "powerlessness", which is identified as a NANDA-I nursing diagnosis, was selected as the test case. A PubMed search was performed on the term "powerlessness" limited to articles in the nursing literature that contained abstracts, resulting in 232 articles published between 1981 to 2010 meeting the criteria. Three-sentence extracts from each abstract were analyzed by applying GATE to identify noun and adjective roots occurring in close proximity to the index word, and then identifying if these proximal words reflected the standardized defining characteristics, adjectives and qualifiers of the diagnostic term. Results: The analysis resulted identification 2,174 unique terms. While a few terms coincided with the NANDA-I defining characteristics of "powerlessness", most of the established defining characteristics were not reflected in the use of the term. Conclusions: Machine language processing techniques are promising in identifying meanings and contextual use of words related to nursing concepts, but the use of such words in published papers does not represent definitions found in standard nursing nomenclature. Nursing writers use terms that are also understood outside the disciplinary domain, making standardization and coding particularly challenging. Future research in Nursing should apply the techniques described to clinical reports and to evaluate the match between clinical usage and standardized meanings.

Keywords. language processing, NANDA-I, nursing diagnosis, powerlessness

Introduction

There have been many arguments put forth for the use of standardized nursing languages, but perhaps none as compelling as the need to provide nursing data in electronic health records (EHRs). In the field of informatics, it is universally understood that standardized, coded terms are essential for the implementation of electronic systems. Nurses have been identified as critically-important stakeholders in development of EHRs [1], yet in the field of nursing, there remains confusion and controversy about the nature of the standardization and the benefits of coded terms over the narrative descriptions [2]. Moreover, current nursing curricula do not include sufficient content to cover essential informatics content, including content about nursing standardized languages [3]. Recent evaluations of 'readiness' for use of standardized systems suggest that practicing nurses [4], nursing faculty [5], nursing doctoral students [6] and graduating nurses [7] have insufficient facility with the standardized nursing systems to make use of them in clinical settings. In spite of years of work developing standardized nursing nomenclature, expert knowledge of such systems to reside with those academics and early adopters who have committed their careers to development and testing of such systems. Given the large number of nursing professionals who are charting and 'thinking' in terms of narrative descriptions, it is reasonable to evaluate whether or not terms captured in the context of narrative data can be matched to terms found in definitions or descriptors and related factors in standardized taxonomies.

There have been prior attempts at capturing data from narrative health records and these have been directed primarily to medical (not nursing) terms. Narratives can be assessed by expert readers and/or by automatic language processing software. Such software uses algorithms to parse sentences, to identify lexical units (e.g. nouns, adjectives, verbs, etc.), and sometimes to relate parsed words and phrases to pre-established lexicons that can identify a given word or phrase as likely belonging to the domain of nursing. In 2005 Bakken [8] and in 2009, Hyun, Johnson and Bakken [9] applied the Medical Language Extraction and Encoding system (MedLEE) to nursing narratives for the purpose of capturing nursing concepts. In both cases, the authors concluded that additional terms and abbreviations need to be added to that program as nursing narratives include descriptions of client status through vocabulary quite specific to the domain of nursing.

The current study takes a different focus, and that is to begin with the nursing terminologies already established in standardized systems and then to determine the degree to which these standardized terms are used in nursing practice or literature in accord with recognized and published definitions. As nursing care becomes documented in EHRs, researchers will have increased access to digital clinical descriptions which can be compared with independently-established nursing diagnostic terms to assess the degree to which there is correspondence between the diagnosis suggested by an expert "gold standard" review and the nurses' descriptors in the clinical record. Benefits of such would be twofold: first, the ability to 'translate' the narrative descriptions into standardized terms that can be coded; and second, the ability to validate that the use of the standardized term is in fact related to the established or accepted definitions of that term for clinical use.

The current study had two objectives: 1) to learn if an open-source natural language processing (NLP) program applied to published nursing documents could capture terms representing nursing autonomous work (e.g. a nursing diagnosis), and 2) to determine if writings concerning a complex nursing concept employed words suggested by the definitions, defining characteristics, and/or related factors in standardized nursing language. Because previous research suggests that nursing faculty may not be teaching students what is necessary to be effective users of standardized language in the EHR era, we wondered how consistently nursing scholars used standardized language to describe fundamental nursing concepts in their own research publications. Furthers, we reasoned that if the application of such language processing techniques proved feasible, we could begin a process of evaluating clinical narrative reports, either to suggest a nursing diagnoses or intervention/outcome term to the clinician writing the narrative, or to extract a codeable term from the narrative account itself.

1. Study Questions

Specifically, our questions were: 1) Could we apply the GATE (General Architecture for Text Engineering) program to published nursing literature to capture the use of an abstract nursing term; and 2) Would there be a match between the words employed in the published nursing literature proximal to the index term and the standardized terms used as defining characteristics or related factors of the index term.

2. Methods

We designed this study around the use of the term "powerlessness" in abstracts accompanying articles published by nursing scholars. We chose to use the term "powerlessness" because the term is a defined nursing diagnosis [10]; it represents a need for autonomous nursing action; and it represents a complex concept that is a human response to a health condition or life process. To obtain narrations about nurses' use of the term, we selected abstracts from a PubMed search of the literature that addressed the subject heading of "powerlessness". For this purpose, the PubMed "limits" function was invoked to include only articles with abstracts published in the nursing literature. Searching was performed on June 27, 2010 using only "powerlessness" entered as a PubMed search term. The resultant automatic Mesh search translation was "powerlessness[All Fields] AND (hasabstract[text] AND jsubsetn[text]. This search identified 232 abstracts published between September, 1981 and May 2010.

Three sentences from each abstract were selected: an index sentence containing the word "powerlessness" and two additional flanking sentences, respectively before and after the index sentence. In a few cases the index sentence was the first or last sentence in the abstract, so it did not lie between the two other sentences chosen. The final compilation of sentences from these abstracts was stored in a MS Word document. This document was further analyzed with GATE (General Architecture for Text Engineering) version 5.2.1 using three components of the "ANNIE" plug-in: English Tokenizer, Sentence Splitter, and POS (part of speech) Tagger along with the GATE Morphological Analyser. All noun forms and adjectives were selected and copied to an external file. The resulting mark-up was further edited in MS Word to include only root words (i.e. proper nouns, plurals, and gerund forms of nouns were reduced to their semantic roots: e.g. *Control, control, controls, controlling* all map to *control.*) The document was loaded into MS Excel 2003 (SP3) and analyzed using pivot tables. Graphs of word frequency were also created.

3. Results

The document had a total of 18,271 words in its initial version and 8,773 in its final version, representing 2,174 unique words. Table 1 presents the most frequently found words.

Table 1. Most frequently-found words associated with "powerlessness" as the index word.

WORD (number of occurrences)		
Patient (134)	Sense (40)	Caregiver (27)
Care (128)	Life (39)	Strategy (26)
Nursing (106)	Group (39)	Anxiety (26)
Feeling (97)	Power (37)	Individual empowerment (25)
Health (77)	Role (36)	Time (23)
Women (70)	Change (30)	Need (23)
Family (47)	Work (29)	Anger (23)
Relationship (44)	Pain (29)	Perception (23)
Control (42)	Support (28)	Frustration (21)
Lack (41)	Violence (27)	Guilt (21)
		Education (21)

The NANDA-I diagnosis of "powerlessness" includes defining characteristics of *passivity, anger, dependence, irritability, dissatisfaction, doubt, frustration, fear of alienation from caretakers, guilt, reluctance to express feelings, resentment, apathy,* and *depression* [11]. Some of the words contained in these defining characteristics do appear in the table above however, most words associated with NANDA-I defining characteristics appear at most twice in the set of abstracts: *reluctance, resentment, alienation, irritability, dissatisfaction,* and *apathy. Dependence* and *doubt* occur five and four times respectively.

4. Analysis/Discussion

A relatively small number of words associated "powerlessness" in standardized nomenclature appeared with high frequency in these abstracts, many of the associated words appeared in less than 10% of the abstracts, and very few of the words that appeared are included in the standardized definition, defining characteristics or related factors. NANDA-I includes *dependence on others* as a characteristic of "moderate powerlessness", and so the observed concept of "relationship*"* might be at least indirectly applicable. However, quite notably, the abstracts did not refer to *apathy* or *depression,* two of three NANDA-I defining characteristics of "severe powerlessness".

This study was conducted to assess the feasibility of using GATE and its ANNIE plug-in for subsequent lexical analysis of nursing clinical records. Even a very large file was analyzed in only a few minutes, and where needed, conversions from XML format were greatly speeded by a VBA macro. An effective search facility within GATE allowed any needed inspection and analysis of words within context. An example was the use of the word *control.* "Verbal expressions of having no control" are in the NANDA-I definition of "severe powerlessness"; however, in many of the abstracts reviewed for this study, "control" was used in the context of an experimental design: i.e. cases and controls. GATE facilitates the employment of semantic ontologies which can allow such variant usages to be identified, though we have not as yet applied such tools to the present dataset.

5. Conclusions

Our pilot evaluation revealed that one can apply the GATE program in the manner described above to capture the context and use of a complex nursing term in the published literature. We found that the words employed in the published literature proximal to the term "powerlessness" do not reflect the NANDA-I defining characteristics or related factors of the nursing diagnostic term.

6. Implications for Future Research

We believe that the method has promise for further testing of use of language processing methods in identifying standardized nursing terms within narrative text created by nurses. An obvious next step would be to apply the GATE program to actual clinical narrative data. A second area of further study would be to determine to what degree nursing complex terms (such as "powerlessness") are used in nursing professional literature and in nurses' work in a manner distinct from the meaning of the term as an actual nursing diagnosis. Nursing, more than other health disciplines, has considerable challenges to standardization of terms and clarity of professional meaning because several nursing diagnostic terms (e.g., the nursing diagnoses of "powerlessness", "hopelessness", "resilience", "comfort", "spiritual distress", "conflict") are both complex and abstract and are represented by words that are used outside the professional disciplinary use.

References

[1] T.J. Watkins, R.E. Haskell, C.B. Lundberg, J.M. Brokel, M.I. Wilson, N. Hardiker, Terminology Use in Electronic Health Records: Basic principles, *Urologic Nursing* **29** (2009), 321–326.
[2] L. Day, What is documentation for? *Amer J Crit Care* **18** (2008), 77-80.
[3] B.N. Thompson, D.J., Skiba, Informatics in the nursing curriculum: A national survey of nursing informatics requirements in nursing curricula, *Nurs Educ Perspect* **29** (2009), 312–317.
[4] J. Klehr, J. Hafner, L.M. Spelz, S. Steen, K. Weaver, Implementation of standardized nomenclature in the electronic medical record, *Int J Nurs Term Classifications* **20** (2009), 169-180.
[5] T. Hebra, L. Calderone, What nurse educators need to know about the TIGER initiative, *Nurse Educ* **25** (2010), 56–60.
[6] B.E. Dixon, C.M. Newlon, How do future nurse educators perceive informatics? Advancing the nursing informatics agenda through dialogue, *J Prof Nurs* **26** (2010), 82–89.
[7] M.S. Fetter, Graduating nurses self-evaluation of information technology competencies, *Journal of Nurs Educ* **48** (2009), 82-89.
[8] S. Bakken, S. Hyun, C. Friedman, S. Johnson, ISO reference terminology models for nursing: applicability for natural language processing of nursing narratives, *Int J Med Inf* **74** (2005), 619- 622.
[9] S. Hyun, S. Johnson, S. Bakken, Exploring the ability of natural language processing to extract data from nursing narratives, *CIN,* **27** (2009), 215-223.
[10] NANDA-International, *Nursing diagnosis: Definitions and Classifications: 2009-2011,* Wiley-Blackwell, Oxford, 2009.
[11] Ibid, p. 190.

International Perspectives in Health Informatics
E.M. Borycki et al. (Eds.)
IOS Press, 2011
© 2011 ITCH 2011 Steering Committee and IOS Press. All rights reserved.
doi:10.3233/978-1-60750-709-3-328

Leveling: An Approach to Advanced Human Simulation which Maximizes Learning and Available Resources

Shannon LANCTOT-SHAH [a,1], Judith FEARING [b], Sandra MORROW [c]

[ab] *Selkirk College* [c] *KBRH*

Abstract. Advanced Human Simulation using computerized mannequin patients has been established as an effective and innovative means of delivering nursing education. Consistent student feedback underscores the value of this teaching approach and the learning gained from it. Students enthusiastically request additional simulated learning opportunities. Instructors acknowledge the additional time and human resources required to provide quality simulated experiences, especially in a small rural college, but consider it worth the effort. As a means of addressing both of these issues, the concept of leveling a simulation scenario involving a client experiencing a cardiac event which can be edited, modified and embellished has been created to provide an on-going learning opportunity across the four years of a baccalaureate degree in Nursing.

Keywords. simulation, nursing education, leveling

Introduction

Baccalaureate nursing education using advanced computerized human mannequin simulation technology provides students with the opportunity to develop critical thinking skills, teamwork and application of theory to practice in a safe and supportive learning environment. Schools of Nursing, especially rural programs are feeling the pressure of increasing student practice needs, coupled with the rapidly changing acute care environment. The literature and our evaluative data support the use of an advanced human simulator as a way of addressing some of these issues; however the investment of time and resources makes it a tremendous undertaking for a small college.

To date a number of simulated learning opportunities have been developed to augment learning in the nursing centre. Traditional teaching methods are brought to life with the use of a simulator that interacts with the student, but does not feel the pain of an invasive intervention. The opportunity to present a cardiac based scenario using a human patient simulator (HPS) to each year of nursing student has allowed us to explore the full spectrum of learning opportunities available by using simulation while reducing the resources required for multiple scenarios. By collecting feedback post

---

[1] Shannon Lanctot-Shah, Selkirk College, Castlegar, British Columbia, Canada; email: sshah@selkirk.ca

scenario using a 5 point Likert scale and narrative notes we have confirmed that our students value the opportunity to use HPS and found leveling of scenario's beneficial.

1. Literature Review

Simulation is defined by Jeffries as "activities that mimic the reality of a clinical environment and are designed to demonstrate procedures, decision-making, and critical thinking"[1]. Simulation provides the opportunity for learners to learn and practice skills within a safe, risk-free environment. It also provides an engaging activity that allows students with different learning styles to experience the scenario in different ways [2]. Brain-based learning provides insight into the nature of learning and gives guidance to the most effective teaching & learning techniques. Experiential learning incorporating multiple senses and positive emotions enables students to interact with knowledge in ways that connects new information with past experiences. This layering builds relational memory and ultimately improves long term memory. Well designed HPS scenarios stimulate student's multiple senses while the emotional intensity of the interactive simulation facilitates relevant and immediate engagement. This engaged state of mind is an opportune time for active learning, critical thinking and reflection, and has strong links to long term memory [3]. Clearly stated learning objectives and goals [4] as well as debriefing and peer observation are integral to the simulation experience, promoting reflective practice, developing critical thinking and aiding in the retention of learning [5-7]. Initial evaluations of the use of HPS for nursing education indicate increased student satisfaction, quicker skill acquisition, increased knowledge retention, enhanced critical thinking and increased self confidence.

2. Educational Methods and Program

The methods for delivering education must address individual learner's needs and take into account the generational factor. The Gen Y (born after 1981) students make's up the bulk of our nursing student population. They are highly adapted to technology, enjoy multi tasking and prefer collaborative, interactive learning activities. They want immediacy and engagement but are less skilled at face to face communication and the ability to go beyond the superficial to develop deeper meaning. Educational activities that facilitate improved listening skills, understanding the impact of personal experiences and working with team dynamics will enhance their capabilities. [8]

Many variables can undermine the process of moving theory to practice and are often identified as gaps in what the students require to be job ready. Within the framework of the Collaboration for Academic Education in Nursing (CAEN) curriculum the simulated situations were designed to demonstrate best practice. As well these experiences identify professional responsibilities and troubleshoot the realities of the clinical setting in which the greatest variable is always the human component. Students are encouraged to draw on their knowledge, explore their resources and respond. The flexibility and the safety of simulation allows for a realistic, unique experience. Students receive feedback from their peers and the facilitators which guides them to try new approaches. Each year students work within the core cardiac simulation to build on their existing skills and challenge themselves to take the next steps towards the roles and responsibilities of a registered nurse.

2.1 Building the Cardiac Simulation Scenario

In conjunction with Nursing Instructors two 4th year students completed an assessment of the use of simulation though the 4 year degree program. The cardiac scenario, with a core template of an individual who experiences distress which advances to cardiac arrest has since been leveled through years 1-4. The shift from standard clients traditionally used in nursing programs now allows for a standard scenario with a variety of clients and situations to challenge the student to cope with the distractions and demonstrate best practice and critical thinking skills.

Using the CAEN curriculum guide, leveling was implemented by: 1) layering more complex data into the scenario as the students advanced through the years of the program and 2) changing the "superficial" characteristics of the patient situation while maintaining the underlying structural similarities. At strategic times in each year of the program students observe and participate in the cardiac event scenario. At each presentation, two students watch through one way glass as two of their colleagues provide nursing care to the HPS patient. The observers are given a list of expected behaviors their colleagues will ideally perform. At the end of the 15 minute scenario both groups spend 5 minutes completing a reflection form that is used during debriefing. Following this, the observers become the nurses in another "cardiac" scenario with a different HPS patient. This repetition ensures that the nursing students carefully assess their patient and develop and implement their plan based on their assessment data while drawing on the knowledge gained through observing the previous scenario and from previous theory. It challenges them to see through the superficial characteristic changes to the underlying similarities.

Simulations work best when the problems are like stories with embedded contextual cues. The more authentic and intense the simulation, the better the learning and student retention. Learning occurs as students become skilled at identifying the salient data and bringing this to the next scenario, building on their clinical skills and strategic pattern identification [9]. Students highly value the opportunity to engage in a second attempt of each simulation [10]. Leveling of scenarios is an important part of successful simulation design. Moving from simple fundamental skill acquisition to more complex skill sets, students are given the opportunity to repeatedly assess and provide care, building their confidence and critical judgment [11]. The complexity of the patient needs, order of the problem presentation and scenario pacing is all part of creating effectively designed scenarios [1,12]. Year 1 nursing students complete a consolidated practice experience (CPE) in a long term care facility. For these students, where institutional policy is for all patients to be no code status, the cardiac event simulation is focused on identifying unresponsiveness, calling for help, opening the patient's airway, moving the patient to a recovery position, and communicating with family members. As the students begin 2nd year and advance to acute care settings, the cardiac event simulation involves assessment and use of safety equipment in the room, understanding the differing expectations for responding to a cardiac event in the acute care setting, understanding code status and preparing the room for the expected arrival of the code team. Following the completion of education on acute coronary syndrome and in preparation for the CPE in acute care, the cardiac event scenario incorporates the initial management of chest pain adding a pain assessment, pharmacological management of the pain, interpretation of vital signs, and communicating with the physician using the SBAR tool. In 3rd year, as the students return to acute care facilities from community practice placements settings the scenario incorporates pharmacological treatment of chest pain which develops into a cardiac arrest necessitating CPR and an opportunity to review the acute coronary syndrome preprinted orders and care pathways. Prior to their 12 weeks of consolidated practice the 4th year students again participate in the scenario working to their professional standards. Documentation and debriefing are part of every simulation scenario.

3. Results

HPS in nursing education provides learning opportunities to both students and instructors to increase proficiency, confidence, and ability to apply and adapt theory to the practice setting in a safe and controlled learning environment. It serves to address the challenge of educating students to develop the wide range of generalist nursing skills needed to prepare them for their roles and responsibilities as new graduates.

3.1. Formative Findings from the Student Survey

Our 5-point Likert scale tool gathered data from 22 questions with the following themes, with their respective mean scores (1 = Strongly Disagree; 2 = Somewhat Disagree; 3 = Undecided; 4 = Somewhat Agree; 5 = Strongly Agree):
1. Student Satisfaction – mean 4.64
2. Realism – mean 4.31
3. Evaluation of Physical Surroundings & Equipment – mean 4.50
4. Development of Critical Thinking Skills – mean 4.11
5. Transference of theory to practice – mean 4.20

3.2. Narratives from the Open-Ended Student Questions.

- Increased my confidence; much easier to play out the scenario with patient feedback – the simulator made it feel 'real' versus pretending. Adds unpredictability, but also adds more pt. related information
- Great to have feedback from client, focusing on clients needs as well as required checks that need to be accomplished. Makes my care more client centered.
- Closer to real life situation- similar intensity – team work
- Seemed more real without the pressure of an emergent situation
- It made the situation more realistic promotes critical thinking and decision-making
- Assisted me with integrating the theory into practice
- There is nothing like hands-on practice to recognize strengths & gaps
- It was nice to experience a complication – allowed us to use our problem solving skills/ knowledge base
- It felt a little intimidating but now that I am used to what its all about I think I will really benefit from the simulator
- To prioritize assessment, care and outcomes. Helped to explain to patients their condition in a way they would understand.
- I wish we could have had this opportunity as we progressed through the program, I think that those who will, will greatly benefit

- Working in a simulated setting is exhilarating, but nerve wracking. It makes me feel nervous about practicing in real life. There is so much to know! And put in a situation that is pressured – with the pt asking for help, trying to coordinate with other team members, trying to do proper assessments & interventions – really makes me see how far I still have to go.
- I would like to see more simulations throughout the program. Great way to practice assessments, team approach, organization, etc.
- Need more practice with it to become more comfortable

4. Discussion

As we move forward to the next level of collecting data and analysis we are responding to the needs expressed by students for increased exposure to the simulator and the opportunity to demonstrate leadership in acute situations. The core scenario is an individual experiencing distress which leads to a cardiac arrest. This scenario was chosen to re-enforce the skills introduced in CPR certification, explore policy and procedure in different areas of care, understand safety, communication and team-work and demonstrate leadership in the clinical setting. Consistently student's feedback indicated that they enjoyed simulation, and that they were becoming more comfortable with each simulated experience. We were able to link students experience in practice and their ability to manage situations and feel confident when situations arose that had been addressed in simulation. We see the opportunity to increase access and build confidence with using technology in nursing education. As we continually strive to link theory to practice and respond to decreasing clinical practice settings, simulation offers our students supported clinical options

References

[1] P.A. Jeffries, A framework for designing, implementing, and evaluating simulations used as teaching strategies in nursing, *Nursf Educ Perspec* **26(2)** (2005), 96-103.
[2] S.H. Campbell, *Clinical simulation,* In K.B. Gaberson & M.H. Oermann (Eds.), Clinical teaching strategies in nursing, Springer, New York, NY, 2007 (2nd ed), 123-140.
[3] J. Willis, Brain-based teaching strategies for improving students' memory, learning, and test-taking success, *Childhood Education.* Retrieved June 25, 2010 from http://www.thefreelibrary.com/_/print/PrintArticle.aspx?id=166187986.
[4] E.A. Henneman., H. CunniJ.P. Roche, M.E. Curnin, Human patient simulation: Teaching students to provide safe patient care, *Nurse Educ,* **32(5)** (2007), 212-217.
[5] K. Lasater, High-fidelity simulation and the development of clinical judgment: Students' experiences, *J Nurs Educ* **46(6)** (2007), 269-276.
[6] C. Kuehster, C. Hall, Simulation: Learning from mistakes while building communication and teamwork, *J Nurses Staff Devel,* **26(3)** (2010), 123-127.
[7] L. Baillie, J. Curzio, Students' and facilitators' perceptions of simulation in practice learning, *Nurse Educ Practice* **9** (2009), 297-306.
[8] C. Schofield, S. Honore, Generation Y and learning, *The Ashridge Journal,* (2009-2010) Retrieved June 25, 2010 from www.ashridge.org.uk/360.
[9] S. Prion, Key note presenter, BC Lab Educators Conference, Vancouver BC, May 15, 2009.
[10] V.A. Ypinazar, S.A. Margolis, Clinical simulators: Applications and implications for rural medical education, *Rural Remote Health,* **6(527)** (2006), Retrieved July 30, 2009 from http://www.rrh.org.au/publishedarticles/article_print_527.pdf.
[11] A.R. Starkweather, S. Karong-Edgren, Diffusion of innovation: Embedding simulation into nursing curricula, *Int J Nurs Educ Scholarship,* **5(1)** (2008), 1-12.
[12] C. Larew, S. Lessans, D. Spunt, D. Foster, B.G. Covington, Innovations in clinical simulation: The application of Benner's theory in an interactive patient care simulation, *Nurs Educ Perspect,* **27(1)** (2006), 16-21.

International Perspectives in Health Informatics
E.M. Borycki et al. (Eds.)
IOS Press, 2011
© *2011 ITCH 2011 Steering Committee and IOS Press. All rights reserved.*
doi:10.3233/978-1-60750-709-3-333

Usability of Electronic Nursing Record Systems: Definition and Results from an Evaluation Study in Finland

Johanna VIITANEN[a,1], Anne KUUSISTO[b], Pirkko NYKÄNEN[c]

[a] *Aalto University, School of Science and Technology, Finland*
[b] *Satakunta Hospital District, Pori, Finland*
[c] *University of Tampere, Finland*

Abstract. Information technologies (IT) are widely used in healthcare, however, little is known about the usability of nursing information systems. This article reports an evaluation study that aimed at researching the usability of four electronic nursing record (ENR) systems and thereby providing guidelines for further IT development. For the purposes of the study the concept of usability was defined to cover the following aspects: nurse-computer interaction in working context, information exchange, and collaboration between healthcare professionals. The study utilized two usability research methods, contextual inquiry and expert review, and was conducted with 18 nurses in Finland. Study results showed that the ENR systems share several usability problems in common, most of them relating to the efficiency of use, intuitiveness, and poor fit for multi-professional needs. Nurses had mainly negative experiences on documenting practices with ENRs: documentation requires a lot of resources, patient information is hard to find, and procedures do not meet the contextual needs. These findings suggest usability problems having significant effects on nurses' documentation practices and nursing work.

Keywords. nursing informatics, usability, electronic nursing record system, human-computer interaction

Introduction

The adoption of information systems has in several ways influenced nursing practices and documentation. Recently, there has been growing interest in exploring nurses' experiences on electronic documentation. These studies have resulted in both encouraging and contradictory findings. According to Törnvall et al. [1], the overall tendency concerning the nurses' opinions on documentation in electronic format seems to be positive. Similarly Kuusisto et al. [2] found that nurses' experiences with electronic nursing discharge summary were mainly positive, though new structures require careful consideration and documentation takes time. Likewise, several studies indicate that in documentation no time-efficiency has been achieved by implementing an electronic nursing or medical record system [3,4,5]. In their studies about the use of

---

[1] Corresponding Author: Johanna Viitanen, Strategic Usability Research Group, Software Business and Engineering Institute, P.O. Box 19210, FIN-00076 AALTO, FINLAND; E-mail: johanna.viitanen@tkk.fi

electronic nursing record (ENR) systems in everyday practice, both Moody et al. [6] and Stevenson et al. [7] find nurses experiencing widespread dissatisfaction because of deficiency of the systems. On the other hand, the use of bedside terminals and mobile solutions in nursing work seem to hold promising opportunities [5,8]. Based on the described results it is unclear how suitable the currently used ENR systems are for nursing work and what kind of use related experiences nurses have. Although some research has been conducted to evaluate the usability of a healthcare information system in clinical settings (e.g. [9, 10]), rather less attention has been paid to examining the usability of nursing information systems.

This article aims to: a) introduce a concept "usability of ENR systems" with related attributes, b) describe a usability evaluation study of four currently used ENR systems in Finland, and c) present summative results from the study. The study to be presented was a part of an empirical research project which incorporated three intersecting themes: 1) the feasibility of the Nationally Standardized Electronic Nursing Documentation model in nursing practices (Finnish nursing documentation is based on the nursing decision making process, nursing core data (NMDS) and Finnish Care Classification (FinCC [11, 12])), 2) the usability of ENR systems, and 3) the role of nursing documentation in multi-professional care work [13].

1. Introducing the Concept "Usability of Electronic Nursing Record Systems"

In the health informatics research field the concept "usability of healthcare information systems" is often mentioned and referred to (e.g. [9,14,15]). Frequently, the term usability is used to indicate the attributes of a system, which make it easy to use. These definitions or criteria of evaluation do not, however, reflect the contextual characteristics of usability or indicate the impacts that usability has on healthcare work.

In usability research literature the widely known definition for usability of interactive systems is by the ISO 9241-210 standard [16]: *Usability is the extent to which a system can be used by specific users to achieve specified goals with effectiveness, efficiency and satisfaction in a specified context of use.* Another widely cited definition is presented by Jakob Nielsen [17]: *Usability has multiple components and is traditionally associated with the five usability attributes, which are learnability, efficiency, memorability, errors, and satisfaction.* Both the definitions emphasize the relation between usability and context of use by stating that the level of usability achieved will always depend on the specific circumstances in which a system is used. These specific circumstances can be described as four elements of context of use: *users, tasks, tools,* and the physical and social *environments* [16].

When applied to the area of nursing informatics, these definitions suggest that the usability of nursing information systems should reflect the characteristics of nurses' work and working environments. The elements of context of use around ENR systems can be described as follows. The *environments* in which ENR systems are used include clinics and wards with different nursing specialties, special and primary healthcare, as well as private and public sectors. ENR systems have several *users*, primary of these being nurses and secondary physicians and other healthcare professionals. ENR systems should serve a number of *purposes or uses*: support documentation, information processing and exchange, and fit for different nursing practices and processes. Technology environments in healthcare organizations consist of hundreds of information systems; however, for the nurses, ENR systems represent the most important daily used *tools* for high-quality and accurate patient care.

General definitions of usability and the illustrated characteristics of nursing context of use, suggest that for the purposes of IT development and evaluation the usability of ENR systems can be described with several context specific attributes. The following definition, indicating five of the most apparent usability attributes, was applied and validated in an empirical evaluation study that incorporated four ENR systems.

Usability attributes of ENR systems:

- *The fluency of reporting practices using ENR systems:* the efficiency and effectiveness of documentation, simplicity of the system, ease of use.
- *Accuracy of documentation:* errors in the performance of documentation, system's support for failure protections and recovery.
- *Learnability:* intuitiveness of use, system's ability to guide new users.
- *Exploitation of documented information within the nurses:* support for nurse's work, exchange of information, manner of representation (content and layout).
- *Support for collaborative care* (nurses and other healthcare professionals): accessibility and readability of documented information, information exchange, and manner of representation compared to multi-professional needs.

2. Usability Study: Procedure and Methods

Evaluation study of four ENR systems was conducted in Finland in spring 2010 with an objective to: 1) evaluate the usability of ENR systems and 2) research how the usability aspects appear in nurses' documenting practices. The evaluated four ENR systems (referred as A, B, C, and D) represented a heterogeneous group of systems that currently contain the implementation of standardized nursing documentation. Systems A and B are used both in special and primary healthcare, whereas C only in primary healthcare. System D is widely used in occupational health, and is especially suitable for private healthcare organizations' needs.

The study incorporated two usability research methods: contextual inquiry [18] and expert review using usability heuristics [17]. Contextual inquires followed the principles of contextual inquiry method and were conducted in Finnish in nurses' real working environments. Altogether 18 nurses from seven healthcare organizations were involved in the study. The criteria for selecting the users was: all four systems as well as public-private sectors and clinic-ward units should be represented, and the nurses need have more than half a year experience in documenting with ENR system according the Nationally Standardized Electronic Nursing Documentation model [13,14]. Table 1 presents a summary of the ENR systems and the users' backgrounds.

Table 1. A summary of the evaluated systems and the involved nurses' backgrounds in the usability study.

ENR system	Number of users in the study	Users' background: healthcare organization	Users' background: working unit:
A	6	Public sector, 4 in special and 2 in primary healthcare	2 clinic / 4 ward
B	5	Public sector, special healthcare	3 clinic / 2 ward
C	4	Public sector, primary healthcare	4 ward
D	3	Private healthcare	3 ward
	Total: 18		

Inquiries lasted about 1 hour each. The predetermined themes for interviews included: a) documentation in nursing work, b) practical documentation exercise based on the written scenario, c) use of patient information for one's own purposes and in collaboration with other professionals. During the inquiry, the documentation exercise was the main theme and incorporated several other topics. Before the data gathering, the researchers had prepared three textual scenarios: one to fit for primary healthcare, others for clinic and special care wards. In the exercise, the nurse was asked to envision a nursing situation described in a scenario, document information as they would normally do, and while working, explain and give reasoning for her actions. For patient information security, interviews and exercises were conducted using educational nursing records. Expert reviews were to supplement the inquiry data and focus on user interfaces and phases of interaction in documentation. The expert reviews were conducted after inquiries by a research group member, who was a usability specialist and based on interviews, had background knowledge about the user's actions with the system. After inquires and reviews, the qualitative data was interpreted and analyzed the content analysis method [19]. While reading through the typed notes, the findings were iteratively classified into several content categories arising from the data and then grouped together with the ENR usability attributes.

3. Results

The usability study revealed mainly negative findings about the usability of ENR systems. On the positive side, nurses seem to prefer electronic documentation and are not willing to go back to paper-based practices. The main reason being the accessibility of information (compared to paper, electronic documentation is easily accessible) and the reuse of documentation (e.g. when a care plan is accurately written, it can be utilized afterwards in care process and documentation). Although the implementation of electronic nursing documentation and related user interfaces were considerably different, all the evaluated systems shared similar usability problems. In the next section, the main results are presented according to the five usability attributes.

The fluency of reporting practices using ENR systems. The ENR systems do not support effective or efficient documentation. Documentation takes a lot of time because of poor user interface design and complicated interaction sequences. Time required for documentation is considerably high because the nurses are forced to take a huge number of unnecessary interaction steps when performing a simple task, for example a new documentation entry. When the nurses are to select classifications for their entries (in Finland the FinCC includes three hierarchy levels and 719 classes [13]) the system does not follow the nurses' mental models or provide intelligent support for search or writing. Instead, the implementation forces a user to proceed top-down (from abstract to concrete). The evaluated systems also poorly supported the use of structured templates or copy functionality, although the contents of patient documentation within a clinic or a ward typically follow the same structure. Additionally, the nurses are required to document the same information several times into different systems because of lack of automatic transfer and integration.

Accuracy of documentation. ENR systems allow the nurses to use a variety of documenting practices, both at content and at technical levels. These practices in healthcare organizations rely on unit's own, commonly agreed instructions and guidelines, and the nurses' own experiences and knowhow. Due to the complexity of the user interfaces, the users can easily make errors in performing the documentation. Generally, the system's support for failure protection is typically insufficient. Accuracy of information is by no doubt endangered because of these facts and the insufficient guidance for users in a documentation process. Especially in a hurry the nurses try use the ENR systems in a simplified and straight forward way, however, knowing that this may reduce the quality of documentation.

Learnability. Nurses felt that learning how to do standardized documentation with an ENR system is demanding and takes a lot of time. Findings from the expert reviews indicated that none of the evaluated four systems are intuitive to use. The systems do not guide the users in information processing. Because of separate systems and lack of integration, the situation is even more complicated for new users.

Exploitation of documented information within the nurses. Nurses argued that based on the documented information it is difficult to get a general view of patient's situation and needs, as well as previous nursing activities. There are several reasons for this: 1) fragmentariness of structured documentation, 2) documentation into separate systems, 3) lack of summaries, and 4) inappropriate manner of information presentation for readers. In addition, differences in documentation practices, both at content and at technical levels, have an effect on information exchange between the units and nurses' abilities in finding and understanding entries written colleagues.

Support for collaborative care. Documented information should be easily accessible and readable for all healthcare professionals involved in patient's care. At present, nurses had difficulties in searching and finding information from ENR systems. Nurses also claimed that physicians experience even more significant problems, and as a consequence, are not willing to use the systems or read the documented patient information. In some healthcare units that were involved in the study, the nurses even felt that physicians may be set against documentation practices with ENR systems.

4. Conclusions

This article provides new information about the usability of ENR systems: a definition with attributes, and summative results to guide the further development. Compared to the widely quoted definitions of usability and the related usability metrics [16,17], the described definition emphasizes the contextual attributes of nursing informatics and thereby increases our understanding about the usability aspects of healthcare information systems. The study indicated that usability problems appear to have effects on nurses' documentation practices and nursing work, and thus reflect to the healthcare professionals' attitudes towards standardized documentation with ENRs. These findings emphasize the need for a good fit between nursing practices and ENR systems as also other researchers field have argued in their articles [e.g. 7, 20, 21]. In conclusion, the presented summative results can be used 1) to determine the current state of usability and 2) to guide the conceptual redesign of ENR systems in the future.

Acknowledgements

We acknowledge the funding of the study by The Finnish Work Environment Fund (Työsuojelurahasto) and the Ministry of Social Affairs and Health (Sosiaali- ja terveysministeriö) in 2010.

References

[1]   E. Törnvall, S. Wilhelmsson, L. K. Wahren. Electronic nursing documentation in primary health Care. *Scan J Caring Sci* **18** (2004), 310-317.

[2]   A. Kuusisto, P. Asikainen, H. Lukka, K. Tanttu. Experiences with the electronic nursing discharge summary. *Stud Health Tech Inf* **146** (2009), 226-230.

[3]   B. Gugerty, M. J. Maranda, M. Beachley, V. B. Navarro, S. Newbold, W. Hawk, J. Karp, M. Koszalka, S. Morrison, S. S. Poe, D. Wilhelm. *Challenges and Opportunities in Documentation of the Nursing Care of Patients. A Report of the Maryland Nursing Workforce Commission*, Documentation Work Group.   [Internet].   2007.   [cited   2010   June   10]   Available   from: http://www.mbon.org/commission2/documentation_challenges.pdf

[4]   R. Verwey, R. A. Claassen, M. J. Rutgers, L. P. de Witte. The implementation of an electronic nursing record in a general hospital in the Netherlands. *Stud Health Tech Inf* **141** (2008), 130-138.

[5]   L. Poissant, J. Pereira, R. Tamblyn Y. Kawasumi. The impact of electronic health records on time efficiency of physicians and nurses: A systematic review. *JAMIA* **12**(5) (2005), 505-516.

[6]   L. E. Moody, E. Slocumb, B. Berg, D. Jackson. Electronic health records documentation in nursing: Nurses' perceptions, attitudes, and preferences. *CIN* **22**(6) (2004), 337-344.

[7]   J. E. Stevenson, G. C. Nilsson, G. I. Petersson, P. E. Johansson. Nurses' experiences of using electronic patient records in everyday practice in acute/inpatient ward setting: A Literature Review. *Health Inf J* **16**(1) (2010), 63-72.

[8]   M. B. Skov, R. T. Hoegh. Supporting information access in a hospital ward by a context-aware mobile electronic patient record. *Per Ubiq Comp* **10** (2006) 205-214.

[9]   J. Kjeldskov, M. Skov, J. Stage. A longitudinal study of usability in health care: Does time heal? *Int J Med Inf* **79**(6) (2008) e135-e143.

[10] L. W. P. Peute, M. W. M. Jaspers. The significance of a usability evaluation of an emerging laboratory order entry system. *Int J Med Inf* **76** (2007), 157-168.

[11] P. Liljamo, P. Kaakinen, A. Ensio. Opas FinCC-luokituskokonaisuuden käyttöön hoitotyön sähköisen kirjaamisen mallissa. Kansallisesti yhtenäiset hoitotyön tiedot -hanke 2007-2008. FinCC-luokituksen käyttöopas. [Internet] 2008. [cited 2010 June 10] Available from: http://www.vsshp.fi/fi/4519

[12] K. Tanttu. *National Nursing Documentation Project in Finland 5/2005- 5/2008: Nationally Standardized Electronic Nursing Documentation*, presentation. [Internet] 2008. [cited 2010 June 10] Available from: http://www.vsshp.fi/fi/dokumentit/15158/National-Nursing-Project-2005-2007.pdf

[13] P. Nykänen, J. Viitanen, A. Kuusisto. Hoitotyön kansallisen kirjaamismallin ja hoitokertomusten käytettävyys, Project report (in Finnish), University of Tampere, Finland, publication D-2010-7. [Internet] 2010. [cited 2010 June 10] Available from: http://www.cs.uta.fi/reports/dsarja/D-2010-7.pdf

[14] J. L. Belden, R. Grayson, J. Barnes. *Defining and Testing EMR Usability: Principles and Proposed Methods of EMR Usability Evaluation and Rating*. HIMMS EHR Usability Task Force. [Internet] 2009. [cited 2010 June 10] Available from: https://mospace.umsystem.edu/xmlui/handle/10355/3719

[15] A. W. Kushniruk, V. L. Patel. Cognitive and usability engineering methods for the evaluation of clinical information systems. *J Biomed Inf* **37** (2004) 56-76.

[16] ISO 9241-210, International Standard: *Ergonomics of human-system interaction – Part 210: Human-centred design for interactive systems*. First edition 2010-03-15. Reference number ISO 9241-210:2010(E).

[17] J. Nielsen. *Usability Engineering*. Academic Press, New York, 1993.

[18] H. Beyer, K. Holzblatt. *Contextual design: Defining Customer-Centred Systems*. Academic Press, San Diego, USA, 1998.

[19] R. P. Weber. *Basic Content Analysis*, (second edition). Series: *Qualitative Applications in the Social Sciences*. SAGE University Paper, Sage Publications, Inc, USA, 1990.

[20] E. Ammenwerth, U. Mansmann, C. Iller, R. Eichstädter. Factors affecting and affected by user acceptance of computer-based nursing documentation. *JAMIA* **10** (2003). 69-84.

[21] E. Reuss, K. Rochus, R. Naef, S. Hunziker, L. Furler. Nurses' Working Practices: What Can We Learn for Designing Computerized Patient Record Systems? in book: *HCI and Usability for Medicine and Health Care* (ed. A. Holzinger). Springer Berlin, Heidelberg, 2007.

Public Health Informatics

International Perspectives in Health Informatics
E.M. Borycki et al. (Eds.)
IOS Press, 2011
© *2011 ITCH 2011 Steering Committee and IOS Press. All rights reserved.*
doi:10.3233/978-1-60750-709-3-341

Design and Testing of an Architecture for a National Primary Care Chronic Disease Surveillance Network in Canada

Karim KESHAVJEE[a] [1], Vijaya CHEVENDRA[b], Ken MARTIN[c], David JACKSON[d],
Babak ALIARZADEH[e], Lorne KINSELLA[c], Raymond TURCOTTE[f], Sarah SABRI[g],
Tao CHEN[h]

[a] *InfoClin Inc,* [b] *University of Western Ontario,* [c] *Queen's University,* [d] *University of Calgary,* [e] *University of Toronto,* [f] *Centre de santé et de services sociaux de Laval (CSSSL),* [g] *Dalhousie University,* [h] *Memorial University*

Abstract. Chronic diseases are a growing concern around the globe. In Canada, chronic disease care is taking an increasing share of health care budgets, and with an aging population, is threatening to overwhelm Provincial budgets where most health care is paid for. A chronic disease surveillance network fills an important gap in current public health surveillance systems. This paper describes the design and feasibility testing of an information technology and privacy architecture to extract, transform and transfer data from 7 electronic medical record systems used by 100 primary care providers in 6 province to a central data repository at the High Performance Computing Virtual Laboratory at Queen's University in Canada.

Keywords. chronic disease, surveillance, primary care, electronic medical records, practice-based research networks.

Introduction

Public health surveillance is important for running an efficient health care system. Chronic diseases have reached epidemic proportions in the developed world and are utilizing increasingly greater shares of health care budgets [1]. A National primary care chronic disease surveillance network will provide an important source of information to an overall public health surveillance system and fill a gap that currently exists in disease surveillance. Surveillance networks are not a new idea. The European General Practice Research Workshop started the European General Practice Research Agenda [2]. There are a number of research networks in Europe, such as the General Practice Research Database in the United Kingdom [3] and the Netherlands Information Network of General Practice [4]. The BEACH project in Australia [5] has been particularly successful in conducting surveillance-based projects. The Distributed Network for Ambulatory Research in Therapeutics in the United States brings together practices with electronic medical records in 8 different organizations [6]. Van Weel and Rosser [7] have argued that primary care networks be supported on a global scale.

---

[1] Karim Keshavjee, InfoClin Inc, 15 Atlantic Ave, Toronto, ON M6K 3E7; e-mail: karim@infoclin.ca.

The College of Family Physicians of Canada (CFPC) in collaboration with several primary care practice-based research networks (PC-PBRNs) associated with university departments of family medicine across Canada and the Canadian Institute for Health Information (CIHI) are collaborating to fully operationalize the Canadian Primary Care Sentinel Surveillance Network (CPCSSN) and its surveillance and research mission and goals. Governance, planning and organization of CPCSSN are described elsewhere [8]. This paper describes the design and testing of an information technology and privacy architecture for capturing chronic disease data from 7 different electronic medical record (EMR) systems used by approximately 100 physicians practicing in 25 clinics in 6 provinces.

1. Development of Surveillance System

1.1 CPCSSN Goals

The founders of CPCSSN are committed to conducting surveillance and research on the impact of chronic diseases on the health and well-being of Canadians. Diabetes mellitus, hypertension, depression, osteoarthritis and chronic obstructive pulmonary disease (COPD) are the first 5 chronic diseases to be studied. Disease definitions have been previously described [8]. To answer research and surveillance questions posed by CPCSSN researchers, a large number of fields are required, including dates of primary care encounters, patient health conditions, vital signs, medications, laboratory results, risk factors, procedures and referrals. The central data repository was designed to capture the data and metadata required to meet the research and surveillance goals [8].

1.2 Privacy and Technical Architecture

To meet the variety of legislative privacy requirements in each province, all EMR data extraction and de-identification work is done independently in each province before data is uploaded to the central repository. To maintain a uniform security environment and uniform security policies for all hardware, all servers are maintained at the Queens University High Performance Computing Virtual Laboratory (HPCVL), which is housed in a secure facility and protected by an active firewall. The server used by a single regional network is contracted to them in their own province, but is housed and maintained by HPCVL. From a legal perspective, the server is considered to be in the province of data origin and all work done on that server is done according to the privacy legislation of that province. Data managers securely access their regional servers remotely through a virtual private network (VPN) connection. All data transfers occur in a secure manner directly over the local HPCVL network from regional servers to a central server which holds the central data repository.

Data extraction in each network is necessarily different, as the various EMR systems are quite heterogeneous. Most physician sites use Client/Server based EMR systems. In some networks, the data manager (DM) is housed in the same building as the clinic from which the data is extracted. In other networks, clinics are far apart and the data manager travels to each clinic to extract data manually or accesses the data remotely. One network utilizes an Application Server Provider (ASP) model EMR system hosted by a provincial government. Data is extracted by the provincial government and provided to the network DM on digital media. In each case, we ensure that there is a secure chain of point to point transfer of data until it reaches the secure regional server at the HPCVL. Where possible, CPCSSN is moving toward an architecture where encrypted data is transferred electronically directly from the physician's clinic to the regional server.

There are two main de-identification needs with the CPCSSN dataset. 1) Several data fields have personal health information (PHI) typed into the field by the clinician. These strings need to be identified and the PHI removed. In the initial data extraction cycles, DMs were asked to suppress any fields with PHI in them. 2) Risk of probabilistic re-identification of individuals using statistical approaches. To reduce the risk of probabilistic re-identification, CPCSSN procured commercially available software for reducing re-identification risk (PARAT, from Privacy Analytics Inc).

Regional networks are in regular communication with their research ethics boards (REBs) and get approval prior to making any changes to the privacy architecture.

1.3 Feasibility Study

From April to November 2008, a feasibility study was conducted to ascertain what would be required to extract, clean and de-identify data for CPCSSN. Data was extracted from 5 different EMRs on a table-by-table basis to identify specific issues and barriers. It quickly became apparent that extracting data would be quite difficult. Of the 6 sites participating in the feasibility study, only one was able to achieve all the feasibility tasks to the level of quality required; this network had already been operational with a DM for the three previous years. We concluded that we would need trained, experienced DMs for the next phase if we were to successfully operationalize a surveillance network. In spite of difficulties, we were able to extract data and demonstrate disease rates that were similar to those observed using other data sources.

Our experience with the feasibility study led us to propose a data extraction and transformation architecture that took into account the unique requirements of the various EMR systems in the various clinics and the heterogeneous data quality issues that each faced. This is described in Figure 1. This process is highly dependent on good quality data managers being in place.

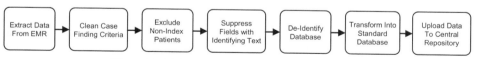

Figure 1. Initial Data Extraction and Processing Approach

1.4 Data Collection and Transformation Processes

In Dec 2008, Phase II of the project was funded whose deliverables included operationalization of the data collection and transformation process developed in Phase I. New data managers with training and experience in computer science or data management were hired. A data manager's 'toolkit' was developed to guide the data managers on how to conduct the processing steps and to ensure uniformity of approach and outcome across all provinces. The data manager's toolkit included documents such as the CPCSSN entity relationship diagram (ERD) and its associated data dictionary, extraction requirements, disease definitions for the 5 chronic conditions, code lists for specific data and a spreadsheet for documenting issues that arose in the process.

Each data manager was also provided with a standard CPCSSN reference database into which they put all relevant data prior to uploading it to the central repository. The plan was to conduct 3 cycles of extraction to iterate and improve the overall process.

2. Findings

Although our initial data extraction and transformation process allowed us to get off the ground relatively quickly (the first data extraction was due on Mar 31, 2009 –3 months after contract signing), it immediately became apparent that the process was not scalable and would not be sustainable over the long term.

The extraction and transformation process required too much human effort and required DMs to standardize clinical data that was not familiar to them.   It was also vulnerable to human error and suffered from a lack of verifiability and lack of uniformity. De-identification of text strings was also difficult to do manually. Because of privacy concerns, it was not possible to review individual network databases to provide appropriate oversight or a second opinion during the actual extraction and transformation process. Each DM worked in isolation from the others and was not able to compare notes to the extent required to ensure standardization and uniformity.

Another roadblock in data collection and transformation was the data heterogeneity that arose from differences in EMR databases and physician data entry habits; physicians do not necessarily use the same medical terms and abbreviations. Heterogeneity of data makes case finding, surveillance and research more difficult. Types of data quality issues have been described previously [8].

3. Discussion

We have revamped the data collection and transformation process to allow for higher levels of automation and standardization. To accomplish this, we are leveraging the strengths of the DM team. DMs can't be expected to do all the work manually –it is too time consuming and prone to error. In the newly designed architecture, DMs only extract data and transform it into the CPCSSN reference database manually. Since the volume of the EMR data makes manual conversion of text strings to standardized terms virtually impossible, developers on the DM team work with clinicians to develop coding and cleaning algorithms and programs to conduct the standardization process using rule-based approaches and information retrieval techniques. The developers also develop de-identification algorithms using open-source tools.   All algorithms are verified independently for accuracy by two experts and reconciled by consensus. The cleaning and de-identification algorithms can be used by DMs at all regional networks to clean and de-identify data.   The aim is to achieve more efficient and effective utilization of our DM resources.

We have adopted standard nomenclatures such as ICD-9-CM (for diagnoses), ATC (for medications), and LOINC (for laboratory results) to address the problem of dirty data. We are also exploring the opportunity of adopting semantic technologies such as LexGrid [9]. The database is designed to ensure that original EMR data are preserved to maintain traceability of the cleaning process.

Even with increased automation, the risk of breach remains finite. To protect against human error, each network director uses a standard checklist to review the process of data extraction and to review the data prior to signing off on uploading the quarterly extraction to the central data repository.

Our experience to date is that the new design is more efficient and risk tolerant. New DMs at sites where there has been DM turnover have been able to climb up the learning curve and deliver high quality data extractions in a very short time. Existing DMs have been able to complete the data extraction process faster and with fewer errors. Except for Quebec where the DM is also the programmer of the EMR software, losing a DM is less likely to lead to loss of EMR specific knowledge. We are currently evaluating the new design and will report on it in the near future.

Acknowledgements

Funding for CPCSSN has been provided by the Public Health Agency of Canada.

References

[1]   D. Drummond, D. Burleton, *Charting a Path to Sustainable Healthcare in Ontario,* TD Economics Special Report, May 27, 2010. [cited 2010 Jun 19], available from: http://www.td.com/economics/special/db0510_health_care.pdf.

[2]   C. Lionis, H.E. Stoffers, E. Hummers-Pradier, F. Griffiths, D. Rotar-Pavlic, J. Rethans, Setting Priorities and Identifying Barriers for General Practice Research in Europe. Results from an EGPRW meeting, *Fam Pract* **21** (2004), 587–93.

[3]   NIHR Clinical Research Network Coordinating Centre, *Primary Care Research Network,* [cited 2010 Jun 19], available at: http://www.ukcrn.org.uk/index/networks/primarycare.html.

[4]   Netherlands Institute for Health Services Research, *Databases and Information Systems: Netherlands Information Network of General Practice,* [cited 2010 Jun 19], available at: http://www.nivel.nl/oc2/page.asp?PageID=8599&path=/Startpunt/NIVEL%20international/Research/D ata%20bases%20and%20information%20systems/National%20Information%20Network%20of%20GP s%20(LINH)

[5]   Australian General Practice Statistics and Classification Centre, *The BEACH Project: Bettering the Evaluation and Care of Health,* [cited 2010 Jun 19], available at: http://www.fmrc.org.au/beach.htm.

[6]   Agency for Health Care Research and Quality. New research: Distributed Network for Ambulatory Research in Therapeutics (DARTNet). [cited 2010 Jun 19]. Available at: http://www.ahrq.gov/about/nac/aafp.htm.

[7]   C. van Weel, W.W. Rosser, Improving Healthcare Globally: a Critical Review of the Necessity of Family Medicine Research and Recommendations to Build Research Capacity, *Ann Fam Med* **2** (2004) Suppl2, S5–16.

[8]   R. Birtwhistle, K. Keshavjee, A. Lambert-Lanning, M. Godwin, M. Greiver, D. Manca, C. Lagacé, Building a Pan-Canadian Primary Care Sentinel Surveillance Network: Initial Development and Moving Forward, *J Am Board Fam Med*, **4** (2009), 412-22.

[9]   J. Pathak, H. Solbrig, J. Buntrock, T. Johnson, C. Chute, LexGrid: A Framework for Representing, Storing, and Querying Biomedical Terminologies from Simple to Sublime, *JAMIA* **16:3** (2009), 305-315.

International Perspectives in Health Informatics
E.M. Borycki et al. (Eds.)
IOS Press, 2011
© *2011 ITCH 2011 Steering Committee and IOS Press. All rights reserved.*
doi:10.3233/978-1-60750-709-3-346

Mandatory Public Reporting: Build It and Who Will Come?

Sigall BELL[a] , James BENNEYAN[b], Allan BEST[c] , David BIRNBAUM[d1]
Elizabeth M. BORYCKI[e], Thomas H. GALLAGHER[f], Chris GOESCHEL[g] ,
Bill JARVIS[h], André W. KUSHNIRUK[e], Kathleen M. MAZOR[i]
Peter PRONOVOST[g], Sam SHEPS[j]

[a]*Harvard Medical School, Boston MA, USA;* [b]*Northeastern University, Boston MA,
US;* [c]*InSource, Vancouver, British Columbia, Canada;* [d]*Washington State Dept. of
Health, Olympia WA, USA;* [e] *School of Health Information Science, University of
Victoria, Victoria, British Columbia, Canada;* [f]*University of Washington, Seattle WA,
USA;* [g]*Johns Hopkins University, Baltimore MD, USA;* [h]*Jason and Jarvis Associates
LLC, Hilton Head Island SC, USA;* [i]*University of Massachusetts Medical School,
Worcester MA, US;* [j]*University of British Columbia School of Population and Public
Health, Vancouver, British Columbia, Canada*

Abstract: Rates of healthcare-associated infections (HAI) are being reported on
an increasing number of public information websites in response to legislative
mandates driven by consumer advocacy. This represents a new strategy to
advance patient safety and quality of care by informing a broad audience about
the relative performance of individual healthcare facilities. Unlike typical
consumer health informatics products, the target audience and targeted health
behaviors are less easily defined; further, the impact on providers to improve care
is unknown relative to other incentives to improve. To address critical knowledge
gaps facing all state agencies embarking on this new frontier, we found it essential
and straightforward to recruit the assistance of university research faculty from a
variety of disciplines. That interdisciplinary group was quickly able to define a 5-
year applied evaluation research agenda spanning a progressive set of crucial
questions.

Keywords: mandatory public reporting; healthcare-associated infections; patient
safety; healthcare quality

Introduction

Years ago, Marshall McLuhan informed us that "the medium is the message" in a
global village, each delivery medium changing the way a message might be perceived
and new forms of delivery media potentially accelerating societal changes [1].
Mandatory reporting on state health department websites to inform the broad public
about hospital infection rates (and eventually about other healthcare settings like

---

[1] Corresponding author contact information: David Birnbaum, Washington State
Department of Health, HAI Program, PO Box 47811, Olympia WA 98504-7811, (360)
236-4153, david.birnbaum@doh.wa.gov

ambulatory surgical facilities, clinics, extended care and nursing homes) is fundamental to a new national strategy in the United States for harnessing information technologies as agents of change. Over a period of just a few years, more than two dozen states have passed legislation requiring this new application of public health informatics – a requirement that propelled state health departments into uncharted territory. Establishing state-wide surveillance over patient records through a secure national network involves ensuring ethical and privacy standards while also better understanding motivations and information needs of patient safety and healthcare quality management. This new national strategy in effect hopes to enlist consumer informatics to motivate institutional improvement. On the consumer end, the message isn't subtle – as the Consumers Union Safe Patient Project website headline says, "End secrecy, save lives" [2].

Consumer health informatics (CHI) has been described as a "new and still evolving" field. There are few evaluation studies and they are inconsistent in use of terminology. Thus, a review published in 2009 states that: "many questions about CHI applications at the patient level remain. The results of our review suggested that the literature is relatively silent on the question of whether or not significant differences in patient preferences, knowledge, attitudes, beliefs, needs, utilization, and potential benefits exists across gender, age, and race/ethnicity. Intuitively, we suspect some differences exist, especially as they relate to the senior population compared to the adolescent population. However, these differences have not been definitively characterized, and the clinical and public health implications of these differences are largely unknown." [3]

All of this presents important knowledge gaps that must be addressed in order for state public health departments to understand the information needs, preferences and influence of key segments of their broad public audience. Without such understanding, it will be difficult to demonstrate that the form and content of information being pushed out in the growing number of mandatory public reporting websites will match the needs of the intended audience. Without that demonstration, it will be difficult to confirm whether this new national strategy is successful in motivating further reduction in infection risks.

Does reporting change consumer choice behavior and incentivize provider improvements? Is informatics clearly the delivery solution, or is this more of an informatics research problem? Informatics itself has been defined in various terms, ranging from narrow technology-focused descriptions ("The study of information and the ways to handle it, especially by means of information technology, i.e., computers and other electronic devices for rapid transfer, processing and analysis of large amounts of data" [4]) to more comprehensive descriptions. The latter is more instructive for the broad range of questions that need to be answered before we can conclude that anyone is delivering the most appropriate information in the most appropriate way to the most appropriate audience. A broader definition from the American Medical Informatics Association (AMIA) states: "Our *working* definition for Consumer Health Informatics (CHI-WG) is "a subspecialty of medical informatics which studies from a patient/consumer perspective the use of electronic information and communication to improve medical outcomes and the health care decision-making process." The working group focuses developing collaboration and academic discussion among members whose diverse interests include: exploring ways informatics can optimize the healthcare partnership of provider and patient, developing technology and software to educate and empower consumer and to allow patients participate in healthcare decisions, identifying factors that the affect the use of technology in the provider-client relationship, and evaluating the effectiveness of health care informatics in patient outcomes. [5]

That range of diverse interests fits the approach that we have taken to develop and refine the Healthcare Associated Infections Program website at the Washington State Department of Health. We recognized the range of academic disciplines needed to aid us in a collaborative venture, starting with initial development of our website through prototyping, moving to evaluation and refinement of its fit to the intended audience, and ultimately to determination of impact or perhaps even cost-effectiveness of this strategy in terms of motivating improvements in patient safety and healthcare quality outcomes. We report here our success in enlisting collaborative support, the reasons that research faculty at several universities wanted to join our group, and the evaluation research plan in which we have engaged.

1. Methods

Washington's Healthcare Associated Infections Program recruited university research faculty to join an interdisciplinary collaborative effort. In university seminars and other venues, key aspects of historical development, program philosophy and strength of evidence underlying fundamental assumptions were described. A conceptual model of an HAI Program's Information Delivery linked to Knowledge Translation and Action to Improve was presented, indicating the range of academic disciplines needed to address this topic (shaded area in Figure 1). Faculty members were recruited to fill the academic disciplines in the model. Their reasons for joining and questions identified by the group were obtained from communications among group members, which also resulted in adding another domain to the model (Patient Expectations & Patient-Provider Communication).

2. Results

Members quickly joined from a comprehensive range of disciplines. Their identities are listed here, along with typical comments about their reason for joining.

Sigall Bell, MD - Assistant Professor of Medicine, Harvard Medical School, and Thomas Gallagher, MD – Associate Professor of Medicine, University of Washington: "*As increasing attention is focused on health care associated infections, little is known about patients' expectations and experiences with communication about these events. We are interested in better understanding the patient perspective on health care associated infections in order to improve communication between patients and providers about these issues. Such understanding can then better inform HAI education strategies (through online reporting venues and at the bedside) that will best match their expectations and needs*".

James Benneyan, PhD - Professor, Northeastern University College of Engineering; Director, Center for Health Organization Transformation; Executive Director, New England VA Healthcare Systems Engineering Partnership:

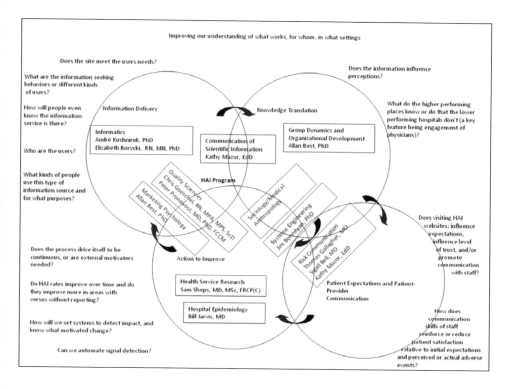

Figure 1. Improving our understanding of what works, for whom, in what settings

"Ultimately what is of interest is whether public reporting, mandatory or not, has a positive impact influencing patient choice, provider performance, and outcomes, especially given the vast amount of information available to consumers and the level of sophistication potentially necessary to make informed sense of it. These effects and system design to maximize them are fundamental to mandatory reporting requirements but to-date largely unknown and untested in this context, in parallel to significant efforts and investments in such systems. This opens up a range of key questions from the most effective manner in which to display such information – in what form and at what level of detail - to the best ways to statistically monitor choice, behavior, and outcomes to test and detect pattern changes."

Allan Best, PhD - Senior Scientist, Centre for Clinical Epidemiology and Evaluation, Vancouver Coastal Health Research Institute; Clinical Professor, School of Population and Public Health, University of British Columbia; Managing Director, InSource. *"The Mandatory Public Reporting collaborative is attractive in several respects: <u>Collaboration and Complexity</u> - The challenge of mandatory reporting requires effective collaboration among many diverse stake-holders in a complex system. <u>Integrated Action Framework</u> - The work requires an interdisciplinary/intersectoral team to build a conceptual framework that effectively blends knowledge with action for large-scale organizational change. <u>Strong Mandate</u> - The risk of pandemics has created a strong mandate for transformative systems change focused on public safety. <u>Strategic Communications</u> - The need for systems solutions* *requires sophisticated, integrated, strategic communications amongst diverse stakeholders. Evaluation - Taken together, these factors provide an excellent opportunity to evaluate and learn from complex systems change."*

David Birnbaum, PhD, MPH - Adjunct Professor, University of British Columbia School of Population and Public Health, and UBC School of Nursing; Adjunct Professor, University of Victoria School of Health Information Science; Principal, Applied Epidemiology; Manager, Washington State Dept. of Health Healthcare Associated Infections Program: *"Mandatory public reporting presents a leading edge of uncharted territory for hospital epidemiology and infection control professionals. Washington state developed its HAI Program website through prototyping, refining prototypes by evaluation-refinement cycles with ever-widening test audiences [6]. All state HAI programs will need the insights that only can come from interdisciplinary applied research, first to help those programs design the most effective communication possible and eventually to assess its impact."*

Elizabeth Borycki, RN, MN, PhD - Assistant Professor, University of Victoria School of Health Information Science, and André Kushniruk, PhD - Professor, University of Victoria School of Health Information Science *"Health Informatics is the science of the study of the effects of health information technology upon creation and use of data, information and knowledge. Health informaticians are involved in the design, development, implementation and evaluation of health information systems. The field itself draws on the information, clinical and management sciences and applies the knowledge gained from research conducted in these areas to the study of health information technology (i.e. including web-based reporting systems such as those currently being developed and used by states to report on healthcare-associated infection rates). As part of this project, health informatics researchers from the School of Health Information Science (i.e. Kushniruk and Borycki) will evaluate the usability of a healthcare-associated infection rate reporting system as well as the effects of the system upon users information seeking and decision-making activities."*

Bill Jarvis, MD - Jason and Jarvis Associates LLC: *"The WSHD (Washington State Health Department) HAI Program's University Council is unique. It brings together experts in a variety of disciplines who can address a multitude of issues related to HAI reporting and improving patient safety in healthcare settings state-wide. These questions that can be addressed range from the validity of the data reported, whether different metrics should be developed and used, the validity of comparison to historical rates (i.e., standardized infection ratios), how the consumer and the reporter access and interpret the reported data, and are the reported data having the result intended - education of the public/consumer and reduction of HAI rates. This University Council should be a model for other State Health Departments and the Centers for Disease Control and Prevention as a method to maximize the potential of the ever-growing transparency in infection control and mandatory reporting of HAIs."*

Kathy Mazor, EdD - Associate Professor, University of Massachusetts Medical School: *"There are two challenges that researchers, including myself, often face: 1) how to get stakeholders to pay attention to the results of our research and 2) how to do research in "real world" settings, in order to determine whether findings obtained under controlled conditions hold up. The partnerships formed through this collaboration will help us to meet both of these challenges. In addition, it will provide opportunities for professional growth, as I anticipate that I will learn from team members from other disciplines."*

Chris Goeschel, RN, MPA, MPS, ScD - Director of Patient Safety & Quality Initiatives, Manager of Operations, Johns Hopkins University Quality & Safety Research Group; Clinical Instructor, Johns Hopkins School of Nursing; Associate faculty, Johns Hopkins Bloomberg School of Public Health, and Peter Pronovost, MD, PhD, FCCM - Professor, Johns Hopkins Schools of Medicine, Nursing, and Bloomberg School of Public Health; Director, Johns Hopkins Quality & Safety Research Group: *"...in background we had, they may also lack technical skills needed and relationship with other entities. My point is that even if the science was clear, this would still be hard for many health departments."*

Sam Sheps, MD, MSc, FRCPC(C) - Professor, University of British Columbia School of Population and Public Health; Director, Western Regional Training Centre for Health Services Research: *"Infectious disease reporting, as any patient safety related issue, is important to know so as to learn from patterns that emerge from such reporting. Most agencies need to develop the capacity to do appropriate analyses of reported events, but generally don't have that capacity. Liaison with university based researchers not only provides an immediate resource for such analyses, but in the longer term, helps to build capacity in state agencies. Thus linkages with university based researchers should be seen as a potential source of assistance with understanding the complex dynamics of infection related adverse events. Better understanding of patterns of hospital induced infection can assist institutions to develop more resilient systems of response. Hospital acquired infections are not rare and thus attention must be paid to their occurrence."*

The group identified a number of questions that need to be addressed in a progressive manner (see Figure). HAI Programs deliver information; there are five questions that address knowing the audience and confirming fit between what is delivered and what is desired. This leads to an unproven assumption that information delivery will lead to knowledge translation by the recipients, whether they be consumers or providers of healthcare. Confirming that the information is trusted and convincing, that it influences beliefs and aligns with the ways that healthcare institutions engage clinical leaders, are additional questions to be explored. The next step leads to two shaded circles – assessing whether knowledge translation motivates institutions to take action to improve directly, and whether knowledge translation on the part of patients influences their expectations, perceptions and actions. Finally, it remains to be demonstrated whether the entire cycle is self-sustaining or requires external support, and whether this provision of public information actually produces improved outcomes (as opposed to other motivators).

3. Discussion

Members identified 8 major reasons for joining. The collaborative is thought to help meet challenges academics face in: 1) getting stake-holders to pay attention to results of their research; 2) extending conduct of research into new areas and "real world" settings, evaluating whether findings obtained under controlled conditions persist in real-world settings; 3) finding opportunities for professional growth, and learning from other disciplines. As allied health professionals, academics also shared state health departments concerns of: 4) building capacity quickly in state agencies to apply sophisticated methods; 5) learning from trends found in patient safety reporting; 6) improved understanding of complex systems change and HAI dynamics (as typical of adverse events); 7) improving information delivery, and 8) finding best ways to make hospitals more resilient "learning organizations" thus confirming universal applicability of optimal organizational development approaches.

The beneficial impact on patient safety and quality of care from state health department HAI programs is indirect, yet to be proven, and based on a series of assumptions that are subject to important knowledge gaps [7, 8, 9]. This model addresses everyone's needs to fill those gaps. In our experience, it has been a useful, productive approach.

References:

[1] The Official Site of Marshall McLuhan [cited 2010 May 19]. Available from: http://www.marshallmcluhan.com/.
[2] Consumers Union Safe Patient Project [cited 2010 May 19]. Available from: http://www.safepatientproject.org/topic/hospital_acquired_infections/.
[3] M. C. Gibbons, R. F. Wilson, L. Samal, C. U. Lehmann, K. Dickersin, H. P. Lehmann, H. Aboumatar, J. Finkelstein, E. Shelton, R. Sharma, E. B. Bass. *Impact of Consumer Health Informatics Applications. Evidence Report/Technology Assessment* No. 188. (Prepared by Johns Hopkins University Evidence-based Practice Center under contract No. HHSA 290-2007-10061-I). AHRQ Publication No. 09(10)-E019. Rockville, MD. Agency for Healthcare Research and Quality. October 2009.
[4] M. Porta, S. Greenland, J. M. Last (Eds.). *A Dictionary of Epidemiology*, 5th Edition. Oxford University Press, 2008.
[5] AMIA, Working Group – Consumer Health Informatics [cited 2010 May 19]. Available from: https://www.amia.org/working-group/consumer-health-informatics.
[6] D. Birnbaum, M. J. Cummings, K. Guyton, J. Schlotter, A. Kushniruk. Designing public web information systems with quality in mind: Public reporting of hospital performance data. *Clin Gov* **15**(4), 272-278.
[7] C. H. Fung, Y. W. Lim, S. Mattke, et al. Systematic review: The evidence that publishing patient care performance data improves quality of care. *Ann Intern Med* **148**(2) (2008),111-23.
[8] P.G. Shekelle, Y. W. Lim, S. Mattke, et al. *Does public release of performance results improve quality of care?* RAND Corporation report published by The Health Foundation, London. 2008. Available from: www.health.org.uk.
[9] D. Birnbaum, J. Van Buren. Applying continuous improvement in public reporting: What should government reports do for quality improvement? *Clin Gov* **15**(2) (2010),79-91.

International Perspectives in Health Informatics
E.M. Borycki et al. (Eds.)
IOS Press, 2011
© *2011 ITCH 2011 Steering Committee and IOS Press. All rights reserved.*
doi:10.3233/978-1-60750-709-3-353

353

Emergence of a New Consumer Health Informatics Framework: Introducing the Healthcare Organization

Paulette REID[a], Elizabeth M. BORYCKI[a]
[a] *School of Health Information Science, University of Victoria, Victoria, British Columbia, Canada*

Abstract. Healthcare consumers are increasingly seeking reliable forms of health information on the Internet that can be used to support health related decision-making. Frameworks that have been developed and tested in the field of health informatics have attempted to describe the effects of the Internet upon the health care consumer and physician relationship. More recently, health care organizations are responding by providing information such as hospital wait lists or strategies for self-managing disease, and this information is being provided on organizational web-sites. The authors of this paper propose that current conceptualizations of the relationship between the Internet, physicians and patients are limited from a consumer informatics perspective and may need to be extended to include healthcare organizations.

Keywords. consumer informatics, health informatics, healthcare organizations, Healthcare Associated Infections, patient safety, transparency, organizational behaviour

Introduction

Consumer health informatics is a subfield of health informatics that focuses upon the study of consumers' health information needs and information seeking behaviours on the Internet [1]. Consumer informatics is at the intersection of other disciplines, such as health informatics, public health, health promotion, and health education [1]. The study of consumer's information needs and information seeking behaviours is a challenging and rapidly expanding area of research [1]. There are a number of reasons for growth in this area of research. Health information technology, has become ubiquitous, and is becoming a desirable way of addressing consumer information needs: patient's, caregivers, or health professionals' needs [2]. Information technology has been incorporated into hospitals in the form of electronic patient records since 1960s. In the 1980s computers were introduced into physician offices. In the 1990s society saw the exponential growth of the availability of health information resources over the World Wide Web (WWW) [2]. Today, health information has become one of the most sought after types of information on the Internet [3]. Recently, there has emerged a demand for transparency in health care. Consumers are demanding more information from healthcare providers and institutions where they receive healthcare. These demands are being recognized by government agencies, private and public sector organizations, hospitals and physician offices. Healthcare organizations' information is becoming more available on the Internet, examples include Healthcare Associated Infection (HAI) rates and waiting times for surgeries or other procedures. In this paper the authors argue for the need to extend and test existing consumer informatics frameworks that include information about healthcare institutions and their ability to provide patients and caregivers with information about institutional processes upon a consumers' health and healthcare.

1. Emergence and Evolution of Health Informatics

Consumer informatics emerged as an area of research in the late 1990's. In 1998, Richards et al. discussed how the Internet rapidly emerged as the most powerful medium of mass communication in this century. Researchers identified that the Internet had the potential to dispense cost-effective, high-quality patient education [5]. In 2002 researchers documented the potential effects of the Internet upon the health professional-patient relationship. According to Jacob (2002)"studies have shown that physicians exchange minimal information with patients during a patient encounter... The deliberative or collaborative model, where the physician helps the patient choose their preferred health-related values, represents our societal norm" [6]. In 2003, we began seeing these changes emerge in the patient-physician relationship. A cross-sectional survey of U.S. physicians (n=1050, 53% response rate) found the Internet had affected the physician-patient relationship. The study revealed 38% of physicians believed the patient bringing in information made the physician visit less time efficient; especially if the patient wanted something considered inappropriate by the physician, or if the physician felt challenged. This study also revealed 85% of physicians had a patient bring Internet information to a visit [7]. In 2004 research began to document patients' desire to acquire information that would address their health needs from their local healthcare organization. A New Jersey study, assessed inner city Emergency Department patients' use of the Internet to obtain medical information. Using a convenience sample of 328 people, it revealed that 33% of those who had previously used the WWW to obtain medical information had difficulty in obtaining **useful** information. 59% of participants were interested or very interested in being provided links to medical sites upon being released from the emergency department [6]. This study suggested patients were interested in being provided with health information by an organization. By 2007 the use of Internet-derived health information within the healthcare encounter had increased. According to Wald et al.'s extensive review, the physician-patient relationship was affected by an emerging consumerist model; 'triangulation' of Patient-Web-Physician [8]. The researchers concluded a 'net-friendly' clinician could be more effective.

2. Emergence of a Consumer Informatics Framework

The traditional view of health information exchange was sequential involving patient, physician and then, if necessary, the healthcare organization (See Figure 1).

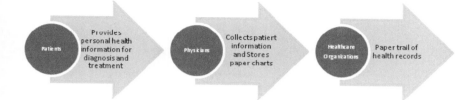

Figure 1. Traditional View of Health Information exchange.

Given the role of the Internet in helping healthcare consumers to seek information, researchers have developed models that describe the impact of the WWW upon the patient-health professional relationship. For example, Lewis et al., developed a model of Shared Decision Making (SDM). The model recognizes the two core players in SDM: the patient and the healthcare provider. Patients use illness experiences, preferences, and health perspectives to participate actively in their own care; the healthcare provider uses research evidence and clinical expertise. Information is exchanged, communication develops, and clinical decisions regarding treatment and care are made [1].

3. Extending Consumer Informatics: The Role of the Healthcare Organization

Earlier in this paper we documented the rise of the Internet and role of the WWW in addressing patient information needs and its impacts upon the patient-provider relationship. By 2004 the literature began to suggest healthcare consumers expected healthcare organizations to provide them with valid and reliable information. One health issue identified as an emerging health information need is HAI. HAI are those infections that are associated with exposure to hospitals or other medical treatments [11]. Patients, and the public in general, are becoming aware of the risk of infection when entering a hospital.

Poor infection control practices in healthcare organizations, hospitals, or physician offices are regarded negatively by patients and their families, regardless of any other superior skills of the practitioner [9]. The organization that accredits hospitals in Canada, Accreditation Canada, supports the position that prevention and control are one of the most effective ways for healthcare organizations to improve the quality of their services [10]. Surveillance and collection to date on 'bug-related' HAI in Canada (e.g. MRSA, c-diff, VRE) are being conducted in hospitals. Some countries have developed methods of data collection for 'procedure-related' HAI and are able to provide this information to healthcare consumers via the WWW . However, Canada does not have a national method of surveillance or reporting for procedural type HAI infection data for healthcare organizations. To take into account this emerging health information need we propose a model that includes the organization where information flows up and down the pyramid between the Healthcare Consumers, Healthcare Providers and Healthcare Organizations using the Internet as the background to provide useful information, and to facilitate information exchange (see Figure 2).

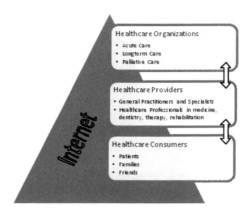

Figure 2. A New Framework for information exchange in Health Informatics.

In various countries, motivated either by political decisions, such as the UK's recent move to post infection numbers of each hospital each week [12], or competitive marketing decisions, hospitals and the associations that represent them have themselves started to post information they feel is appropriate to their target markets. As more invasive care procedures became provided by ambulatory facilities outside the traditional hospital setting, it was widely assumed that patient safety would be among the highest priorities regardless of setting. Experience has shown that inspection was infrequent, lapses in technique became normal cost-cutting measures, and compromised patient safety was compounded by billing fraud (e.g. recent CMS study of ambulatory care facilities [4] and the Las Vegas outbreak report [13]). There are many factors driving a trend toward increased transparency, with more sources of information becoming available from providers as well as government programs. The challenge facing consumers is to determine which of these sources meets the information needs of the intended audience; whether all are providing equally credible and trustworthy information; and the extent to which event rates can be simplified into "plain talk" without losing essential context and meaning. It also important that providers and consumers recognize how information fits into the concepts of quality care and patient safety, so that informed decisions weigh all pertinent information rather than base judgment on too narrow a perspective.

4. Conclusion

With healthcare consumers growing need to seek health information, health informatics has the ability to capture, collect, and process information to satisfy this demand for knowledge. Healthcare consumers and providers now demand more specific health information - of a higher quality. It has become commonplace for patients, when visiting health care providers, to bring questions with them from their Internet research. In response to consumer health information needs, using HAI data as an example, it has been identified that some countries are successfully reporting HAI data on the WWW based upon individual healthcare organizations' data. Healthcare organizations are becoming a source of information on a variety of health topics enabled with the use of the internet. Consequently, frameworks for consumer health informatics need to extend to include the relationships between the Internet, physicians and patients, and healthcare organizations.

References

[1] D. Lewis, G. Eysenbach, R. Kukafka, P.Z. Stavri, H. Jimison. *Consumer health informatics: Informing consumers and improving health care*, 2005.
[2] A. Otto, A. W. Kushniruk. Incorporation of medical informatics and information technology as core components of undergraduate medical education: Time for change! *Stud Health Tech Inform* **143** (2009), 62-67.
[3] M. McMullan, Patients using the internet to obtain health information: How this affects the patient-health professional relationship. *Pat Ed Counse* **63**(1-2) (2006), 24-28. doi:10.1016/j.pec.2005.10.006
[4] Regarding the CMS study: M. K. Schaefer, M. Jhung, M. Dahl et al. Infection control assessment of ambulatory surgical centers. *JAMA* **303**(22) (2010), 2273-2279
[5] B. Richards, A. W. Colman, R. A. Hollingsworth. (1998). The current and future role of the internet in patient education. *Int J Med Inf* **50**(1-3) (1998), 279-285.
[6] D. Salo, C. Perez, R. Lavery, A. Malankar, M. Borenstein, S. Bernstein. Patient education and the internet: Do patients want us to provide them with medical web sites to learn more about their medical problems? *J Emerg Med* **26**(3) (2004), 293-300. doi:10.1016/j.jemermed.2003.09.008
[7] E. Murray, B. Lo, L. Pollack, K. Donelan, J. Catania, K. Lee, K. Zapert, R. Turner. The impact of health information on the internet on health care and the physician-patient relationship: National U.S. survey among 1.050 U.S. physicians. *J Med Internet Res* **5**(3) (2003) e17. doi:10.2196/jmir.5.3.e17
[8] H. S. Wald, C. E. Dube, D. C. Anthony, Untangling the web--the impact of internet use on health care and the physician-patient relationship *Pat Ed Counsel* **68**(3) (2007) 218-224. doi:10.1016/j.pec.2007.05.016.
[9] J. K. Ferguson, Preventing healthcare-associated infection: Risks, healthcare systems and behaviour. *Internal Med J* **39**(9) (2009) 574-581. doi:10.1111/j.1445-5994.2009.02004.x
[10] W. Nicklin, G. Lanteigne, P. Greco, Strengthening the value of accreditation: Qmentum - one year later *Healthcare Quart (Toronto, Ont.),* **12**(3) (2009) 84-88.
[11] N. M. M'ikanatha, R. Lynfield, C. A. V. Beneden, H. Valk, *Infectious disease surveillance* Wiley-Blackwell.
[12] Website accessed June 2010: www.dh.gov.uk/en/MediaCentre/Speeches/DH_116643
[13] B. Labus. Large outbreak of healtcare-acquired hepatitis C in Las Vegas, NV. 2010 Council of State & Territorial Epidemiologists Annual Conference, 6-10 June, Portland Oregon, presentation #5114.

Safety and Quality Management

International Perspectives in Health Informatics
E.M. Borycki et al. (Eds.)
IOS Press, 2011
© *2011 ITCH 2011 Steering Committee and IOS Press. All rights reserved.*
doi:10.3233/978-1-60750-709-3-361

Evaluation of Alert-based Monitoring in a Computerised Blood Transfusion Management System

Omid SHABESTARI [a 1], Philip GOOCH [a], Kate GODDARD [a], Kamran GOLCHIN [a],
Jonathan KAY [a], Abdul ROUDSARI [a,b]

[a] *Centre for Health Informatics, School of Informatics, City University, London, UK*
[b] *School of Health Information Science, University of Victoria,*
British Columbia, Canada

Abstract. Blood transfusion is a critical and multi-step process that can be life-saving. At the same time, any mistakes can be life threatening. An electronic blood transfusion system has been designed to ensure the correctness and safety of the blood transfusion process. The standards for the system include notification mechanisms to inform system managers of any errors in the process. Analysis of system alerts has been used to evaluate the performance of the system. The majority of alerts were classified as 'moderate' in terms of risk (i.e. operational rather than affecting clinical safety) and tended to result from user error. The process of alert acknowledgement and resolution by the system administrator acted as a bottleneck whenever the alerts increased above 100 items per month. Although there was no statistically significant correlation between the number of alerts and the number of transfusions or number of the new users of the system, relatively similar patterns were observable in their charts. A major benefit is that the alerts automatically provided information that would not be captured in a manual transfusion process.

Keywords. blood transfusion, evaluation studies as topic, medical informatics applications

Introduction

Blood transfusion is the process of transferring blood or blood-based products from one person into the circulatory system of another [1]. Indications for blood transfusion include massive blood loss due to trauma; surgical operations; and blood diseases such as severe anaemia, thrombocytopenia haemophilia, and sickle-cell disease. Recent advances in medicine have allowed the transfusion of whole blood to be replaced with transfusion of individual blood components such as red blood cells or platelets, depending on requirements.

Thousands of routine and emergency blood transfusions take place every day in the UK. Although the vast majority of them are carried out safely and without adverse incident, the complex sequence of activities means that occasionally mistakes do occur.

---

[1] Corresponding Author: Dr. Omid Shabestari, Centre for Health Informatics, City University, Northampton Square, London, EC1V 0HB, UK   Email: omid.shabestari.1@soi.city.ac.uk

In 2006, the National Blood Transfusion Committee (NBTC) along with the National Patient Safety Association (NPSA) and Serious Hazards of Transfusion (SHOT) issued recommendations for improving the safety of blood transfusions, including the Electronic Clinical Transfusion Management System (ECTMS) guide [2]. Blood transfusion is a multi-step process that involves many actors from different professions. There are many opportunities for mistakes and errors to occur during this process. Such errors can result in serious harm or even the death of the patient [3]. An electronic transfusion management system can identify potential problems and report them to the key actors in a timely fashion to prevent serious adverse incidents from occurring. These alerts can go far beyond the types of errors that can be picked up during normal manual operation [4]

The Centre for Health Informatics at City University has been commissioned by NHS Connecting for Health (CfH) to undertake a full, independent evaluation of a new electronic blood tracking system, developed in accordance with ECTMS guidance and using barcode technology and Radio Frequency Identification (RFID), at the Mayday Healthcare NHS Trust. This paper considers one of the performance indicators evaluated in this project. A similar evaluation in the US reported no incidences of blood transfusion mismatch following implementation of an electronic system [5].

1. Methods

The electronic blood transfusion management system at Mayday Healthcare NHS Trust monitors 132 different types of potential error and records the events causing them in its database. The system assigns a unique identifier to each new blood unit and records the result of the patient blood-type cross match test, in order to maintain a link between the patient and the compatible blood units assigned to them. Additionally, the system tracks each blood unit as it is moved from the blood bank to wards.

System events are recorded in the following checkpoints during the clinical workflow:

- Checking new blood units into the blood bank: user authentication and blood unit identification;
- Returning unused blood units or transferring blood units from another fridge: user authentication, unit expiry date and blood unit transit time (i.e. how long unit has been out of the fridge);
- Checking blood units out from the kiosk: user authentication and patient— blood unit compatibility;
- Commencing bedside transfusion: user authentication, patient—blood unit compatibility and blood unit transit time and start transfusion;
- Completing post-transfusion: user authentication and end transfusion

The research team was provided with a daily database dump from the system. System alert data from the checkpoint events covering the period 13/11/2008 to 18/05/2010 was extracted from the daily database feed. The data used in this study were: the type of the alert; date and time of the alert; date and time of acknowledging the alert; and the date and time of alert resolution.

As there was no separate training data set in the system, a data cleaning process was required to exclude data produced during staff training and system testing. The blood units used for training were identified and all the corresponding transactions and alerts were deleted from the extracted data before the final analysis.

Using data mining techniques, data cubes were developed in Microsoft SQL Server 2008 to study the alerts in the extracted data. Data on the number of transfusions and the number of new users of the system in each month was extracted from the database. The correlation between these variables and the number of alerts were evaluated. SPSS v. 17 was used for statistical analysis.

2. Results

In total 12,540 blood units have been used in the hospital during this evaluation period. System alerts were recorded from different sources including the issue fridges, kiosks, management console and portable computers used at the bedside. The products used in the blood bank are of different types. The type and count of these units are presented in Table 1.

Table 1. Type and count of blood units used during the evaluation

Type	Count
Fresh frozen plasma	1791 (14.3%)
Platelets	1036 (8.2%)
Red blood cells	9703 (77.4%)
White blood cells	10 (0.1%)

1559 instances of system alerts had been recorded during the evaluation period. The alerts consisted of 24 of the possible alert types. The frequencies of the most commonly recorded alerts are listed in Table 2.

Table 2. Frequency of the alerts

Type	Count
Transport time exceeded configured limit	248 (16%)
User logged out without scanning	243 (16%)
Blood unit moved out of wrong storage location	224 (14%)
Expired blood unit	159 (10%)
Invalid blood unit condition	118 (8%)
Blood unit de-reservation date has passed	105 (7%)
Other alerts	462 (29%)

The reason for each alert being raised was explored from the resolution notes recorded in the database. Reasons were classified as alerts of blood handling procedures, system failure and user errors. The relative frequency of these groups is presented in Table 3.

Table 3. Relative frequency of reason for alerts per severity of the alerts

Type	Mild	Moderate	Severe	Total
Procedure reports	7.62%	0.53%	1.47%	9.62%
System failure	1%	3.09%	2.27%	6.36%
User errors	10.83%	40.84%	32.35%	84.02%
Total	19.45%	44.46%	36.09%	100%

Alerts were classified to three groups based on the potential impact of the error on the patients and the system using recoding in SPSS. Table 3 also shows the relative frequency of the alerts based on this classification.

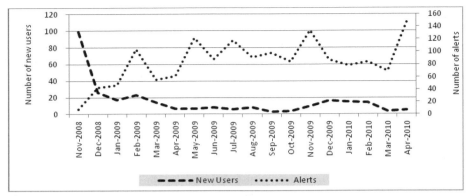

Figure 1. Comparison between number of new users and number of alerts

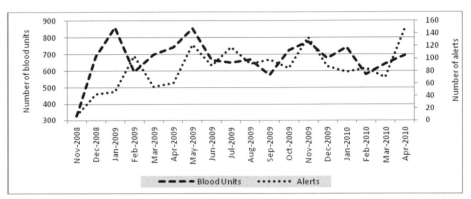

Figure 2. Comparison between number of blood units and number of alerts

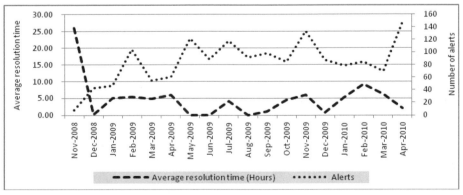

Figure 3. Comparison between average resolution time and number of alerts in each month

The daily distribution of the alerts showed peaks during mid-day between 10:00 AM to 1:00 PM and another peak at 5:00 PM corresponding to the change in work shifts. Pivoting the alerts based on the day of the week showed that they were more common during mid-week; this period also had more transfusions performed.

New users could be expected to follow a learning curve while becoming familiar with the system, and this may result in more alerts. However, the data used in this evaluation did not show a significant correlation (P = 0.149) across months although a relatively similar pattern between these two variables was observed (Figure 1).

A comparison was performed between the number of blood units used in the system and the number of alerts. These two variables showed no significant correlation (P=0.825) (Figure 2). The number of new users had a high correlation (P < 0.00) with the resolution time.

The latency between time the alert was recorded in the system and the time of resolution by the user was calculated for each alert across months. This variable can be viewed as a measure of responsiveness of the system users. Comparison between this variable and the number of alerts in each month is presented in Figure 3. A rapid change in number of alerts was observed in April 2010. This coincided with the start of using the system at the bedside in the wards.

3. Discussion

The alerting module in the blood transfusion management system facilitates recording of important events in the system. This can be used both for immediate problem resolution and future audit. As with any computer system, the electronic blood transfusion management system can itself be a source of the error in the process. Although system failures contributed to only 6% of the alerts they have a higher impact on the system and in some cases they even stopped the whole system from working; examples include kiosk hardware failure, interface or kiosk restart, and a major fire incident which occurred in the hospital.

Some aspects of the blood transfusion process can be controlled by manual procedures in a timely fashion, but in most cases an electronic system is much more suitable for managing alerts. In this evaluation only 29% of the alerts were found to be identifiable via a manual process equivalent to checks in the electronic system.

Although the system can identify such issues, it needs an expert operator to rectify them. However, the expert operator can be a bottleneck in the system performance. This problem of excessive amount of alerts and the reaction from the system users was previously studied in the physician order entry systems [6], but there was no evidence about blood transfusion management systems. The difference between this system and the order entry system is that the alerts cannot be overridden in blood transfusion management system. They should be acknowledged and resolved and increased number of alerts can cause lowered performance. As can be seen in Figure 3, in most instances when the number of alerts rose above 100, a considerable delay in the resolution of the alerts occurred. Pearson test showed a significant correlation between these two variables (P=0.18).

As the system consists of distributed applications, it should be possible to configure the system to notify the supervisor via on-screen warnings on any PC running the management console or blood kiosk, or via PDA, email, voice mail or text message. An expert operator could be alerted by different methods even if the system supervisor is not in the blood bank. Implementation of such a feature may improve the performance of the system supervisor.

4. Conclusion

The error alerting feature of the electronic blood transfusion management system enables users to manage any problems that may arise before they become critical. As this paper has demonstrated, useful insights into to the transfusion process and clinical workflow can also be gained.

The issues identified by this system go far beyond the types of errors that can be handled by a manual process. It should be emphasised that the system is not fully automatic and that problems detected must be rectified by a system supervisor. However, the system supervisor can be the bottleneck in the performance of the system when there are a large number of alerts.

Acknowledgement

This research was commissioned by NHS Connecting for Health Evaluation Program (CfHEP). The researchers acknowledge the continuous support of Shanaz Sohal (project manager at Mayday Healthcare NHS Trust) and Dr. Tony Newman-Sanders (chairman of the project board).

References

[1]   Wikipedia. Blood Transfusion. 2010 [cited 20/06/2010]; Available from:
       http://en.wikipedia.org/wiki/Blood_transfusion
[2]   NPSA. Electronic Clinical Transfusion Management System 2006.
[3]   C. Hillyer, F. Strobl, K. Hillyer, L. Jefferies, L. Silberstein. *Handbook of Transfusion Medicine.*
       Orlando: Academic Press, 2001.
[4]   Murphy MF, Staves J, Davies A, et al. How do we approach a major change program using the
       example of the development, evaluation, and implementation of an electronic transfusion management
       system. *Transfusion* May **49**(5) (2009), 829-37.
[5]   R. K. Aulbach, K. Brient, M. Clark M et al. Blood transfusions in critical care: improving safety
       through technology and process analysis. *Crit Care Nurs Clin North Am* Jun;**22**(2) (2010) 179-90.
[6]   H. van der Sijs H, J. Aarts, A. Vulto, M. Berg. Overriding of Drug Safety Alerts in Computerized
       Physician Order Entry. *JAMIA* **13**(2):138-47.

International Perspectives in Health Informatics
E.M. Borycki et al. (Eds.)
IOS Press, 2011
doi:10.3233/978-1-60750-709-3-367

Data that Makes a Difference in Quality Improvements in Primary Health Care: Approaches through a Pan-Canadian Voluntary Electronic Medical Record Source

Patricia SULLIVAN-TAYLOR, Shaheena MUKHI,
Michelle MARTIN-RHEE, Greg WEBSTER
Canadian Institute for Health Information

Abstract. Primary Health Care (PHC) is the most common health care experienced by Canadians and is an important source of chronic disease prevention and management; however, PHC providers say they have little information about their patient populations, especially groups of patients with multiple conditions. The Canadian Institute for Health Information in collaboration with 50 PHC providers examined the ability to extract and use a subset of PHC EMR data from four disparate environments in an agreed and privacy sensitive manner. Findings describing the feasibility of clinician engagement, EMR data extraction, EMR content standards and data utility gaps, information system requirements, and systemic enablers and barriers are described in this paper. Ability to collect and use discrete and standardized clinical and administrative information is fundamental to improving practice efficiency, optimal use of information, and patient quality of care. Improving quality of EMR data captured at the point of service will considerably enable our ability to measure and understand PHC across Canada; promote dialogue to identify priority information needs; and support health system information uses for clinical program and health system management, research, and population surveillance.

Keywords. EMR content standards, EMR data gaps, PHC data utility, PHC patient centered care, PHC quality improvement, PHC data makes a difference

Introduction

Today, more than half of Canadians report receiving routine or ongoing care in a primary health care (PHC) setting and it is the most common health care experienced by Canadians. It is also an important source of chronic disease prevention and management; 76% of seniors in Canada have a least one chronic condition[1]. However, PHC providers often say they have little information about their patient populations, especially in groups of patients with multiple conditions. Electronic medical record (EMR) systems are used by 37%[2] of PHC providers with the intention to capture, track and use critical information for prevention, monitoring and management of health conditions on a patient by patient basis.

In Canada, the current EMR environments capture patient service events mostly through open text fields, thus posing challenges to information utility. As such, the quality and effective use of clinical information for patient care and practice operation is suboptimal, leading to inefficiencies and limitations that impede our ability to measure and understand aspects of patient-centered care. International efforts within PHC context focus on improving the management of patients with chronic diseases in order to improve care outcomes. Promoting efficiency through effective use of decision support systems has been shown to improve PHC practice capacity to provide high-quality care management and promote coordination of care through team collaboration[3]. For example, in Denmark, 98% of the physicians are able to electronically manage patient care—including ordering prescription, drafting patient visit notes, and sending appointment reminders[4,5].

Since early 2009, the Canadian Institute for Health Information (CIHI) has worked with interested PHC providers across Canada and with the Canadian Primary Care Sentinel Surveillance Network in the pan-Canadian EMR Voluntary Reporting System (VRS) Prototype to collect a subset of PHC EMR data from disparate environments in an agreed and privacy sensitive manner. Findings describing the feasibility of clinician engagement, EMR data extraction, EMR content standards and data utility gaps, information system requirements, and systemic enablers and barriers are described in this paper. Ability to collect and use discrete and standardized clinical and administrative information is fundamental to improving practice efficiency, optimal use of information, and patient quality of care. Collection of standardized data will make a difference and a significant contribution for the country by promoting pan-Canadian use and understanding of population-based information along the continuum of care in the areas of clinical program (quality, coordination of care and outcomes of care), health system management (access, utilization, and resources), research, and population surveillance.

1. Objectives

In collaboration with clinicians, jurisdictions and researchers, CIHI's pan-Canadian EMR VRS Prototype successfully demonstrated the following objectives:
- The current state of the EMR environment and EMR data utility for patient care activities;
- EMR content standards and utility gaps, and future information system requirements;
- Systemic enablers and barriers to improving availability and use of EMR data for primary and secondary purposes; and
- Immediate and long-term steps in increasing availability and use of EMR data.

2. Methods

In collaboration with 50 clinicians across two provinces, the pan-Canadian EMR VRS Prototype pilot tested the EMR Content Standards V 1.1 (112 data elements)[4] using four diverse EMR environments and demonstrated the feasibility of extracting, transforming, analyzing and reporting to inform and support patient-centered care.

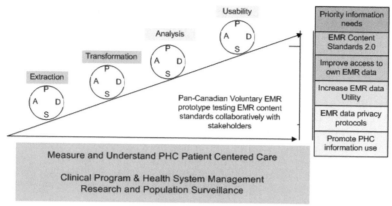

Figure 1. Illustrates the use of continuous improvement cycle (Plan, Do, Study and Act) in demonstrating the feasibility.

3. Results

Discharge abstracts are a rich source of data to assist in better understanding aspects of population hospital service events and outcomes in Canada. Similarly, in PHC settings, EMRs are a rich source of information. However, their potential for use is challenged by the structure in which clinical, demographic and administrative data is captured. Structurally, an EMR allows narrative and free text entry with no validity checks built-in. Such a design results in data collection variation and misinterpretation, and multiple capture points. Lack of interoperability has resulted in manual entry of test results and medications, and scanning of referral and consult notes. Though rich in content, the current EMR data structure poses severe data utility challenges to understand access, outcomes, and population needs, and efficiently use clinical decision support systems in EMRs.

Of the content, 112 data elements[6] were extracted of which approximately 56 data elements are captured by PHC providers. In most cases there was a lack of correspondence between the front end content naming convention and the back-end storage system. It took between 3 to 10 days to extract EMR data where local EMR servers were available. In cases where provider EMR data was stored in application service provider (ASP) server, extraction involved vendor intervention and a considerable cost and time for PHC providers to get access to their own data; therefore, it was excluded from the scope of feasibility work.

To help clinicians gain access to their patient data, six priority data elements were analyzed in depth (codes, description and value sets) to draw out cases of diabetes, coronary artery disease, hypertension and depression. The elements included listed health issues or diagnoses, risk factors, labs, medications, and when available billing information. Text parsing methodology using SAS and CIHI's data quality assessment framework was systematically applied to examine dimensions of relevance, accuracy, comparability, usability and timeliness. This work led to further consult with the clinicians to verify targeted disease cases and confirm reporting needs to inform and support patient-centered care activities. Clinicians spent on average a day to verify disease cases. The verification process allowed them first hand exposure to the quality of their EMR data, and provided opportunities to make corrections if needed. For example, diagnostic ICD-9 codes used for insulin resistant and when antidepressants were prescribed to treat pain were corrected.

Provider feedback reports (sample shown in Figure 2) on four priority chronic diseases and a subset of PHC clinical quality of care indicators in the areas of chronic disease primary and secondary prevention and management, patient safety and outcomes were generated and shared with clinicians. Out of the 12 indicators, the calculation of risk factor screening was not possible to generate as data for risk factors is not captured discretely. Risk factor is encompassed in the clinical progress notes, which also holds patient sensitive information. For privacy reasons, a collective decision was made not to extract this information. This reporting cycle took the dedicated time of four analysts over three months to parse, analyze, and verify the data, and generate reports for 50 clinicians. Beyond the feasibility phase, the same level of effort and resource intensity is not scalable.

Figure 2. Provider Feedback Report on Diabetes Prevalence and A1C tests

Canadian Institute for Health Information Primary Health Care Voluntary Reporting System Physician-Specific Patient Profile DIABETES		PHC Practice ID:			A01
		Number of Physicians in the Practice:			3
		Physician ID:			12345
		Physician-Specific Patient Count:			495
		Report Release Date:			Jul 1, 2009
		Reference Period:		Apr 1, 2008 - Mar 31, 2009	
	Physician 495 (%)	Practice 4,905 (%)	Regional N (%)	Provincial N (%)	National N (%)
Diabetes Diagnoses					
Prevalence	35 (7%)	407 (8%)			
On Insulin, Metformin, Glyburide, or other anti-diabetic drugs*	19 (54%)	247 (61%)			
Diabetes Care Management and Prevention					
Blood Glucose Control					
Met A1C ≤ 7 %	23 (66%)	239 (59%)			
Unmet A1C > 9 %	2 (6%)	19 (5%)			

 By 2010

Lessons learned included:

- Priority list of EMR data elements for the next iteration of pan-Canadian PHC EMR Content Standards;
- Requirements to bridge data capture and usability gaps
- Systematic enablers and barriers to improve EMR data availability and usability informed by clinicians, vendors and jurisdictions
- Priority needs to expand data utility and promote efficiency and effectiveness by capturing standardized data

Clinicians increasingly expressed the need for smart systems to avoid duplication of data entry efforts, efficiently use clinical decision support systems and effectively make health system planning decisions with evidenced-based information. Getting to smart systems, they recognize the integral role of introducing standardized capture of EMR data subset within PHC setting and of nationally coordinating efforts to uniformly address EMR standards for technical and content infrastructure, and vendor certification process. In Denmark, both national overarching policies linking health information technology enhancements to quality, efficiency and patient-centeredness, and engagement of clinicians in determining precise content of the EMRs and in setting standards for data made significant contribution to its success[7].

Within the scope of EMR Content Standards project, CIHI in collaboration with Canada Health Infoway facilitated a pan-Canadian cross collaboration between jurisdictions and broadened engagement of clinicians and field expert to develop a common set of PHC EMR Content Standards (scheduled for release in late 2010).

Beginning 2010-11, data elements and value sets described in the pan-Canadian PHC EMR Content Standards will be further tested using 11 EMR environments and involving 250 PHC providers through the pan-Canadian EMR VRS Prototype. Our goal is to strengthen collaboration with a broad range of stakeholders and achieve the following objectives:

- Increase utility of EMR data for health system uses
- Improve EMR data quality by identifying tools
- Establish pan-Canadian EMR data source – VRS
- Inform future iteration of PHC EMR Content Standards
- Generate comparative provider and provincial reports by 2015 and gather benefits experienced by information users

4. Conclusion

Improving availability of and access to EMR data may promote use of information in ways that can increase knowledge awareness and dialogue among PHC providers, policy makers and Canadian and set clear directions for delivery of service and performance of PHC system. Improving quality of EMR data captured at point of service through tools that allow consistent capture of priority content will considerably enable our ability to measure and understand PHC across Canada; promote dialogue to identify priority information needs; and support health system information uses for clinical program and health system management, research, and population surveillance.

References

[1] *Canadian Survey of Experience with Primary Health Care*, 2008, Statistics Canada; Canadian Institute for Health Information.
[2] C. Schoen, R. Osborn., *The Common Health Fund 2009 International Health Policy Survey of Primary Care Physicians in Eleven Countries*.
[3] Y. Engels et al., Developing a Framework of, and Quality Indicators for, General Practice Management in Europe, *Family Practice* 22, **2** (2005) 215-222.
[4] D. Protti, I Johansen, *Widespread Adoption of Information Technology in Primary Care Physician Offices in Denmark: A Case Study*, Commonwealth Fund 1379, 80 (2010), 1-11.
[5] *100% of Primary Health Care Doctors in Denmark Use Electronic Medical Records.* New Commonwealth Fund Profile Points to Lessons for the U.S. and Health Care Reform. March 11, 2010. Retrieved on June 17, 2010 @ 3 pm.
[6] CIHI 2009, Primary Health Care Indicators Electronic Medical Records Content Standards Version 1.1.
[7] CIHI 2010, *Lessons Learned Piloting Primary Health Care Electronic medical Record Content Standards: Areas of Opportunity.* Retrieved on June 18, 2010 @ 2 pm. www.cihi.ca.
[8] D. Protti and I. Johansen, *Widespread Adoption of Information Technology in Primary Care Physician Offices in Denmark: A Case Study*, Common Wealth Fund 1379, 80 (2010), 1- 11.
[9] WHO Regional Office for south-East Asia and WHO Regional office for the Western Pacific. *People at the Center of health care: harmonizing mind and body, people and systems.* Geneva, World Health Organization, 2007

International Perspectives in Health Informatics
E.M. Borycki et al. (Eds.)
IOS Press, 2011
© 2011 ITCH 2011 Steering Committee and IOS Press. All rights reserved.
doi:10.3233/978-1-60750-709-3-372

Situation Awareness and Risk Management Understanding the Notification Issues

Plinio P. MORITA [a], Catherine M. BURNS [a]

[a]*Department of Systems Design Engineering – University of Waterloo*

Abstract. Healthcare institutions are known to be risky environments that still lag behind other industries in the development and application of risk management tools. Awareness of risk is an important aspect of a risk management program. People depend on high awareness to take precautions to manage risk. The Situation Awareness framework describes how a person perceives elements of the environment, comprehends and projects its actions into the future, and analyzes the cognitive process used. Consequently, it allows the integration of the cognitive model and the risk assessment model into one single framework, provides a means of examining if the risk awareness is calibrated to the true risk levels of the institutions, and a better understanding of the issues with adverse events notification systems. In this paper we discuss how the situation awareness model can be used in the assessment of risk awareness, for understanding risk awareness and safety culture, and finally, for designing more effective risk management systems. For the purpose of this paper, we focus on the adverse event notification system.

Keywords. situation awareness, adverse events, detection, healthcare

Introduction

Healthcare institutions are known to be risky environments that lag behind other industries in the development and application of risk management (RM) tools [1]. Awareness of risk, however, is a very positive thing. It is only with a good awareness of risk that people can take precautions to manage it [2,3]. Without appropriate awareness of risk, personnel are likely to inadvertently take inappropriate and dangerous actions [2]. The degree to which workers are properly aware of and calibrated to the risks in their environment is an important factor in having an effective safety culture in an organization, and vice versa. While the terms "risk awareness" and "safety culture" are commonly used and tacitly understood, there is a need to integrate these concepts. In this paper we argue that the concept of "Situation Awareness," developed by Endsley [4] may provide a unique way of understanding these ideas. Furthermore, with a situational awareness (SA) understanding we should be able to discuss whether an organization has developed an appropriate safety culture and whether its personnel hold appropriate awareness of the risks in their environments. Finally, we discuss how these concepts could lead to the design of more effective RM systems for healthcare. As a working example for this publication, we will discuss the improvements for an adverse event (AE) notification system.

1. The Situation Awareness Model

Endsley's [5] definition of SA is one of the more widely adopted and is the one we will use in this paper. In particular, Endsley breaks down the human cognitive process of SA into three distinct levels, each one with different characteristics and effects on the overall awareness:

- Level 1 – Perception: this level describes how people perceive elements of the environment within the restrictions of a known space and period of time.
- Level 2 – Comprehension: this level describes how people process the information collected in Level 1 to gain an awareness of the current situation. With Level 2 situation awareness, people understand how the current situation will impact their goals and objectives.
- Level 3 – Projection: this level focuses on how people can predict future events and actions in their environment. To do this, people must already have appropriate Level 1 and 2 situation awareness and, through knowledge of the dynamics of their world, can extrapolate from this information to predict future states and future courses of action (COA).

When people have good and appropriate SA they operate effectively in their environments, properly interpreting information and taking necessary actions to prevent future problems. When people have inadequate SA they may misunderstand the state of the system or inappropriately predict future events [5].

While there is a wide body of research that examines risk perception [2] (similar to Level 1 SA) and risk comprehension [6, 7] (similar to Level 2 SA), little can be found regarding risk prediction (similar to Level 3 SA). Therefore, the strength of Endsley's model [5] is in three potential contributions. First, this model integrates other known concepts relating to the cognitive assessment of risk into a single model. Secondly, Endsley's model can be used to examine whether the awareness of risk is properly calibrated to the true risk levels of the environment. Third, this model can be used to examine different awareness of risk at the institutional level and the level of personnel, allowing a better understanding of the issues found when using notification systems for detecting AE. Therefore, it is possible to say that the SA model provides a framework from which risk managers can better understand the environment of the institution, and the cognitive process of the staff, adjusting the RM tools to better fit them.

2. SA in Healthcare – Awareness of Risk and Safety Culture

Awareness of risk is deemed as one main factor for the success of RM programs [3]. A high level of risk awareness within the institution's administrative structure will result in a more successful RM program [3]. Safety culture and risk awareness are directly connected, where a more developed safety culture will result in greater risk awareness due to investments in training, cultural change, and better support for the RM team [8]. The inverse is also valid: greater risk awareness will result in a quest for a better RM program. Many of the RM endeavors focus on raising awareness of risks – such as through training and campaigns – and efforts in creating a safety-focused culture.

The RM team is responsible for training the staff to be able to detect, briefly analyze, and decide if they should notify the RM team of risks and AE (Personnel SA) [9]. This training improves staff awareness both by facilitating the perception of occurrences and by giving a better understanding of AEs – focus on SA Level 1 and 2. In the same perspective, changing the safety culture in institutions can benefit the notification process by changing the attention level and perception of occurrences, and by changing the staff's mental model of the institution regarding the notification process, highlighting the benefits of successful notification.

3. SA in Healthcare – Institutional SA, Personnel SA and the Institutional SA Gap

The SA model allows a more in-depth analysis of the AE notification process in healthcare institutions, creating a better understanding of the reasons why notification systems sometimes fail in raising the RM team's awareness of AEs, even while the personnel SA is high. Since notification systems are the mostly commonly used AE detection systems, it is necessary to understand them in order to design new systems that improve the institutional awareness of AEs.

Institutional SA - An institution's RM team needs to gain awareness about AE before investigating them and creating RM projects. Even though an institution is not a person, we have adapted the SA framework to understand the process used to detect AEs. The diagram shown in Figure 1 shows how the SA model can be expanded to an institutional perspective. The perception mechanisms used by the institution to gain awareness of AEs range from passive notification systems to active registry scouting systems [10]. Related personnel SA is also described in the diagram. Some parallels can be drawn between the RM processes and the SA model [5]: the AE detection systems correspond to institution's perception mechanisms, the AE investigations correspond to the comprehension mechanisms, and the RM projects based on investigations correspond to the projection of those findings into measures that would reduce the risks in the future. By understanding the SA framework [5], a mapping of the links between each SA phase would highlight possibilities for improvement. Focusing on the perception mechanisms, the notification link provides most of the perception regarding AEs. If the safety culture of the organization does not support notification, the perception of AEs is severely hindered [11]. Since the later stages of SA (comprehension and projection) rely on perception, this further hinders the institution SA of AE.

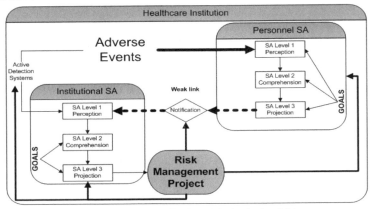

Figure 1. Graphical visualization of the institutional SA gap.

Personnel SA – Most AEs are detected by one or more staff members (SA Level 1) as they participate directly in the situations where AEs take place. The COA taken from this point – notify the institution of the AE or not – depends on an individual's goals, training, and motivation towards safety. Some examples of factors that can prevent hospital staff from submitting an AE notification are: lack of comprehension of the risk to patients and peers (Level 2 SA) and fear of reprisal, a negative projected COA, which could be considered Level 3 SA. In contrast, personnel with a strong understanding of the risk of the AE (Level 2 SA), who can accurately estimate the future risk of the AE to patients and are optimistic about that the institution will take effective action (Level 3 SA), are more likely to submit an AE notification. This model clearly identifies two key issues – first, that personnel must have a strong comprehension of what AEs mean in terms of patient risk. Secondly, the safety culture of the institution is critically influential in a person's assessment of the future events that will follow their AE notification. In this way, the decision to submit an AE notification can be directly related to the staff member's SA regarding a particular event. To influence this SA, personnel must have adequate knowledge to comprehend the event and the institution must have a healthy safety culture so that the person is confident the AE will be handled effectively.

Institutional SA Gap – Since the only link between personnel SA and institutional SA is the notification system and given the fact that most of the perception of AEs by the institution comes from the notification system, whenever a staff member decides not to submit a notification for an AE, the chances of the RM team gaining awareness about that event are drastically reduced. Since the SA process is guided by goals, without the solid depiction of safety as a main goal inside the institution, it is difficult to promote notification. As discussed by other authors [12,13], safety culture is one of the most challenging, yet simultaneously most rewarding aspects of change in an organization. Implementation of a healthy safety culture would result in the alignment of the institutions safety goals and the needs of a successful AE detection system, improving the likelihood of proper AE notification.

One critical issue that can be identified by the SA model [5] is that in all cases, the goals and objectives of the staff and those of the institution may not be properly aligned. When institutions are driven towards safety programs, the objective can often be to increase the quality of care, but also to reduce the costs associated with AEs. In contrast, personnel may be driven by pressures to maintain tight schedules, manage high workloads, and maintain good relationships within their team and their managers. In some situations, depending on how much the institution is perceived to value safety, personnel goals and institutional goals may be misaligned.

The model shown in Figure 1 describes this institutional SA gap. The notification link is shown as the most used, but least robust, as poor personnel SA can weaken this link. This link can be improved with better designed AE notification systems that contribute to better personnel SA by promoting comprehension and ensuring effective COAs. In contrast, active detection systems are shown as a robust but less common link. This link is more robust, as it does not rely on personnel SA to same degree as the notification link; it is less common, because active AE detection systems are still not commonly deployed. Due to the challenges that can occur with personnel SA, however, active detection systems should be considered as an opportunity to bridge the institutional SA gap, by making institutional SA more resilient

4. Conclusion – Bridging the Gap

To improve the detection of AEs it is necessary to bridge the institutional SA gap between personnel SA and institutional SA. Some solutions to this problem include:

Improve the notification systems in place – improving the current notification system towards a more automated, easier to notify system may increase the number of notifications. These changes should occur in concert with general improvements to personnel risk comprehension (Level 2 SA) and a healthy safety culture [11] (Level 3 SA). Ways to improve these systems include simple usability changes so that notifications are straightforward and less time consuming, protecting anonymity so that personnel are confident that the COA will not negatively impact them, and giving feedback on how the AE has resulted in positive changes in the organization.

Develop a safety culture – this technique is the most effective approach, although it is a long-term endeavor and requires effort, patience, and resources [11]. An example of successful safety culture development is the Veterans Association [12], which consists basically of changing the culture to one that encourages notification, investigation, and modifications that improve safety in all processes in the institution.

Use active detection systems that are not based on peer notification – these systems can improve the detection of AEs without using personnel notification systems by actively scouting through the institution records, video detection systems, registry scouting systems, and RM brokers [10]. These systems are more effective than personnel notification systems because they are less reliant on personnel SA.

Overall, in order to increase the number of AEs detected, the institutional SA gap must be avoided. The described alternatives focus both on reducing or avoiding the gap, always with the intent of increasing institutional SA.

References

[1]   R. L. Helmreich. On error management: Lessons from aviation. *BMJ (Clinical Research Ed.)*. **320** (7237) (2000), 781-785.
[2]   P. Slovic. *The Perception of Risk*. London: Earthscan Publications Ltd.; 2000.
[3]   T. Rundmo, A. R. Hale, Managers' attitudes towards safety and accident prevention. *Saf Sci*. **41** (2003), 557-574.
[4]   M. Endsley. Toward a theory of situation awareness in dynamic systems, Human Factors. *J Human Factors Ergon Soc*. **37** (1995), 32–64.
[5]   M. Endsley, B. Bolté, D. Jones, *Designing for situation awareness: an approach to user-centered design*. Florida: Taylor and Francis Group; 2003.
[6]   J. Adams. *Risk*. London: Routledge; 1995.
[7]   N. Luhmann. *Risk: a sociological theory*. New York: Aldine de Gruyter, Hawthorne; 2005.
[8]   J. Harvey, G. Erdos, H. Bolam, M. A. Cox, J. N. Kennedy, D. T. Gregory. An analysis of safety culture attitudes in a highly regulated environment. *Work & Stress*. **16**(2002), 18-37.
[9]   P. P. Morita, S. J. Calil. The importance of a safety culture in healthcare facilities for the development of an incident investigation system, In: *World Congress on Medical Physics and Biomedical Engineering*. 2009: 20-23.
[10] N. Leroy, E. Chazard, R. Beuscart, M. C. Beuscart-Zephir. Toward automatic detection and prevention of adverse drug events. *Stud Health Technol Inform*. **143**(2009), 30-35.
[11] V. Nieva, J. Sorra. Safety culture assessment: A tool for improving patient safety in healthcare organizations. *Qual Saf Health Care*. **12**(2003), 17-23.
[12] W. Weeks, J. Bagian. Developing a culture of safety in the Veterans Health Administration. *Eff Clin Pract*. **3** (2009), 270-276.

International Perspectives in Health Informatics
E.M. Borycki et al. (Eds.)
IOS Press, 2011
doi:10.3233/978-1-60750-709-3-377

Design of Adverse Drug Events-Scorecards

Romaric MARCILLY[a,1], Emmanuel CHAZARD[b], Marie-Catherine BEUSCART-
ZÉPHIR[a], Werner HACKL[c], Adrian BĂCEANU[d],
Andre KUSHNIRUK[e], Elizabeth M. BORYCKI[e]

[a] *Evalab INSERM CIC-IT, Lille ; Univ Lille Nord de France ; CHU Lille;
UDSL EA 2694 ; F-59000 Lille, France*
[b] *CERIM, Univ Lille Nord de France ; CHU Lille ;
UDSL EA 2694 ; F-59000 Lille, France*
[c] *Institute for Health Information Systems, UMIT - University for Health Sciences,
Medical Informatics and Technology, 6060 Hall in Tyrol, Austria*
[d] *Ideea Advertising, Bucharest, Romania*
[e] *School of Health Information Science, University of Victoria, Victoria, Canada*

Abstract. This paper presents the design of Adverse Drug Event-Scorecards. The
scorecards described are innovative and novel, not having previously been
reported in the literature. The Scorecards provide organizations (e.g. hospitals)
with summary information about Adverse Drug Events (ADEs) using a Web-
based platform. The data used in the Scorecards are routinely updated and report
on ADEs detected through data mining processes. The development of the ADE
Scorecards is ongoing and they are currently undergoing clinical testing.

Keywords. adverse drug event, scorecards, user-centered design, data mining

Introduction

Improving the quality of health care is an important aspect of healthcare administrator
work. In order to improve healthcare quality and safety, managers and health
professionals require information to inform their decision-making. In recent years we
have seen a significant increase in the amount of data that is being collected by health
information systems. One possible approach is to collect data gathered in electronic
patient record systems and provide decision makers with information using a Scorecard
approach. Scorecards have been used in a variety of industries. More recently, they are
being used in healthcare as a method of providing hospital unit decision makers with
information that can help them design interventions that can improve their
organizational processes [1]. Scorecards are organizational performance management
frameworks that have strategic and non-financial performance measures to provide
managers with a top level view of the organization's performance [2]. Scorecards are
considered to be a tool that can help decision makers to improve the quality of the
organization's performance and as a strategic management tool (e.g. helping managers
to make decisions about the types of interventions they wish to undertake that may
address issues in quality or organizational performance) [3].

---

[1] Corresponding Author: romaric.marcilly@univ-lille2.fr

An important area that healthcare organizations worldwide are focusing upon is adverse drug event (ADE) reduction. Presently, there is a need for new methods for reporting about ADEs that would allow health care administrators and professionals to work together and identify strategies for reducing the frequency and types of adverse events that are occurring at a unit level. This paper reports on the development of a novel type of scorecard (which has not previously been reported in the literature) designed to report on adverse drug events at hospital and hospital unit levels. This work is part of a large EU project entitled "PSIP - Patient Safety through Intelligent Procedures in Medication" which has provided the unique opportunity to link results of data mining about ADEs with Scorecard reporting. The PSIP project aims to:

- Innovatively produce knowledge on ADEs (to identify within hospitals, their number, type, consequences and causes by data and semantic mining methods) and
- Investigate different possibilities for reducing ADEs (e.g. developing contextualized decision support, rules and solutions supporting patients' compliance, using Human Factors engineering).

In this paper one of the possibilities emerging from the PSIP project is explored - the development of ADE-Scorecards to provide a novel way of reporting on ADEs.

1. ADE-Scorecards Development

1.1. Background

In the frame of the PSIP project, several hospitals provide a data-mining team with their Electronic Health Records (EHR) through a common data model [4]. A common repository currently contains 90,000 stays from 6 hospitals. Those data are analyzed thanks to methods such as decision trees and association rules. This allows discovering ADE detection rules. Those rules are made of a set of conditions (e.g. drug administration, lab abnormalities, patient condition etc.) that can lead to adverse effects. The rules are then reviewed and validated by a group of pharmacists, pharmacologists and physicians. For now, 236 rules are validated and used for ADE detection [5].

Each month, the hospitals involved make available anonymized data from the previous month. Each new set of data is screened using all the available rules, providing information about adverse effects and their potential causes. This information is uploaded to the web-based ADE-Scorecard website (described below).

The ADE-Scorecards' aim is to provide healthcare professionals with detailed information about the ADE cases (type and cause of ADEs, statistics) that occurred previously in their department in order to help them learn about how to avoid such ADEs in the future. These regular monthly reports of contextualized ADE statistics are displayed through a website that is updated monthly with new data.

1.2. Interface Design and Development

The website for displaying scorecards was designed using user-centered design principles [6]. From the beginning of this work, an ergonomist was integrated in the designers-developers team to support cooperative design. Moreover, a sample of final users (4 physicians, 2 pharmacists, 3 head nurses, 6 nurses, 1 health care quality manager), participated in the design by commenting on the first mock-ups and the first version of the prototype, choosing features among parallel versions, and proposing new features and/or facilities. Results from the participatory design supported the recommendations used by the developers. A continuous evaluation procedure ensures that recommendations are taken into account.

2. ADE-Scorecards

The ADE-Scorecards aim at being used by different categories of professionals (e.g. physicians, head nurses, nurses, pharmacists and may be quality management). By logging in, users are identified (thus, the interface's language is automatically adapted and only the user's department data are displayed). This section illustrates the design of the ADE-Scorecards displays for both the summarized data and detailed statistics.

2.1. "Synthesis and Edition of Detailed Statistics" Page

The "Synthesis and Edition of detailed statistics" page contains (see figure 1):
- A table and a graph, for each kind of ADE, and for each month, the number of cases.
- A drop down menu allowing users to choose the period for which they want to get ADE statistics. A choice in this menu immediately changes the data displayed in the previous table/graph.
- Next to every adverse effect's name, check boxes allow for selecting the effects for which "detailed statistics" pages will be generated.

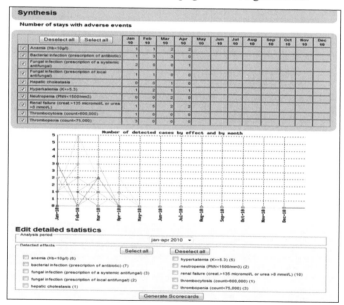

Figure 1. Screenshot of "Synthesis and Edition of detailed statistics" page.

2.2. *"Detailed Statistics" Page*

For each selected adverse effect a page is generated which presents (see figure 2):

- The characteristics of identified stays, all rules together, that describe the sample of stays presenting the adverse effect, including: number of patients concerned, average age, gender proportions, proportions of diseases that might have impact on ADEs (e.g. alcoholism, cancers, renal insufficiency) and the death rate (these deaths are not necessarily due to the adverse effect).

The conditions (rules' premises: patients' conditions, administered drugs) potentially leading to an adverse effect with their confidence (percentage of stays for which the event occurs among the stays meeting the conditions), their median delay (from the moment when all conditions of the rule are met, the period from which over 50% of events appeared) and the number of stays they target.

- A chart representing the distribution of the number of effects per month during the current year.
- Description of the conditions, which may contain a longer description of the rules, scientific explanations and references, and advice.
- Access to a synthetic view of the patients' record using an EHR visualization tool named "Expert Explorer" [7].

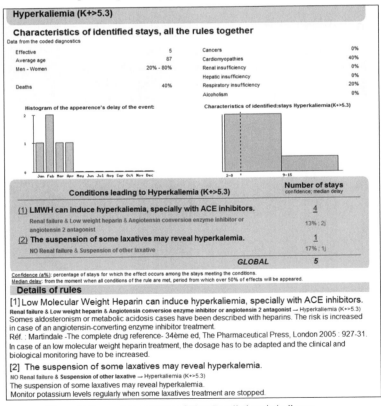

Figure 2. Screenshot excerpts of The "Detailed statistics" page.

3. Discussion

Currently, the ADE-Scorecards contain information about 27 classes of ADEs (e.g. anemia, hyperkaliemia, hyponatremia, renal failure, hemorrhage hazard due to vitamin K antagonists) which are detected automatically by 236 PSIP-rules. The scorecards already allow physicians from 6 hospitals to view their statistics and to explore the corresponding ADE cases. For a clinical test, the scorecards are currently being implemented in three departments at Denain's Hospital, a 300-bed hospital in northern France. Their impact, in terms of ADEs' appearance and monitoring, is being evaluated in a longitudinal observational study and by the mean of observations of changes in ordering/monitoring policy. Another clinical test is under preparation in hospitals in the Capital Region of Denmark and will start soon. These tests aim at carrying out a clinical validation of the PSIP-rules and follow-up of the user-centered design approach using an iterative design method. Moreover, in parallel, a second ergonomist team is currently evaluating the interface. The results of the clinical validation, the iterative design and the interface's evaluation will support the follow-up refinement of the scorecards website, with the objective of increasing its usability, reliability and utility.

References

[1]   R.S. Kaplan, D. P. Norton, *The balanced scorecard: Translating strategy into action.* Harvard Business School Press, Boston, 1996.
[2]   M.C. Kocakulah, D. Austill, Balanced scorecard application in the health care industry: A case study. *J. Healt Care Finance* **34**(1) (2007), 72-99.
[3]   H. Atkinson, Strategy implementation: A role for the balanced scorecard? *Manage Dec* **44**(1) (2006), 1441-1460.
[4]   E. Chazard, B. Merlin, G. Ficheur, JC. Sarfati & R. Beuscart, Detection of adverse drug events: proposal of a data model. *Stud Health Tech Inf* **148** (2009), 63-74.
[5]   E. Chazard, G. Ficheur, B. Merlin, M. Genin, C. Preda & R. Beuscart, Detection of Adverse Drug Events Detection : Data Agregation and Data Mining, *Stud Health Tech Inf* **148** (2009), 75-84.
[6]   ISO 13407:1999, Human-centred design processes for interactive systems.
[7]   A. Băceanu, I. Atasiei, E. Chazard, & N. Leroy, The Expert Explorer: A Tool for Hospital Data Visualization and Adverse Drug Event Rules Validation, *Stud Health Tech Inf* **148** (2009), 85-94.

Acknowledgment

The research leading to these results has received funding from the European Community's Seventh Framework Program (FP7/2007-2013) under the Grant Agreement n°216130-the PSIP project.

Standardization and Interoperability

International Perspectives in Health Informatics
E.M. Borycki et al. (Eds.)
IOS Press, 2011
doi:10.3233/978-1-60750-709-3-385

Development of a Draft Pan-Canadian Primary Health Care Electronic Medical Record Content Standard

Patricia SULLIVAN-TAYLOR[a], Tanya FLANAGAN[a],
Ted HARRISON[a], Greg WEBSTER[a]
[a]Canadian Institute for Health Information

Abstract. In collaboration with a broad range of stakeholders, the Canadian Institute for Health Information (CIHI) led the development of the draft pan-Canadian primary health care (PHC) electronic medical record (EMR) content standard to be used in EMR applications across the country to support PHC data capture and information use and improved health system management. To achieve this goal, CIHI initiated the following activities: stakeholder engagement, information requirements gathering and adoption and implementation promotion of the common content standard for wide-spread use. The resulting pan-Canadian standardized data set will allow consistent data capture that will improve understanding and ability to report on PHC utilization and access, chronic disease prevention and management, health promotion, medication usage, patient safety, quality of care including patient safety and outcomes. The standard will improve patient care information by providing the structured comparable information needed to care for patients over time and across the continuum of care. Standards support clinical practice reminders and alerts, improvements in operating efficiencies, onscreen feedback reports to PHC providers and the ability to look at clinical trends over time. This standard will improve the flow of information by providing standardized information to providers at points on the continuum of care leading to better coordination of care and a reduction of repeat tests. Lastly, a common content standard will improve the health system use of data; by enabling aggregation and analysis of comparable standardized health information, clinicians, jurisdictions, and regions can benefit from using this data for more effective planning and policy decisions. The jurisdictions and clinicians, supported by CIHI and Canada Health Infoway will continue to work together with other key stakeholders, such as vendors to support the adoption and implementation of this standard into future jurisdictional EMR vendor specifications.

Keywords. electronic medical record, content standard, data, health information, improvement, panCanadian, primary health care, quality improvement

Introduction

Primary health care (PHC) has been described as the foundation of Canada's health care system and is the most common type of health care experienced by Canadians. Ninety-four percent of Canadians aged 15 and over use "first contact" services each year[1] and Canada's First Ministers agreed that PHC is one of the priority areas for improvement.[2] Despite the importance of PHC in the overall management of Canadians' health and the health system, it is an area lacking comparable, standardized data to support system-level analysis to better understand and inform delivery. With the increasing use of electronic medical record (EMR) applications in PHC settings across Canada, the use of a common EMR content standard in PHC is necessary in order to have relevant and standardized data to support decision making related to key elements of care such as access, quality and outcomes.

In 2006, the Canadian Institute for Health Information (CIHI) released a set of 105 pan-Canadian PHC indicators in a series of reports[3,4] that were developed with support from national, provincial/territorial representatives, clinicians and researchers. After this release, CIHI conducted an environmental scan to assess the feasibility of collecting data on these indicators from a variety of data sources including data from EMRs, existing CIHI databases, other administrative databases, as well as patient, provider, and organizational surveys.

In 2009, to facilitate the collection of EMR data and in response to provincial and territorial requests, CIHI released version 1.1 of the *PHC Indicators Electronic Medical Record (EMR) Content Standards*[5]. This common EMR content standard included 56 data elements related to the patient, provider, encounter and outcomes of care and supported consistent, comparable data capture for 12 CIHI PHC clinical indicators. CIHI worked with PHC providers across Canada in the Voluntary Reporting System (VRS) Prototype to pilot test the collection of this data from provider EMRs. Information from the pilots demonstrated enormous gaps in the way that the data is collected. For example, much of the EMR data collected in the pilots was unstructured, non-standardized and really designed for single patient care delivery, not population-based care planning and management.

In 2010 at the request of the jurisdictions, CIHI led the development of a pan-Canadian EMR content standard for priority PHC data elements. This work, led by the jurisdictions and Canada Health Infoway (Infoway), and informed by key stakeholders across the country, was intended to support consistent data capture in EMR applications to improve PHC and health system management.

1. Objectives

The objectives of the pan-Canadian PHC EMR content standard were to:
1. develop and release a common pan-Canadian EMR content standard that could be used in PHC EMR applications to support PHC data capture, information use and improved health system management;
2. align this standard with jurisdictional needs and priorities and pan-Canadian EHR/EMR standards where appropriate;
3. promote the adoption and uptake of the pan-Canadian PHC EMR content standard for use in EMRs by a wide range of stakeholders.

2. Methods

To lead the development of a pan-Canadian PHC EMR content standard that is clinically relevant, aligned with existing standards where appropriate, meet the needs of stakeholders and are implementable, CIHI initiated a strategy that included:

1. Stakeholder Engagement
2. Information Requirements Gathering
3. Promotion, Adoption and Implementation

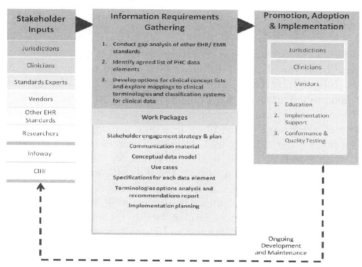

Figure 1. Strategies toward achieving a pan-Canadian PHC EMR Content Standard

2.1. Stakeholder Engagement

In an effort to develop a common PHC EMR content standard, CIHI required input and buy-in from a variety of key stakeholders including jurisdictions, clinicians, Infoway, standards experts, EMR vendors, EHR standards specialists and researchers.

A stakeholder engagement strategy guided the project's understanding of the needs and priorities of its key stakeholders, the best approaches to working with each and the potential risks and mitigation strategies to ensure the initiative's success.

A jurisdictional advisory group (JAG), co-chaired by a jurisdictional representative and CIHI, was formed with senior representatives from each province and territory, including Infoway and the Federal Healthcare Partnership. The JAG operated as a single coordination point for jurisdictional engagement and approved workplans, the consultative process and outputs.

To support promotion of this work, a communication tool kit was developed, which included a single information sheet about the goal of the initiative, an electronic frequently asked questions document that grew over time as the project and stakeholder awareness and understanding evolved, a PowerPoint slide presentation and video presentation overview of the initiative for use and repurposing by the jurisdictions and a variety of testimonials, video and audio impacts stories to be used as promotional material. All of the written materials were available in English and French.

Some of the key engagement activities included stakeholder specific workshops, meetings, teleconferences, web conferencing including for example, jurisdictional meetings and vendor workshops. Other examples of engagement included stakeholder participation on expert review committees, conference plenary or subjects of impact stories championing the value of the content standard. Throughout the initiative, the jurisdictions managed clinical engagement with their respective PHC providers and associations and CIHI supported their efforts by making the communication tool kit available to the jurisdictions for customization for specific clinical audiences.

2.2. Information Requirements Gathering

A pan-Canadian Content Standards Working Group (CSWG) with JAG-appointed representatives from jurisdictions, Infoway, PHC clinicians, standards experts and CIHI, was established to reconcile stakeholder requests for data elements for inclusion against a predetermined inclusion and exclusion criterion set by the JAG early on in the project. To be included for consideration in the content standard, the data elements had to have both a clear primary use and health system use application. Primary use was defined as supporting the delivery and, or administration of care. Health system use was defined as supporting public health surveillance, health system management, research and clinical program management. The data elements had to also be captured in the normal course of the delivery and, or administration of care by PHC providers. In addition, the data elements had to align with existing standards and jurisdictional priorities and relevant EMR and electronic health record (EHR) initiatives where appropriate. Finally, the data elements had to be implementable in the Canadian PHC context. Figure 2, provides an illustrative example of the initiative's inclusion criterion.

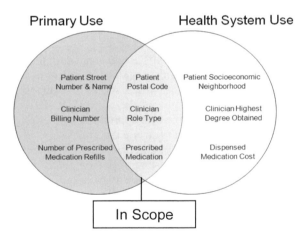

Figure 2. Primary Use and Health System Use Inclusion Criterion

The scope of the standard did not include detailed clinical notes or other information that was not required to support at least some health system use purposes. Furthermore, the focus of this project was on data to be standardized; recommendations on system functionality such as prompts and alerts were out of scope. Similarly, recommendations on changes to provider work flow and clinical guidelines were out of scope.

The CSWG had three comprehensive review cycles. After each review cycle the CSWG reconciled requests against the inclusion/ exclusion criteria and refined the list of elements going forward for consideration in the next review. It is important to note that once a request was rejected from the list, the stakeholder that made the request was notified and given the rational for exclusion. Once a specific request was rejected, it would not be included for consideration in subsequent review cycles. Based on the expertise of the CSWG and their rigorous review process, the final set of recommended data elements to be standardized in PHC EMRs were forwarded to the JAG for consideration. The JAG reviewed the CSWG recommendations and came to a consensus on the minimum data set to be included in the pan-Canadian PHC EMR content standard.

2.3. Promotion, Adoption and Implementation

The JAG not only functioned as the ultimate decision makers on what data elements were to be included in the final content standard, they were also responsible for recommending promotion, adoption, implementation, governance and maintenance strategies for the standard. The JAG-led approach was an efficient and effective strategy that offered leadership, coordination and logistical support, shared development of implementation resources and an opportunity for common conformance testing. To assist the promotion of this pan-Canadian PHC EMR content standard, CIHI presented the collaborative work at numerous conferences and workshops across the country. CIHI also supported the production and dissemination of the printed pan-Canadian PHC EMR content standard in both official languages. To aid adoption and implementation, CIHI conducted a clinical terminologies and classification systems options analysis for six important concepts, including "reason for visit" and "health issue." Unlike other recommended data elements that require less complex value sets, these concepts were identified as potentially benefitting from the use of a terminology or classification system. The options analysis determined which clinical terminologies and classification systems could be used for each of the six data elements, based on their ability to meet four criteria: clinical relevance and level of detail; costs of adoption to all those affected; the quality of the standard; and the clinical terminology's ability to incorporate new Canadian needs. The analysis provided insight on how to input value sets in EMRs in a way that supports clinicians. Future work is underway to develop terminology value sets and mapping terminology classification standards at the point of care delivery while supporting coded data capture in the back-end for interpretation and analysis at the practice and system level.

3. Results

Between December 2010 and June 2010, the CSWG received over 11,000 suggestions on data elements for inclusion in the standard from a variety of stakeholders or queries and comments on their attributes. The CSWG had three comprehensive review cycles over this period, including an initial face-to-face meeting where the working group deliberated over the inclusion of the 56 data elements in version 1.1 of the *PHC Indicators Electronic Medical Record* (EMR) Content Standards. In June 2010, 106 data elements were forwarded to the JAG for consideration.

Based on the expertise of the CSWG and their rigorous review process, the JAG considered the 106 CSWG recommended data elements for inclusion. In August 2010, the JAG approved and endorsed the 106 data elements as the normative content of the draft pan-Canadian PHC EMR content standard. Table 1, provides a simplified view of the data elements with their common names. Where possible, the elements were aligned to pan-Canadian and international EHR/EMR standards, and jurisdictional needs and priorities. This standardized data set will allow consistent data capture that will improve understanding and ability to report on PHC utilization and access, chronic disease prevention and management, health promotion, medication usage, patient safety, quality of care practices and outcomes.

Table 1. Simplified view of the draft pan-Canadian PHC EMR content standard (106 data elements with their common names).

Demographics						
Patient			**Clinician**		**Clinic**	
Identifier			Identifier		Identifier	
Identifier Type			Identifier Type		Name	
Identifier Assigning Authority			Identifier Assigning Authority		Type of Services	
Date of Birth	Status		Last Name		Postal Code	
Gender	Date of Death		First Name			
Highest Education	Rostered (Start / End Date)		Middle Name			
Housing Status	Ethnicity		Role			
Primary Language	Postal / Zip Code		Expertise			
Patient Care Activities						
Patient						
	Health Concern(s) (Date of Onset / Resolution Date)					
	Social Behaviour(s) (Date of Onset / Resolution Date)					
	Allergy / Intolerance Type	Agent	Severity	Status (Date of Onset / Resolution Date)		
	Vaccine Administered	Date Administered		Lot #	Reason Not Given	
Encounter Specific						
	Appointment Requested Date	Reason for Visit		Visit Date	Visit Type	
	Systolic / Diastolic Blood Pressure			Site	Position	Representative
	Height *	Weight *		Waist Circumference *		
	Intervention (Treatment)	Date		Reason for Refusing Intervention		
	Clinician Assessment	Payment Source		Payment Type		Billing Code
Medications						
	Prescribed		Prescribed Date	Estimated Completed Date	Stop Date	Repeat
	Strength *		Dosage *	Form	Frequency	Route
	Reason Not Prescribed		Medication Compliance	Medication Dispensed	Dispensed Date	
Lab						
	Lab Test Name Ordered	Order Date	Performed Date	Result Name	Result Value*	Low/High Range *
Diagnostic Imaging						
	Diagnostic Imaging Test Ordered	Order Date	Performed Date			
Referral						
	Referral Service	Request Date	Occurred Date			
Family History						

Relationship to Patient	Ethnicity	Deceased Date	Cause of Death
		Health History Concern(s) (Age at Onset or [Start / End Date])	
		Social Behaviour(s) (Age at Onset or [Start / End Date])	
		Intervention (Treatments) (Age at Onset or [Start / End Date])	

* These data elements are associated with additional data elements to express the Units of Measures (e.g. cm, kg, etc.).

The published document, *Draft Pan-Canadian Primary Health Care Electronic Medical Record Content Standard*⁶, was disseminated electronically in December 2010 and posted on the CIHI website. Each jurisdiction was provided with printed copies in both official languages. Supporting documents were also produced for jurisdictional use, including business view documentation, implementation and data extraction guides, and the evaluation of the terminology report.

4. Conclusion

By working together and seeking input from key stakeholders across the country, the jurisdictions, clinicians, vendors, standards experts, CIHI and Infoway have demonstrated an efficient process for developing and implementing content standards in Canada; standards that support interoperability of EMRs with EHR systems and meet the needs of stakeholder use and application.

A pan-Canadian PHC EMR content standard will be very valuable for PHC in Canada because it will support the improved collection of standardized information needed to care for patients and monitor their status over time. Standards support clinical practice reminders and alerts, improvements in operating efficiencies, onscreen feedback reports and give providers the ability to look at clinical trends over time. This standard will improve the flow of information by providing standardized information to providers at points on the continuum of care leading to better coordination of care and a reduction of repeat tests. Lastly, a common standard will improve the health system use of data by enabling aggregation and analysis of standardized health information, clinicians, jurisdictions, and regions can benefit from using this data for more effective planning and policy decisions. The jurisdictions, clinicians, vendors, standards experts, CIHI and Infoway will continue to work together, with other key stakeholders to support the adoption and implementation of this standard into jurisdictional EMR vendor specifications in the future.

References

[1] C. Sanmartin et al, *Access to Health Care Services in Canada 2001* (Ottawa, Ont.: Statistics Canada, 2001) catalogue number 82-575-XIE2002001 (2001).

[2] Health Council of Canada, *Health Care Renewal in Canada: Accelerating Change*, (Toronto, Ont.: Health Council of Canada, 2005).

[3] Canadian Institute for Health Information, *Pan-Canadian Primary Health Care Indicators*, Report 1 Volume 1 and 2, (Ottawa, Ont.: Canadian Institute for Health Information, 2006)

[4] Canadian Institute for Health Information, *Enhancing the Primary Health Care Data Collection Infrastructure in Canada*, Report 2. (Ottawa, Ont.: Canadian Institute for Health Information, 2006)

[5] Canadian Institute for Health Information, *Canadian Institute for Health Information Primary Health Care Indicators Electronic Medical Record Content Standards, Version 1.1.* (Ottawa, Ont.: Canadian Institute for Health Information, 2009)

[6] Canadian Institute for Health Information, *Draft pan-Canadian Primary Health Care Electronic Medical Record Content Standard.* (Ottawa, Ont.: Canadian Institute for Health Information, 2010)

International Perspectives in Health Informatics
E.M. Borycki et al. (Eds.)
IOS Press, 2011
© 2011 ITCH 2011 Steering Committee and IOS Press. All rights reserved.
doi:10.3233/978-1-60750-709-3-392

Data Encryptions Techniques for Electronic Health Record Exchange

David SHIN[a], Tony SAHAMA[a,1], Steve (Jung Tae) KIM[b], Ji-Hong KIM[c]
[a]Computer Science Discipline, Faculty of Science and Technology (FaST)
Queensland University of Technology (QUT)
PO Box 2434, Brisbane 4001, QLD, Australia
[b]Department of Electronic Engineering, Mokwon Univerisity, Republic of Korea
[c]Department of Info.& Commu. Eng., SeMyung University, Republic of Korea

Abstract. Simulation approaches on data encryption techniques to improve health care decision making processes are presented in this paper. Database-as-a-Service model (DAS) was utilised to employ the databases and related records for the scenarios selected. Data that was used for the simulation process ranged from 10,000 to 2 million records. When the bucket indexing model incorporated partitioning fields and bloom filters in a Singleton design pattern, it effectively provided faster responses in the range query. The results showed that query response time in the bucket indexing model is approximately 3.32 times faster than the normal range query response time in the encrypted database.

Keywords. data encryption, electronic health record, DAS, bucket index, bloom filter.

Introduction

Health care is an information-intensive business. Trusted health care outcomes are crucial to patients. Requirements to ensure both quality and sharing of patients' health records are an important factor for better clinical decision making and sustainable health care service deliveries. In the view of maintaining a quality of life, the sharing of data and information between professionals and patients is critical when the data is revealed. This information sharing process is a challenge and costly if patients' trust between professionals' and institutional accountability are not established. Data and information exchange in the health care decision making process is vital in order to make an informed decision. E-health is a combination of information technology and communication for supporting decision-making processes using electronic health records. The widespread adoption of E-health is essential for the sharing of knowledge, safety and quality in healthcare. However, health information and communications technology (HICT) will not dramatically improve care nor reduce costs for health care services individually. Even though information is available electronically, it is not always shared across organisational boundaries freely due to multiple constraints,

---

[1] Dr. Tony Sahama, Computer Science Discipline, Faculty of Science and Technology (FaST), Queensland University of Technology (QUT), PO Box 2434 Gardens Point, Brisbane, QLD 4001, Australia. t.sahama@qut.edu.au

barriers and the culture of information sharing. There is already a significant investment in the electronic health data and information exchange all over Australia. At present, information security and privacy in the health care system is required to improve synergies and further research between professionals and patients. Unfortunately, despite successful application of information technology in other information-intensive industries, the current situation to share information across systems and between care organisations encounters many obstacles with efficiency and cost-effectiveness in health care[1].When information is shared in a health care delivery processes, particularly the major concern is information security and privacy for the patients' records. Such concerns emphasises security issues and requires addressing techniques for security from the point of data extractions and/or retrievals. In this connection, realisation of data structure is a must. The simulation comprises databases ranging from 10,000 to 2 million records in different scenarios selected in this paper. These records were encrypted, indexed and retrieved with query optimisation. Bucket indexing including conventional AES (Advanced Encryption Standard) and Bloom filter in Singleton design pattern with Database-as-a-Service model (DAS) was adopted for the simulation.

1. Concepts of the Service Model

A. DAS Model and Query Processor: Wei et al.[2] highlighted that the Database-as-a-Service model is a new data management model that allows users to outsource their data to database service providers (DSP). Since data is stored in cryptographic form at DSP, query efficiency becomes a critical problem. Existing solutions for this problem concentrate mostly on cryptograph index technology. The outsourcing database to a third party aims at decreasing the cost of maintenance of DBMS.

B. Bucket Index: The Bucket index is identical for character type data. The construction of the index should follow two principles; firstly the index should filter false records efficiently and secondly it should be safe enough not to leak the true value. Numeric data needs equations and a range query with "between", "and" terms. An index supporting all computations does not exist, thus, it is possible to create different types of indexes according to the data type and their purposes. The index tries to translate the character string into numeric data on which the primary query will be processed to filter the records roughly. Only the rest of the records need to be decrypted and it will save a considerable amount of time.

C. Bloom Filter Algorithm: Zhong et al.[3] indicated that bloom filters are compact set representations that support set membership queries with small, one-sided error probabilities. Standard bloom filters only support elemental insertions and membership queries. The Bloom filter is used to speed up answers in a key-value storage system.

D. Secured Electronic Medical Records (EMR) Requirements and Design Under the DAS Model: According to Essin & Lincoln[4], the EMRs (Electronic Medical Record) should have certain requirements such as atomicity, authenticity, persistence, flexibility of representation and retrieval, semantic integrity, interoperability, process ability, performance and security. In the context of security, there are legal and ethical requirements that the records should be kept secure and confidential so that each individual's privacy is preserved.

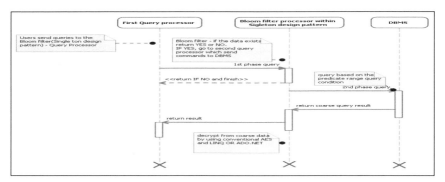

Figure 1. Main Simulation Design -Sequence Diagram for Query Flow in Bucket Index using Bloom filter under AES-DAS model

The main idea behind the bucket indexing engine is to use predicate key information that has already been physically partitioned in tables. It also initially loads bucket key information into Bloom filter as a Singleton design pattern as shown in Figure 1.

Table 1. List of experimental databases

DB Name	Encryption(Y|N)	DAS model(Y|N)	Details of the Records.
Plain_Hospital	N	Y and N	Plain data, 10,000 records
Enc_Hospital	Y	N	MS Built-in Encryption scheme, 10,000 records
Enc_Hospital2	Y	Y	Conventional AES, 10,000 records
Enc_Hospital3	Y	Y	Conventional AES, semi-bucket, 10,000 records
Enc_Hospital5	Y	Y	Conventional AES, Bucket, Bloom filter,10,000 records
Enc_Hospital6	Y	Y	Conventional AES, Bucket, Bloom filter and other collection classes,2 million records

Table 1 depicts the lists of experimental databases. Under DAS models, there are three stakeholders such as database owners, professional data service providers and clients. In the case of a semi-DAS model, the database owners are in charge of preserving security on their data sets. The Bucket index is identical to numeric data such as birth date Year – nvarchar data type (string data type).

We designed a proto-type EMR on the SQL Server. The simulation environm00000ent Before generating the random data, we inserted indispensable base records including information about doctors, researchers and nurses. We managed the random data generator with a range of 10,000 records to 2 million records. And we checked the inserted data and the count of the records. In the case of the 2 million-records database, we ran the index tuning advisor to get a faster result. We analyzed SQL files in the database query window in a built-in encryption scheme and checked the codes inside the random data generator which is based on the DAS model and conventional AES. Finally, we evaluated the response time of the queries from simulation results.

Table 2. Simulation Environment

Software	Hardware
Windows XP	32-bit Intel Core2duo (3GHz processor)
C# (.NET 3.5 Framework)	4GB RAM
Microsoft SQL Server 2008	500GB HDD
Bloom Filter (From an open source - http://bloomfilter.codeplex.com/releases/view/25930)	

Table 3. Simulation Results and Analyses - Response Time of Selection Test

Query Response Time (milli second)	String 1 (Address)	String 2 (medica reNo)	Range query (BirthDate) (>=)/ (count)	Range query (Semi bucket index)	Range query (Bucket index ,Bloom filter)	Aggregate function (Blood Type -group by)
Plain_Hospital	23	23	80/0	not available		6
Enc_Hospital (MS built-in Encryption scheme)	113	26	200/40	not available		80
Enc_Hospital2 (AES, DAS model)	156	156	140/140	not available		31
Enc_Hospital3 (AES, semi-bucket, DAS model)	156	156	156/156	16	not available	31
Enc_Hospital5 (AES, Bucket & Bloom filter)	156	156	156/156	16	47	31
Enc_Hospital6 (AES – 2 million record)	249550	2250	31049/31049	3703	not tested	4860

Table 3 shows key results taken from the simulation that measures select query response times on each different maintenance model. The simulation is under 10,000-record-sized databases: Plain-text, MS built-in and AES-DAS models. As a result of the simulation, most plain-text queries show the fastest response time in each category of queries. In the case of retrieving string type and numeric type, MS built-in encryption is faster than AES-DAS model whereas in the case of range query, AES-DAS model is faster than MS built-in. However, there is more to investigate in order to bring about more efficient secured EMR from the simulation. AS an example, string-typed data encryption / decryption show slower response time than numeric-typed data encryption / decryption in MS built-in security compared to result in AES-DAS model. Internally, MS built-in security combines both symmetric keys and asymmetric keys. Nevertheless, Microsoft does not fully open its schemes to public. For this reason, while using MS built-in security, numeric-typed data encryption/decryption performance is much more efficient than string-typed data.

In the case of range queries based on category: Normal range, Semi-Bucket and Bucket index, Semi-Bucket shows the fastest response time among them. For the simulation, Bloom filter in application memory using Singleton design pattern is used for the first coarse query. If Bloom filter contains the wanted data, then the real second query is passed to DBMS. The coarse data works by taking the results from the partitioning data or grouping data based on the characteristics of the queries. Thus, Bucket index saves decryption processing time due to the narrower coarse results. There are two types of Bucket index: Semi-Bucket and Bucket index. The concept of Semi-Bucket is that a DBA can make logical assumptions of where the readable data will be partitioned to the partitioning field. In contrast, the Bucket index contains hardly-any readable versions of partitioning information that uses binary operation which means conversion to bits and changes its positions reversely similar to Vigenere Cipher. For the simulation, patients' birth date are used and compared. However, if Bucket index is more complicated, it also takes additional time to calculate arithmetic or binary operation. As a result, the Bucket index performs around 3.32 times faster than a normal range operation.

In the case of group by functionality, if the query does not utilise bounded index, then, it does not show better performance compared to MS built-in or AES-DAS model. But if the query utilises index scanning, it shows much better performance compared to encrypted models. On the other hand, it depends on the SQL Server query processor to adopt the indexes or there are different aggregate query schemes in accordance with the content of the aggregate query conditions. When retrieving encrypted alphabetical datafields in the 2 million record database with the DAS model, the performance with nvarchar(max) type as the field 'Address' is significantly lower than when using other techniques whereas it is not as prevelent when retrieving numeric data such as 'medicareNo'.

2. Conclusion

Data-sharing techniques provide many benefits to health care services. As e-health data sharing is promising, illegal data leakage and data theft in the DAS model would become a major issue to preserve patients' privacy. This work focuses on the impact of data encryption techniques under a DAS model for effective decision-making.
The 'Bucketization' using bloom filter in the application memory shows the improvement for a range of query response times. For the encrypted databases, querying in real time is an important issue to fulfill requirements such as shorter response times, separated roles and maintenance under DAS models.

References

[1]   J. Grimson, W. Grimson, W. Hasselbrin. The SI Challenge in Health Care. *Comm ACM* **43**(6) (2009) 49-55.
[2]   Z. Wei, et al. *A tuple-oriented bucket partition index with minimum weighted mean of interferential numbers for DAS models*. in *Computer and Automation Engineering (ICCAE), 2010 The 2nd International Conference on*. 2010.
[3].   M. Zhong, et al., *Optimizing data popularity conscious bloom filters*, in *Proceedings of the twenty-seventh ACM symposium on Principles of distributed computing*. 2008, ACM: Toronto, Canada. p. 355-364.
[4].   Essin, D.J. and T.L. Lincoln, *Healthcare information architecture: elements of a new paradigm*, in *Proceedings of the 1994 workshop on New security paradigms*. 1994, IEEE Computer Society Press: Little Compton, Rhode Island, United States. p. 32-41.

Telehealth

International Perspectives in Health Informatics
E.M. Borycki et al. (Eds.)
IOS Press, 2011
doi:10.3233/978-1-60750-709-3-399

Teleoncology Uptake in British Columbia

Melissa CLARKE [a,b,1], Jeff BARNETT [a,b]

ᵃ BC Cancer Agency, Victoria, BC, Canada
ᵇ University of Victoria, Victoria, BC, Canada

Abstract. Telehealth enables the delivery of specialized health care to patients living in isolated and remote regions. The purpose of this analysis is to determine the current uptake of teleoncology in mainland British Columbia. Patient appointment data was extracted from the Cancer Agency Information System (CAIS) for the 2009 calendar year. Three types of practitioners used teleoncology in 2009: Medical Oncologists, Genetic Counsellors and Medical Geneticists. In total, 712 telehealth encounters were conducted; Medical Oncologists conducted 595 encounters (83.6%), Genetic Counsellors conducted 112 encounters (15.7%) and Medical Geneticists conducted 5 encounters (0.7%). The most common oncology appointments were Gastro-Intestinal (11.4%) and Lymphoma (11.0%) follow-up appointments with a Medical Oncologist. Telehealth encounters were conducted by 46 individual health care providers however, a single Medical Oncologist conducted 418 encounters and this accounts for more than half (58.7%) of all telehealth appointments in 2009. Radiation Oncologists on the mainland up to this point are not using the technology. The Local Health Areas with the highest number of oncology telehealth appointments were: Kamloops: 203 encounters (34.1%), Penticton: 84 encounters (14.1%), Cranbrook: 58 encounters (9.7%) and the Southern Okanagan: 33 encounter (5.5%). Use of telehealth in rural and remote areas of BC is limited and there is significant room for growth. Further research will be required to identify barriers and restrictions to the use of telehealth in order to increase teleoncology adoption in British Columbia.

Keywords. telehealth, teleoncology

Introduction

The BC Cancer Agency is the organization responsible for providing cancer care for residents of British Columbia and the Yukon. The BC Cancer Agency has integrated the use of telehealth into oncology care to reduce the patient burden associated with travelling for specialized cancer care. The purpose of this paper is to examine the current uptake of teleoncology in British Columbia. The BC Cancer agency has five regional cancer centres that provide comprehensive oncology health care. The regional centres are located in southern regions of the province and most cancer specialists (oncologists) work and provide care out of one of these facilities. Patients living in rural and remote areas must travel great distances in order to access specialty care.

Telehealth technology connects cancer care providers to patients living in isolated and remote regions. Telehealth uses video-conferencing technology to conduct patient consultations when the patient and health provider are not located in the same

---

[1] Corresponding author, Melissa Clarke: mcclarke@uvic.ca

geographic location. This technology has been implemented for use in multiple health disciplines such as cardiovascular diseases, mental health, inflammatory bowel disease, pediatric oncology, cystic fibrosis [1]. Teleoncology in B.C. began as a pilot study lead by Weinerman et al. (2005) [2]; this study assessed the use of telehealth to conduct oncology consultations on Vancouver Island. The pilot study determined that telehealth was acceptable to both patients and health care providers as an alternative method to deliver cancer care. To assess the uptake of oncology telehealth in mainland British Columbia, an analysis of telehealth records extracted from the Cancer Agency Information System (CAIS) for the 2009 calendar year was conducted.

1. Objectives

To assess the current level of oncology telehealth uptake in British Columbia, several key questions were asked, including: "What types of appointments are occurring via telehealth?", "How many health practitioners are using the technology?" and "Which regions of B.C. are using telehealth?" To provide a comparison for this analysis, appointments that were conducted in person that could potentially be held via telehealth were also examined. This study builds on previous research conducted on Vancouver Island [2] and to limit overlap between these studies, 2009 telehealth records for Vancouver Island were not selected for this analysis.

2. Methods

Telehealth records were extracted from CAIS and organized into Excel spreadsheets. The types of appointments selected for a qualitative analysis were: "Follow-Up", "New Patient" and Genetic Counselling appointments. Weinerman et al. (2005) [2] identified "Follow-Up" and "New Patient" encounters as suitable oncology appointment types to be conducted via telehealth. Other appointment types such as Radiation Treatment and Imaging appointments are not suitable as a patient must physically be present to conduct these types of appointments. The health providers using telehealth on Vancouver Island are Medical and Radiation oncologists [2]. Genetic counselling appointments conducted by Genetic Counsellors and Medical Geneticists via telehealth were also included in the analysis.

The evaluation of telehealth uptake included telehealth encounters that originated from 4 BC Cancer regional centres: Abbotsford Centre (AC), Fraser Valley Centre (FV), Vancouver Centre (VC), and the Centre for the Southern Interior (SI). The analysis excluded telehealth encounters that originated from the Vancouver Island Centre (VIC).

2.1. Potential Telehealth Data

Appointments that were conducted in person that could potentially be held via telehealth were identified as potential telehealth if they had an activity type that had been successfully conducted by telehealth in the 2009 calendar year. Potential telehealth data did not include genetic counselling appointment, as the primary focus was oncology telehealth. Potential telehealth would generally be considered for patients that are living further than a 50km drive away (or greater) from one of the BC Cancer Agency facilities. For example a Lymphoma Chemotherapy Follow-Up appointment would be considered a potential telehealth encounter for a patient living in Kamloops. Lymphoma Chemotherapy Follow-Ups had been successfully conducted via telehealth in 2009 and Kamloops is a city that is more than a 50km drive away from the nearest regional facility.

3. Results

712 telehealth encounters were conducted in the 2009 calendar year. These encounters fell into one of three activity classes: New Patient appointments, Follow-Up appointments or Genetic Counselling appointments. Follow-Up appointments were the most common class of appointment with 492 (69.1%) telehealth encounters conducted. Gastro-Intestinal and Lymphoma cancer patients were the most common cancer types seen via telehealth. Gastro-Intestinal and Lymphoma patients accounted for 393 encounters, which is slightly more than half (55.2%) of all telehealth encounters conducted.

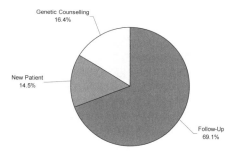

Figure 1. Percentage of telehealth by appointment class.

There were 43 different types of health care activities successfully conducted via telehealth. Genetic Counselling Videoconference (GENECV) was the most common activity type performed via telehealth in the 2009 calendar year with 115 records. This type of activity was conducted by Genetic Counsellors and Medical Geneticists. The next most common appointments conducted via telehealth were Gastro-Intestinal and Lymphoma Follow-Up appointments with a Medical Oncologist. There were 81 Gastro-Intestinal Follow-Up appointments and 78 Lymphoma Follow-Up appointments conducted via telehealth.

The telehealth and potential telehealth encounters were grouped by cancer site to determine if uptake of telehealth varied by cancer site. Table 1. summarizes the data captured for the cancer sites that were performed via telehealth. This table indicates that certain activity sites have a higher percentage of telehealth uptake than other activity sites.

Telehealth encounters were carried out by 46 individual health care providers. There were 3 types of health care providers using telehealth appointments: Medical Oncologists performed 595 encounters (83.6%), Genetic Counsellors performed 112 encounters (15.7%) and Medical Geneticists performed 5 encounters (0.7%). There were no telehealth appointments recorded for Radiation Oncologists. There were 37 individual Medical Oncologists that used telehealth; however, a single Medical Oncologist conducted the majority of the telehealth encounters. This individual conducted 418 encounters and most of these encounters were Gastro-Intestinal (171 encounters) and Lymphoma patients (163 encounters). This oncologist also saw Breast, CNS, Genito-Urinary, Head & Neck, Lung, Sarcoma, Primary Unknown and Skin cancer patients via telehealth

Table 1. Oncology telehealth uptake by cancer site

Cancer site	Telehealth Encounters	Potential Telehealth	%Uptake
Lymphoma	175	6616	2.6
Breast	72	6555	1.1
Gastro-Intestinal	218	6540	3.2
Lung	69	3049	2.2
Genito-Urinary	17	2043	0.8
Sarcoma	26	382	6.4
Head & Neck	6	334	1.8
Gyne	2	318	0.6
CNS	4	275	1.4
Melanoma	1	82	1.2
Primary Unknown	1	58	1.7
Skin	4	23	14.8
Totals	**595**	**26275**	n/a

%Uptake= (Telehealth Encounters/(Telehealth Encounters + Potential Telehealth)) x100

712 telehealth encounters were recorded by 48 Local Health Areas (LHAs) in the 2009 calendar year. The LHAs with the highest number of oncology telehealth appointments (greater than 30 records) were the following: Kamloops: 203 encounters (34.1%), Penticton: 84 encounters (14.1%), Cranbrook: 58 encounters (9.7%) and the Southern Okanagan: 33 encounters (5.5%). The number of oncology telehealth encounters was compared with potential telehealth encounters to investigate levels of uptake by LHA. Telehealth uptake varied by LHA and is relatively low for all LHAs. Table 2. summarizes telehealth and potential telehealth data by LHA.

Table 2. Comparison of oncology telehealth and potential oncology telehealth encounters by LHA.

Local Health Area	Telehealth Encounters	Potential Telehealth	%Uptake
Kamloops	203	3736	5.2
Penticton	84	2091	3.9
Cranbrook	58	488	10.6
Southern Okanagan	33	915	3.5
Kimberley	26	236	9.9
Summerland	20	454	4.2
Keremeos	19	281	6.3
Windermere	18	88	17.0
Creston	18	227	7.3
Fernie	17	183	8.5
Cariboo-Chilcotin	14	218	6.0
Merritt	12	319	3.6
Princeton	10	243	4.0
100 Mile House	9	243	3.6
Totals	**541**	**9722**	n/a

Summerland (<50km from regional centre) appointments were included in the potential data set because of the high number of telehealth encounters that occurred in 2009.

4. Discussion

Medical Oncologists, Genetic Counsellors and Medical Geneticists were the health care providers that used telehealth to conduct oncology appointments in 2009. According to this data, Radiation Oncologists did not use telehealth to conduct appointments in 2009. Out of 46 individual health care providers that used telehealth, one single Medical Oncologist conducted 418 of the 712 encounters. This oncologist provided care for a diverse group of patients via telehealth, which included: Breast, CNS, Genito-Urinary, Head & Neck, Lung, Sarcoma, Primary Unknown, and Skin cancer patients. Since the majority of telehealth encounters were conducted by this individual the result of the analysis has a significant bias, as it is driven by the pattern of practice of this one oncologist.

In 2009, New Patient appointments accounted for 103 telehealth appointments in comparison to 492 Follow-Up appointments conducted via telehealth in BC. Follow-Up appointments were more commonly seen via telehealth and are likely to be more acceptable to oncologists because the patient has already been seen in a "face-to-face" appointment type and have already begun/finished treatment.

There were 43 different activity types conducted via telehealth. Gastro-Intestinal and Lymphoma follow-up appointments with a Medical Oncologist were the most common oncology appointments performed. These results reflect the pattern of practice conducted by the medical oncologist conducting the majority of the telehealth appointments. The two most common cancer patients seen by this oncologist were in fact Gastro-Intestinal and Lymphoma patients.

Comparison of telehealth and potential telehealth by cancer disease site suggests that the level of telehealth uptake is relatively low for almost all cancer sites. It was also observed that certain cancer sites had higher uptake levels than others. The most likely explanation for higher uptake levels is that the type cancer sites seen via telehealth will be based on the preference or specialty of the provider.

Telehealth encounters were recorded by 48 Local Health Areas. The highest numbers of oncology telehealth occurred in Kamloops, Penticton, Cranbrook, and the Southern Okanagan. The oncologist that conducted the majority of telehealth encounters, works primarily out of the Centre for the Southern Interior (CSI), which is located in Kelowna. This would account for the high numbers of telehealth encounters seen in and around this area. CSI has 4 satellite clinics in Vernon, Penticton, Cranbrook and Kamloops. Teleoncology has become important to this region for a variety of reasons. There have been staffing issues at the satellite clinics resulting from unfilled positions, resignations, illness, maternity and sabbaticals [3]. Telehealth provides an alternative way to meet staffing challenges by "lending out" an oncologist to an area experiencing a shortage. There were closures to the Summerland highway beginning in the fall of 2008 and Okanagan fires in the summer of 2009 [3]. These events would have presented challenges for cancer patients trying to access cancer care in Kelowna and could explain the higher numbers of telehealth encounters seen for these areas that are geographically close to a regional facility.

Comparison of telehealth and potential telehealth by Local Health Area indicate that uptake levels are low for most LHAs and the highest uptake recorded did not exceed 20%. There were a handful of LHAs that did not have any telehealth encounters occurring. For example: Stikine, Telegraph Creek, Snow Country, Nisga'a, and Burns Lake LHAs did not record telehealth encounters. These LHAs could be potential gaps in telehealth service.

5. Conclusions

Use of telehealth in rural and remote areas of BC is limited for now and there is significant room for growth. There are numerous New Patient and Follow-Up appointments for a variety of cancer types that could potentially be conducted via telehealth. The same type of specialized services rendered at regional cancer centres could be achieved for patients living in rural areas.

A significant barrier for adoption is physician acceptance; this is clearly indicated in this analysis as one oncologist conducted the bulk of telehealth appointments. There are currently no incentives for health providers to use telehealth. For some oncologists, it is easier from their own perspective, to have patients travel for face-to-face visits than to deal with the perceived challenges of using this technology. With only one individual conducting the majority of the appointments it raises concerns over the longevity of the adoption of telehealth. If this one individual retires or relocates to a different province then the use of teleoncology will decrease significantly. Further investigation into the factors that are preventing other oncologists from using this technology must be determined and addressed.

A second potential barrier to telehealth adoption is the issue of resources, as there are a finite number of tele-conferencing units available to conduct appointments. This issue has surfaced at the Vancouver Island Centre where telehealth units on the island are utilized by multiple disciplines and this has resulted in competition over the receiving units that are used by patients (B. Weinerman, personal communication, March 30, 2010). Future research will need to identify other barriers and restrictions to the use of telehealth in order to propose solutions that will facilitate higher uptake of teleoncology in British Columbia.

6. Acknowledgements

The authors would like to thank Dr. Brian Weinerman and Dr. Kong Khoo for their expertise and constructive comments, Sandra Dillabough for extracting the raw data from CAIS and Erin Gibbs for her previous research in teleoncology.

References

[1] K. Tran, J. Polisena, D. Coyle, K. Coyle, E-H. W Kluge, K. Cimon, S. McGill, H. Noorani, K. Palmer, R. Scott, *Home telehealth for chronic disease management* [Technology report number 113]. (2008) Ottawa: Canadian Agency for Drugs and Technologies in Health

[2] B. Weinerman, J. Den Duyf, A. Hughes, S. Robertson, Can Subspecialty Cancer Consultations Be Delivered to Communities Using Modern Technology? – A Pilot Study. *Telemedicine Journal & E-Health* **11(5)** (2005), 608-615.

[3] K. Khoo, *Telemedicine in the Southern Interior (2004-present).* [PowerPoint slides]. BCCA Rounds presentation March 9, 2010

International Perspectives in Health Informatics
E.M. Borycki et al. (Eds.)
IOS Press, 2011
© *2011 ITCH 2011 Steering Committee and IOS Press. All rights reserved.*
doi:10.3233/978-1-60750-709-3-405

Strengths and Weaknesses of Using Conferencing Technologies to Support Drug Policy Knowledge Exchange

Mowafa Said HOUSEH[1,a], Andre W. KUSHNIRUK[b],
Malcolm MACCLURE[b], Bruce CARLETON[d], Denise Cloutier-FISHER[c]

[a] *College of Public Health and Health Informatics, King Saud Bin Abdul Aziz University for Health Science, Riyadh, Kingdom of Saudi Arabia*
[b] *School of Health Information Science, University of Victoria, Victoria, British Columbia, Canada.*
[c] *Department of Geography, University of Victoria, Victoria, British Columbia, Canada.*
[d] *Department of Pediatrics, University of British Columbia, Vancouver, British Columbia, Canada.*

Abstract. This paper outlines the experiences with and lessons learned from the use of conferencing technologies in supporting knowledge exchange groups. We discuss the strengths and weaknesses of these technologies when used to support distant knowledge exchange activities within drug policy groups. The strengths and weaknesses of face-to-face meetings are also discussed.

Keywords. conferencing technologies, strengths and weaknesses, knowledge exchange

Introduction

As collaborative healthcare research groups increasingly communicate at a distance, information and communication technologies play a more important role in supporting such interactions. When these interactions occur between clinicians, academics, and policy makers in a collaboration and information-sharing network, they are referred to as knowledge exchanges [1]. The benefits of knowledge exchange occur when decision-makers incorporate research evidence into the decision-making process as a result of the knowledge exchange process. Drug policy is one of several domains that have been successful in forming knowledge exchange groups.

For years, knowledge exchange groups within the drug policy domain have been working together in face-to-face and distant environments to support group interactions. The existence of knowledge exchange networks within drug policy is not new. For example, in 1997, Soumerai et al. published a paper on various factors that influence

---

[1] Corresponding Author: Dr. Mowafa Househ, Assistant Professor, King Saud Bin Abdul Aziz University for Health Sciences, College of Public Health and Health Informatics, Riyadh, Kingdom of Saudi Arabia; Email: househmo@ngha.med.sa

drug-cost-containment policies within the United States [2]. The authors found that one of the factors influencing drug policy decision-making was the information sharing that occurred among various stakeholders around certain Medicare policies. Similarly, a study examining drug policy knowledge exchange practices within six different countries found that knowledge exchange networks involving academics and drug policy decision-makers helped influence various drug policies within each country.[3]

These results demonstrate the benefits of creating face-to-face knowledge exchange networks involving academics, clinicians, and drug policy makers. To date, little is known about the impacts of knowledge exchange interactions when they move from a face-to-face setting to a virtual setting. The purpose of this paper is to describe the strengths and weaknesses of face-to-face and distant interactions among drug policy group members within the context of knowledge exchange.

1. Methods

The findings outlined in this paper were part of those of a larger case study on the use of conferencing technologies to support drug policy exchange groups that took place between 2004 and 2007.[4]   For this case study, three drug policy groups were observed over a three-year period between 2004 and 2007. There was an education task group, a research task group, and a decision-making task group. The education task group consisted of academic detailers who worked collaboratively to produce research reviews focused on new drugs to disseminate to physicians. Of the 26 potential participants in the education task group, 20 were included in the study, comprising researchers, educators, and decision-makers.

The research task group was charged with the task of evaluating the cost savings of physician educational interventions. This task involved collaborations between researchers and decision-makers working on the evaluation of education for quality improvement in patient care. Of the 17 potential participants in the group, 14 researchers and decision-makers were included in the study. For the drug policy task group, decision-makers and their staff met on a monthly basis, using live teleconferencing as a communication method. A designated researcher would disseminate research information on the latest drug policy research trends. Of the 32 potential participants in the decision-making task group, 27 were included. The 27 participants included in this task group were researchers, decision- makers, and staff from provincial Canadian drug plans.

A conceptual framework was designed to guide the study, and was built from the information and communication technology ICT and knowledge exchange literature. This framework is composed of various inputs, processes, and outputs that can influence knowledge exchange within a distant environment, the details of which have been published in our previous work.[5] Important components of the framework are the processes that are relevant to distant knowledge exchange: facilitation, social interaction, and information sharing. These three processes were found to be relevant to both the ICT and knowledge exchange literature.[5] The findings related to this paper are based on post-interviews conducted with various participants from the groups and on researcher observations recorded over the course of the study.

2. Technologies Used

Both web-conferencing and teleconferencing technologies were used in this study. Elluminate Live V-Class edition was the web-conferencing tool used in the study. This version of the technology allows for half-duplex audio communication that permits users to speak one at a time. Elluminate also allowed users to upload the agenda to a whiteboard, share documents via application sharing, use instant text messaging, vote/poll participants, use emoticons, raise hands, and see participants' names. These were the most relevant features used by the groups in the study. The education and research task groups used Elluminate. The decision-making task group did not use the web-conferencing tool.

For teleconferencing, the education and decision-making task groups used audio teleconferencing technology. The technology used audio-only communication where multiple participants could speak at the same time. There was no video or other media for communication. A participant simply dialed a telephone number, entered a conference code, and responded to a prompt requesting his or her name. A beep sound let other participants know that someone had joined the meeting. To use this technology, group members needed access to e-mail and a telephone. E-mail was necessary to inform the participants about the meeting details (time, numbers to dial, and the agenda). The decision-making task group completed one pre-recorded teleconference. In a pre-recorded teleconference, the researcher would present his or her findings during the teleconference, and the recording of the teleconference would be distributed via e-mail to the decision-makers.

Only the research and education task groups met in face-to-face meetings. The education task group met once a year in a face-to-face session, and the research task group discontinued the use of web-conferencing and returned to face-to-face meetings that occurred once a month. During face-to-face meetings, group members met in a designated room where the chairs were arranged around a space or a table. An image projector connected to a computer was placed in the middle of the meeting setup. The image projector projected items onto a screen; the agenda and other related meeting documents were projected throughout the meeting.

3. Strengths

The strengths inherent in face-to-face, teleconferencing, and web-conferencing meetings helped facilitate knowledge exchange within drug policy groups. Face-to-face meetings were the preferred method of communication because participants were more able to discuss original topics and carry out complex discussions. In face-to-face meetings, interactions were much more immediate, spontaneous, and richer than in web-conferencing or teleconferencing meetings. In face-to-face meetings, participants were less distracted and participated more frequently. Face-to-face meetings had an established culture and were already a well-accepted method of meeting.

Generally, teleconferencing provides a simple and convenient method of meeting for groups whose members are located far from one another or for groups with very busy members. Participants can be on the road, on the street, at the airport, in another city, or in another country, but as long as they have access to a phone, they can join the meeting. The study found that teleconferencing maintained the immediacy and spontaneity in discussions that were available in face-to-face meetings. Pre-recorded teleconferencing meetings had an advantage over live teleconferencing meetings because they allowed the participants to listen to recordings at their convenience. However, comparisons of live vs. pre-recorded teleconferencing suggest that live teleconferencing was the preferred method of communication because it offered interactions through live discussions and, in this study, provided a communication link between decision-makers and researchers. The advantages of teleconferencing included general comfort with the medium and teleconferencing's long history and reliability.

Web-conferencing meetings offered strengths with regard to facilitating knowledge and exchange between groups. In general, when the groups needed to collaborate, yet were restrained by a limited budget and were geographically dispersed, web-conferencing meetings improved knowledge exchange. Groups with such characteristics found web-conferencing to be a much more valuable medium than teleconferencing because web-conferencing provided a much richer forum for interaction through its voting/polling, whiteboard, application sharing, and display of participant information functions. Furthermore, web-conferencing tools improved meeting interactions by making them more disciplined, helping to keep group members focused on the same topic, making the meetings less time consuming, and facilitating democratic decision-making during meetings.

Regarding facilitation, face-to-face meetings allowed the facilitator to see and read non-verbal cues from group participants. Non-verbal cues played a large role in helping the facilitator manage group interactions. Because non-verbal cues were not available in web-conferencing (unless video transmission is a component of the meeting; video transmission was not included in this study) and teleconferencing, the facilitator might interject more often into group discussions to keep the group focused on the agenda. One advantage of web-conferencing over teleconferencing was that web-conferencing allowed the facilitator to see the participants' names and to recognize who was interested in speaking through the hand-raising feature. This was not possible in teleconferencing meetings.

4. Weaknesses

Weaknesses were found in the use of face-to-face, teleconferencing, and web-conferencing meetings when facilitating knowledge exchange within drug policy groups. Face-to-face meetings were found to be very time consuming and costly. For large groups that were geographically dispersed and had a limited budget, such as the education task group, face-to-face interactions were difficult to schedule often. Therefore, the exclusive used of face-to-face meetings limits the frequency of knowledge exchange interactions for large geographically dispersed groups with limited budgets.

Weaknesses were also evident in the use of teleconferencing to facilitate knowledge exchange. The conduct of teleconferencing meetings was found to be distracting because there were no explicit phone etiquette norms introduced within the group. For example, participants shuffled papers, spoke out of turn, listened to music, audibly typed, or did a host of other activities that could distract other participants during a meeting. With teleconferencing, participants were passive, possibly because group members felt disconnected from the group. For an audience interested in obtaining the latest research information, teleconferences were more anonymous because individuals were not required to participate in the meeting; they joined and logged off at any time. The weakness of teleconferencing is that it limited social interaction and did not provide opportunities for social relationships.

Weaknesses emerged as well when web-conferencing was used to facilitate knowledge exchange. The use of web-conferencing enforced a communication structure on the group. Because of the imposed structure (e.g., the inability to interrupt a speaker and enforced turn taking in speaking), web-conferencing was found to suppress spontaneity, group social interactions, and free-flowing conversation. Another weakness of web-conferencing was that participants had to surmount a learning curve in order to use the web-conferencing interface. For example, group members who wanted to share a slide or a document had to learn how to use the application-sharing feature of the technology. Therefore, a group that is not highly collaborative, not geographically dispersed, and not interested in learning new technologies may not want to use web-conferencing to facilitate knowledge exchange despite the potential advantages for working on shared documents.

For facilitation, it is important to note that face-to-face meetings lasted longer than teleconferencing and web-conferencing meetings because of the higher level of social interactions. Group members in face-to-face meetings were usually more talkative and focused less on the agenda. Therefore, the facilitator needs to place more effort on keeping the group focused on the task at hand. In teleconferencing and web-conferencing meetings, the facilitator felt disconnected from the group due to the inability to see facial expressions and body language, which provide a rich source of information for facilitators. The ability to read these non-verbal cues was found to be important in helping the facilitator manage group interactions. Concerning information exchange, the use of live teleconferencing to disseminate research information did not cause a change in policy; it functioned more as a news service or a dissemination tool. Regarding web-conferencing, the technology limited the amount of information that could be shared. For instance, group members could not share large documents via web-conferencing because of screen size limitations.

5. Conclusions

This paper discussed the experiences of three drug policy groups using conferencing technologies to facilitate distant knowledge exchange and outlined the various strengths and weaknesses of these technologies.

References

[1] Canadian Health Services Research Foundation (CHSRF) . Knowledge Exchange. 2010. Available at: http://www.chsrf.ca/knowledge_transfer/index_e.php.
[2] S. Soumerai, D. Ross-Degnan, E. Fortess, B. Walser. Determinants of change in medical pharmaceutical cost sharing: Does evidence affect policy? *The Milbank Quarterly*. **75**(1) (1997), 11-34.
[3] The Cochrane collaboration: Informing judgment: Case studies of health policy and research in six countries. Milbank Memorial Fund, 2001.
[4] M. Househ, A. Kushniruk, M. Maclure, B. Carleton, D. Cloutier-fisher. A Case Study Examining the Impacts of Conferencing Technologies in Distributed Healthcare Groups. *Electronic Healthcare*. **8**(2) (2009), 10-14.
[5] M. Househ, A. Kushniruk, M. Maclure, B. Carleton, D. Cloutier-Fisher. Technology Enabled Knowledge Exchange: Development of a Conceptual Framework. *J Med Sys*. (2009). Available at: http://www.springerlink.com/content/x82042876822g465/fulltext.html.

410

International Perspectives in Health Informatics
E.M. Borycki et al. (Eds.)
IOS Press, 2011
© 2011 ITCH 2011 Steering Committee and IOS Press. All rights reserved.
doi:10.3233/978-1-60750-709-3-410

Functional Safety in Telecare: A Proposal for Implementation and Joint Validation

Juan ADRIANO[a, d, 1], Alejandro TORRES-ECHEVERRIA[b, 2], Abdul ROUDSARI[a, c]

[a]Centre for Health Informatics, City University London, London, UK
[b]ABB Limited, Process Automation, St Neots, UK
[c]School of Health Information Science, University of Victoria, BC, Canada
[d]Information Systems, Carnegie Mellon University in Qatar, Doha, Qatar

Abstract. The introduction of telecare systems represents an inherent risk which can potentially result in patient harm. Given the importance of patient safety, in this paper, we address safety from the functional safety point of view.

Keywords. healthcare, functional safety, telecare

Introduction

In recent years, the global tendency has been to consider ehealth as a key service for the future delivery of care. While telemedicine involves the intervention of a whole range of health professionals and patients geographically separated (but usually located within healthcare facilities), telecare describes any service supported by Information and Communication Technologies that facilitates the delivery of health and social care directly to users at home.

In general, healthcare organisations are usually complex in nature; this partially explains why the design, implementation and evaluation of telecare systems is not an easy task. For successful implementation, this innovative care delivery process must ensure that the new system meets the criteria of being safe, reliable, acceptable, and ergonomic by design.

In this paper, we address telecare safety from the functional safety point of view. This is the first criteria to meet during the formative evaluation within the overall evaluation process described by Cramp and Carson [1], and its achievement is relevant for the adoption of new safety critical systems such as telecare.

1. An Overview of the IEC 61508 Standard

The International Electrotechnical Commission has developed the IEC 61508 [2] standard which aims to provide a means of ensuring that safety is effectively reached based on the functionality of electrical, electronic or programmable electronic (E/E/PE)

---

[1] Corresponding Author: Juan Adriano, Centre for Health Informatics, City University, Northampton Square, London EC1V 0HB, UK; E-mail: J.J.Adriano-Moran@soi.city.ac.uk
[2] This article reflects the opinion of the author and not the views of his institution of affiliation.

systems. This is a generic document non-specific to any industry sector and can be relevant to a number of different sectors (e.g. aircraft, process, nuclear).

IEC 61508 comprises seven parts, being mandatory the first 3 sections. Part 1 provides the overall framework, including technical and management requirements; part 2 deals with technical requirements for hardware realisation, and part 3 for software realisation. The most important features of the standard are: (1) the establishment of a safety life cycle to functional safety; (2) the formulation of Safety Integrity Levels (SIL) to be complied by the safety related system, and (3) the approach for addressing systematic failures, especially in software.

The safety lifecycle is a sequence of all necessary activities to implement safety-related systems. Although compliance with the safety lifecycle is not a simple task, this can be implemented by putting in place a Functional Safety Management System (FSMS) built upon a company's quality system.

The standard requires that every safety function achieve a specific SIL. The SIL is an index that indicates the acceptable probability of failure that a system can have in order to be considered appropriate for a given specific safety integrity requirement. In addition to this, the hardware is also limited by architectural constraints, detailed in IEC 61508 Part 2. These constraints are the Hardware Fault Tolerance (HFT) and the Safe Failure Fraction (SFF). The architectural constraints aim to provide additional hardware safety to the failure rate estimation. This prevents the claim of unrealistically high SIL levels for designs without an adequate level of redundancy.

There are two main categories of failures (Figure 1): random failures and systematic failures. Random failures are caused by the hardware components' ageing degradation, whereas systematic failures are caused by any other causes but degradation (i.e. stress, design, and operation). Thus, when demonstrating achievement of a specific SIL, both random and systematic failures must be addressed. Random hardware failures are quantified to establish that for a specified safety function the required failure measure for the target SIL has been achieved. However, since software does not degrade, it is only affected by systematic failures. But systematic failures cannot be quantified, and the only way to claim a specific SIL is to implement "state-of-the-art" qualitative measures that help to avoid systematic failures in a proportional way to the SIL effort [3].

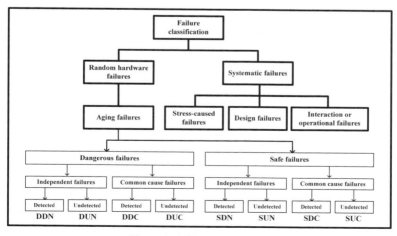

Figure 1. Failure classification.

The standard introduces the concept of "systematic capability". Although systematic failures cannot be quantified to demonstrate SIL achievement, if all requirements established by the standard are fulfilled, it can be claimed that the systematic safety integrity corresponding to a specific SIL has been achieved; this is its systematic capability. In addition to the safety requirements for software, the Annexes in Part 3 indicate a series of measures and techniques to be used for ensuring that the required software's systematic capability is achieved. These annexes are mandatory and the measures and techniques depend on the effort needed by a specific SIL requirement.

As for the hardware, there is a lifecycle for development of the software. The standard recommends the use of the V model (IEC 61508-3), which can also be adapted to a required SIL effort. The V model helps to ensure that software development is subject to a management process, from safety requirements specifications, to design and coding. Safety requirements for software include not only functional specification (what the software has to do), but also safety integrity requirements (likelihood with which the software will perform its intended function). It is important to highlight that the model calls for verification of all stages and final validation of the product.

In addition, the standard also intends to make sure that software and hardware integrate correctly, perform the required safety functions, and behave without unintended effects. To achieve this, it establishes requirements for integration testing.

Another interesting requirement is that a safety manual has to be developed for a safety system. The safety manual should specify, among other things, functional specification, configuration, installation instructions, constraints of use, modification control, competence of the user, and compatibility with other systems. The safety manual is, in summary, a document that describes all the conditions to be met during the useful life of the system in order to preserve its specified safety integrity.

Finally, the safety lifecycle requires verification of each stage through examination of the outputs produced, a final validation of the completed safety system, and an investigation of the functional safety assessment based on evidence. These activities are very important since they provide recorded evidence of the safety system functionality and safety integrity.

2. The IEC 61508, DSCN 18/2009 and Their Relation to Telecare

The guidance DSCN 18/2009 [4] challenges the lack of standards governing clinical safety management for health and social care IT systems; that is the domain of telecare. Its aim is to manage and mitigate clinical risks associated with the production of software and systems through documentation and agreed level of risk. It addresses the required processes for risk management focused on healthcare organisations in order to ensure safety of patients. The guidance [4] proposes as stages of the lifecycle: (a) concept development and requirements capture; (b) detailed design; (c) software development; (d) software verification; (e) software release/marketing; (f) system validation and deployment; (g) use; and (h) decommissioning.

The intention of [4] is to cover the safety lifecycle stages of deployment, use and decommissioning. Stages (a) to (c) are manufacturers' responsibilities and covered by DSCN 14/2009 [5]. However, it is not clear where the responsibility for verification and validation lies. Although it would be logical to place the responsibility on the manufactures, nowadays, it seems to be a common practice to leave such responsibility in the hands of healthcare institutions [6].

Ref. [4] also includes the recommendation for the creation of a risk management plan that includes lifecycle. This requires the establishment of an iterative ongoing process for clinical risk management; i.e. risk identification, analysis and control based on clinical cases. It requires decisive commitment of the top management function which meets some basic requirements of [2] for establishment of a Functional Safety Management Plan.

By comparing the IEC 61508 and the DSCN 18/2009 lifecycles, it can be noticed that there is a reasonable inclusion of the former into the latter. However, in the DSCN document, some important requirements are left unattended. These are: (1) to produce the evidence that a FSMS has been put in place; (2) the overall planning of validation, maintenance, installation and commissioning; (3) production of a safety manual; (4) the functional Safety Audit; and (5) the functional Safety Assessment.

To overcome these gaps, a group of outputs have been identified in order to provide good evidence for the implementation of the FSMS:

- *Verification* must be done in every stage of the lifecycle. For this, a verification specification (e.g. test specification) has to be written and records should be generated subsequently.
- *Validation* requires a written specification, which aim is to ensure that the safety requirements have been achieved.
- The *functional safety audit* intends to ensure that all procedures established by the FSMS have been followed.
- The *functional safety assessment* aim is to judge whether functional safety has been effectively achieved or not. This is based on the analysis of produced evidence at every stage of the lifecycle, having as evidence records and reports of verification, validation and audit activities. This is perhaps the ultimate and most important output of all the process.

3. Discussion

Given that the first activities of the lifecycle in [2], from conceptualisation to realisation (design and development), are performed by the manufacturers or system integrators, the process of verifying these stages shall, certainly, rely on them in compliance with [5]. Nevertheless, in DSCN18/2009 is not clearly stated who is responsible for performing validation and deployment. Due to the fact that the users may not be aware of the proper techniques and methods for deployment, the authors of this paper suggest that for telecare, such stages should be a joint responsibility between manufacturers, systems integrators and users. Most important, validation of the system requires specific technical and detailed knowledge of the system's intended function and integrity requirements which the user may not have. Therefore, the validation specification (e.g. final system test) should be produced by manufacturers or systems integrators as well as execution of the validation, and overseen by the user, or ideally, with a joint active participation of the user and the manufacturers/integrators.

As part of the user's FSMS or clinical risk management process, management for supplier assessment shall be included. In addition, a functional safety assessment of the manufacturer's product should be demanded by the user, employing if necessary an independent third party (e.g. a safety consultant). As part of this assessment, the user can require from the manufacturers the specifications and records of, at least, the validation activity. The manufacturer should also have in place a FSMS. Consequently, the manufacturer must perform its own functional safety assessment and the report generated from this should be available to the user.

4. Conclusions

It is undeniable that the introduction of new products and services in health consumer markets represent an inherent risk which can potentially result in patient harm. This risk is of course not only particularly latent in the health informatics arena. However, if the expectations are that telecare helps to provide not only equal health access to underserved populations but also to keep people living independently and supported in their own places of residence, it is essential that adequate measures for ensuring good design, performance and safety of telecare systems are in place. To achieve this, the deployment and validation of safety systems in telecare should be a shared responsibility among the users, manufactures and systems integrators, and not exclusively rely on health institutions as the contractual and legal "hold harmless" clause (which shifts liability and remedial burdens to users) [6] implies for information technology vendors in the United States.

In addition, to ensure that the minimum requirements of the safety lifecycle have been met by the manufacturers and system integrators, and that the specified functional safety has been actually achieved, the user should be able to request as part of the contractual obligations, not only evidence of the manufacturer's FSMS, but also the product's safety manual, as well as the evidence of the execution of verification, validation and the assessment stages. Having met these requirements would certainly help to ensure the patient's safety when interaction with telecare occurs.

References

[1]   D. G. Cramp, E. R. Carson. The evaluation of information and communications technologies in health care: The role of a multi-dimensional value criterion model. In: *4th International IEEE EMBS Special Topic Conference on Information Technology Applications* in Biomedicine. Birmingham, UK; 2003: 47-50.

[2]   International Electrotechnical Commission. *IEC 61508 Functional Safety of Electrical/Electronic/Programmable Electronic Safety-Related Systems.* Parts 1-7. Ed. 2.0. Geneva, Switzerland; 2010.

[3]   D. Smith, K. Simpson. Functional Safety. *A straightforward guide to applying IEC 61508 and related standards.* 2nd edition, Elsevier Butterworth-Heinemann. Oxford, UK; 2004.

[4]   NHS Connecting for Health, Health informatics - *Guidance on the management of clinical risk relating to the deployment and use of health software* (formerly ISO/TR 29322:2008(E)) – DSCN18/2009. Ver. 1.0. UK; 2009.

[5]   NHS Connecting for Health, Health Informatics — *Application of clinical risk management to the manufacture of health software* (formerly ISO/TS 29321:2008(E)) – DSCN14/2009. Ver. 1.0. UK; 2009.

[6]   R. Koppel, D. Kreda. Health care information technology vendors' "hold harmless" clause. *JAMA* 301(12) (2009), 1276-1278.

International Perspectives in Health Informatics
E.M. Borycki et al. (Eds.)
IOS Press, 2011
doi:10.3233/978-1-60750-709-3-415

Robots, Multi-User Virtual Environments and Healthcare: Synergies for Future Directions

AJung MOON [a,1], Francisco J. GRAJALES III [b], H.F. Machiel VAN DER LOOS [a]

[a] *Department of Mechanical Engineering, University of British Columbia, Canada*
[b] *eHealth Strategy Office, Faculty of Medicine,*
University of British Columbia, Canada

Abstract. The adoption of technology in healthcare over the last twenty years has steadily increased, particularly as it relates to medical robotics and Multi-User Virtual Environments (MUVEs) such as Second Life. Both disciplines have been shown to improve the quality of care and have evolved, for the most part, in isolation from each other. In this paper, we present four synergies between medical robotics and MUVEs that have the potential to decrease resource utilization and improve the quality of healthcare delivery. We conclude with some foreseeable barriers and future research directions for researchers in these fields.

Keywords. multi-user, virtual environments, human-robot interaction, medical robots.

Introduction

Over the last two decades, the adoption of technological solutions in healthcare has steadily increased. For example, between 2007 and 2009 the number of robot-assisted medical procedures more than doubled from 80,000 to over 205,000 [1]. Both robots and multi-user virtual environments (MUVEs) contributed to this trend by improving quality of care in a number of ways, such as providing tireless mechanical platforms for otherwise labor intensive movement therapy and minimizing surgical invasiveness [2, 3]. In general, however, robots and MUVEs have developed as separate fields, with little overlap as to how their synergy can further improve quality of care while decreasing resource utilization. In this paper, we outline how these two fields can work in synergy, and postulate some of the likely barriers in this synergy and some future research directions.

This paper is structured in four sections: 1) historical background; 2) similarities and differences between robots and MUVEs; 3) present and future synergies; and 4) barriers and future directions.

---

[1] Corresponding Author: Department of Mechanical Engineering, University of British Columbia, 6250 Applied Science Lane, Vancouver, BC, Canada V6T 1Z4; E-mail: ajung@amoon.ca

1. Historical Background

Medical and healthcare robots have been used for over forty years to improve patient care. The first medical robot was the Case Western University arm (1962), a computer controlled prosthesis for a paralyzed person's arm [4]. Today, the majority of medical robots on the market continue to target applications for short patient interactions (e.g., surgery), and applications requiring frequent or continuous supervision of a physician. Intuitive Surgical's da Vinci System, for example, is seen as the gold standard for minimizing surgical invasiveness and maximizing recovery time in a number of surgical interventions [3].

On the other hand, MUVEs are virtual immersive environments that serve as a type of 3D wiki, allowing the interaction between people through the use of avatars to create and innovate [5]. Historically, these emerged from text-based role-playing computer games that evolved to include realistic graphics, similar to those of flight simulators used in aviation. In medicine, MUVEs have been used for cognitive behavioral therapy, post-traumatic stress disorder rehabilitation, medical education, and simulations [2, 6].

2. Robots and MUVEs – Similarities and Differences

2.1. Cost

Due to the intrinsic differences between medical robots and MUVEs, their R&D and implementation costs differ by orders of magnitude. For instance, a new medical robotic platform (e.g., hardware), incurs not only the costs of prototypes, materials, manufacturing, and assembly, but also those of testing and refining the concept from the lab to the bedside.

In comparison, MUVEs are much simpler and safer to implement. Once a working prototype is complete, for example, the system can be tested for usability and congruency with information safety standards (e.g., HIPAA).

The clinical trials process of MUVEs and robots are also distinct. Robots may have the "new gadget factor" advantage; however, they are limited by the geographical location of the device and the number of clinicians and patients who can use them at any given time. Human-subject trial costs are also greater due to the need for specialized, and often patented, disposables (e.g., video catheters) that are only available from a single vendor. On the other hand, MUVEs can be used by a large number of patients and clinicians from the comfort of their own homes, and with a minimal need for specialized training or equipment (such as a broadband Internet connection).

2.2 Interaction

At present, medical human-robot interaction (HRI) is mainly physical and, in certain cases, psychological [7]. Healthcare robots are generally built to provide a physical advantage (e.g., operate in crowded spaces) or assistance (e.g., remove operator hand tremors) to clinicians and patients. Neuro-rehabilitation robots for post-stroke motion therapy are exemplars of medical robots with a physical HRI. These robots use direct physical contact with patients to help guide their impaired limbs in prescribed movement tasks, such as reaching and grasping, for upper-limb motor recovery. Psychotherapy robots such as Paro, the huggable baby harp seal robot designed for use in pediatric and geriatric wards, are most analogous to MUVEs in that they aim to stimulate psychological, social, and emotional responses via expressive behaviors similar to a pet but with the added benefit of disease transmission prevention and caregiver burden reduction [8, 9].

In comparison, medical applications of MUVEs aim to change cognitive processes through the virtual manipulation of a 3D character, i.e., an avatar. Research has shown that manipulating an avatar can elicit social responses, although this character exists in a "fictional" world that is manipulated by standard computer input devices (a mouse and a keyboard) [10]. This also means that although physical harm may not be enacted upon an avatar's operator, psychological and physiological harm may occur [11, 12]. A recent study also showed that user tendencies in positioning avatars for virtual interaction with other avatars are congruent with real-life social norms [13].

3. Robots and MUVEs: Present and Future Synergies

Based on recent research [1, 5, 7], we postulate the following four synergies between MUVEs and robotics. Regardless of their timeliness in implementation, we believe that these can work both individually and collectively to improve the efficiency, efficacy, and equity of healthcare over the next decade.

First, MUVEs can provide a platform for pilot testing medical robots and their user interfaces prior to physical development. Cyberknife, for example, is a robotic radiosurgery system that allows the treatment of cancerous tumors by delivering a targeted beam of high-dose radiation. Cyberknife and similar robots operate with interfaces that are familiar to and well-adapted by trained users, and changes to preexisting platforms, such as modifications to control interfaces, can have a significant impact on the usability and user acceptability of the device. Conducting a pilot test or user study to gauge user-device dynamics traditionally requires prototyping of the physical platform. Such traditional iterative design processes can be expensive and time-consuming. The use of MUVEs can improve the efficiency of this process by decreasing R&D costs, improving user-centric design, and allowing clinicians and engineers to virtually test (and simulate) a new device prior to its physical construction.

MUVEs can facilitate patient empowerment prior to real-life robot interactions. The Royal Sussex County Hospital, for example, uses Linden Lab's Second Life [14] to acquire informed consent from patients with disabilities prior to a surgical procedure [15]. In the same manner, MUVEs can educate patients about their options for medical interaction with a robot in advance, thereby promoting a better informed clinician-patient medical decision (e.g., Which type of surgery would you prefer?). MUVEs can also better accommodate patients' personal needs and preferences, such as religious or cultural obligations to interact only with physicians and avatars of a particular gender. An added advantage is that this can take place without the physical presence of a physician, saving valuable resources.

MUVEs can improve medical education by decreasing the cost of surgical simulation while increasing the throughput of trainees for a given procedure. MUVEs have been used as an effective multi-user education tool for paramedic students who virtually engage in a variety of real-life medical scenarios in Second Life [16].

Extensions of such initiatives could provide immersive multi-user simulation environments for robot-assisted surgical procedures. Improving current MUVE experiences with haptic and other high fidelity interface systems can also help standardize surgical training to aviation-like standards by allowing clinicians to experience the capabilities and limitations of a robot without damaging the robotic system, or even make critical mistakes without causing physical harm to a human [5].

MUVEs can be used to elucidate some of the ethical issues surrounding medical robotics. The implications of HRI, particularly as it relates to vulnerable populations, are a new and emerging discipline [17]. Philosophers and engineers are beginning to raise ethical concerns regarding the increased use of robots for the care of older persons and children [18, 19]. In contrast to easily quantifiable and familiar problems of physical safety, psychological and social impacts of HRI, such as psychotherapy robots [20], are harder to predict, quantify, and address in real life. By taking advantage of human-avatar congruency, we postulate that MUVEs can provide the platform to quantify such impact. Analogous versions of real-world HRI studies can be conducted in MUVEs to stimulate and collect avatar responses to robots in virtual worlds. We posit that this could lead to a better understanding of moral consequences of medical HRI and promote socially conscious design decisions.

4. Barriers and Future Directions

A number of barriers have historically impacted the adoption of MUVEs [21]. We foresee these to continue in the near future and include: fear of the unknown, usability, lack of Continuing Medical Education accreditation, and technical requirements (e.g., 3D graphics cards, new physical human-robot interface devices).

In addition, due diligence must be exercised whenever the results of avatar responses to robots are analyzed to maximize transference and safety. Although avatars exhibit human-like behaviors, analysis of their responses to a stimulus may not be analogous to human responses. For instance, avatars participating in an experiment inside Second Life may reasonably respond by flying, which is obviously an unlikely response to be expected of human subjects in real life.

We recommend that future research investigate the differences and similarities between real and virtual interactions and evaluate the transferability of the synergies discussed in the preceding section.

5. Conclusion

In this paper, we presented a background on the medical applications of MUVEs and robots. These two disciplines have historically evolved in parallel and offer different healthcare advantages. Robots, intrinsically requiring physical platforms, are costly to develop and implement, but offer significant physical assistance and advantage to patients and clinicians. Medical practices are much cheaper to develop and implement in MUVEs; however, the current limitations of standard computer interfaces are slowing the medical application of MUVEs to education, simulation, cognitive therapy and psychological rehabilitation. We posit that MUVE-robot synergy can collectively improve R&D, patient empowerment, medical/surgical education, and elucidate some of the ethical issues of medical HRI in the years to come.

References

[1] Barbash GI, Glied SA. New technology and healthcare costs - the case of robot-assisted surgery. *N Engl J Med.* 2010;363(8):701–704.

[2] Van der Loos HFM, Reinkensmeyer DJ. Chapter 53: Rehabilitation and health care robotics. In: Siciliano B, Khatib O, eds. *Springer Handbook of Robotics.* Berlin, Heidelberg: Springer; 2008:1223-1251.

[3] Sung GT, Gill IS. Robotic laparoscopic surgery: a comparison of the da Vinci and Zeus systems. *Urology.* 2001;58(6):893-898.

[4] James R, Mergler K. Medical Engineering Progress Report on Case Research Arm Aid - *report number: EDC 4-64-3*; 1962.

[5] Bainbridge WS. The scientific research potential of virtual worlds. *Science.* 2007;317(5837):472-476.

[6] Beard L, Wilson K, Morra D, Keelan J. A survey of health-related activities on second life. *J Med Internet Res.* 2009;11(2):e17.

[7] Okamura A, Matarić, M, Christensen H. Medical and health-care robotics. *IEEE Robotics & Automation Magazine.* 2010;17(3):26-37.

[8] Wada K, Shibata T, Saito T, Tanie K. Effects of robot-assisted activity for elderly people and nurses at a day service center. *Proceedings of the IEEE.* 2004;92(11):1780-1788.

[9] Shibata T, Mitsui T, Wada K, Tanie K. Subjective evaluation of seal robot: Paro – tabulation and analysis of questionnaire results. *Journal of Robotics and Mechatronics.* 2002;14(1):13-19.

[10] Yee N. *The Proteus effect: Behavioral modification via transformations of digital self-representation* [Doctoral thesis]. Palo Alto: Department of Communication, Stanford University; 2007.

[11] Wolfendale J. My avatar, my self: virtual harm and attachment. *Ethics Inf Technol.* 2006;9(2):111-119.

[12] Slater M, Antley A, Davison A, et al. A virtual reprise of the Stanley Milgram obedience experiments Rustichini A, ed. *PLoS One.* 2006;1(1):e39.

[13] Yee N, Bailenson JN, Urbanek M, Chang F, Merget D. The unbearable likeness of being digital: the persistence of nonverbal social norms in online virtual environments. *Cyberpsychol Behav.* 2007;10(1):115-121.

[14] Linden Lab. Second Life. [Internet]. 2010. [cited 2010 Oct 15]. Linden Lab, San Francisco, CA. Available from: http://secondlife.com/

[15] The Economist Group. Informed consent and virtual worlds: The avatar will see you now. [Internet]. 2009 Jun 25. [cited 2010 Oct 15]. Available from: http://www.economist.com/node/13899038.

[16] Conradi E, Kavia S, Burden D, et al. Virtual patients in a virtual world: training paramedic students for practice. *Med Teach.* 2009;31(8):713-720.

[17] Capurro R, Tamburrini G, Weber J. Emerging technoethics of human interaction with communication. *bionic and robotic systems (Ethicbots).* Naples; 2008.

[18] Sharkey A, Sharkey N. Granny and the robots: ethical issues in robot care for the elderly. *Ethics Inf Technol.* 2010:1-14.

[19] Tanaka F, Kimura T. The use of robots in early education: a scenario based on ethical consideration. In: *RO-MAN 2009 - The 18th IEEE International Symposium on Robot and Human Interactive Communication.* IEEE; 2009:558-560.

[20] Nomura T. Robots in mental therapy: its possibility and danger. In: *RO-MAN 2009 - The 18th IEEE International Symposium on Robot and Human Interactive Communication.* IEEE; 2009:569-572.

[21] Kashani RM, Roberts A, Jones R, Kamel Boulos MN. Virtual worlds, collective responses and responsibilities in health. *Journal of Virtual Worlds Research.* 2009;2(2):4-7.

Acknowledgements

This work was supported by the University of British Columbia Institute for Computing, Information and Cognitive Systems (ICICS) and the Western Regional Training Centre for Health Services Research (WRTC-HSR).

International Perspectives in Health Informatics
E.M. Borycki et al. (Eds.)
IOS Press, 2011
© *2011 ITCH 2011 Steering Committee and IOS Press. All rights reserved.*
doi:10.3233/978-1-60750-709-3-420

Tele-ICU - A Canadian Review

Reza SHAHPORI[a, 1], Andre KUSHNIRUK[b,] Marilynne HEBERT[b, c], Dan ZUEGE[a]

[a] *Department of Critical Care Medicine, Alberta Health Services, Calgary, Canada*
[b] *School of Health Information Science, University of Victoria, Canada*
[c] *Community Health Sciences, Faculty of Medicine, University of Calgary, Canada*

Abstract. Based on the learnings and experiences from implementations in the United States, telemedicine may offer certain advantages to help address some of the challenges faced by the Canadian critical care community resulting from staff shortages and increasing demands for quality care. The initial and operating costs of the technology and its impact on direct bedside care are perceived to be significant drivers of resistance to its wide spread implementation. This qualitative review of the available literature summarizes the opportunities and challenges with the potential use of telemedicine to enhance the delivery of critical care services in Canada.

Keywords. Tele-ICU, telemedicine, telehealth, critical care

Introduction

There is compelling evidence that shortages of experienced human resources are impacting the delivery of critical care services in North America. Underlying contributing factors include an increasing demand for critical care resources, given a growing and aging population, relative to a retiring human resources and a decreasing supply of new expertise. A rising public awareness and professional focus on quality of care and patient safety issues, augmented from health care quality improvement institutions such as the Institute for Health Improvement and the Canadian Patient Safety Institute, has required critical care staff to dedicate increasing amounts of time to participate in quality improvement initiatives intended to reduce adverse events resulting from medical errors and preventable complications. These important initiatives further complicate the delivery of critical care services. Tele-ICU or use of telemedicine in critical care has been suggested as one potential solution to aid some of these challenges. In this study we searched the published literature to understand the pros and cons of such a system, in particular within a Canadian environment.

Tele-ICU refers to the concept of monitoring large numbers of remotely-located ICU patients in order to detect early signs of deterioration and to provide consultation to the bedside caregivers. Tele-ICU generally consists of real time remote access to patient data, extracted from physiologic monitors and ventilators, as well as laboratory results, radiographic images, medication histories, orders and clinical notes. Complex decision support systems apply algorithms and pre-defined rules to this data to provide

---

[1] Corresponding Author: Reza Shahpori, Phone: 1-403-944-2857, Fax: 1-403-283-9994, email: Reza.Shahpori@AlbertaHealthServices.Ca

alarms and alerts, calculate scores and prioritize tasks. Staff in Tele-ICU center survey patient data and respond to alerts, communicating with the direct care providers as appropriate using audio and video means. Each team member has a workstation made up of multiple computer monitors, each of which is typically dedicated to a special purpose. A master monitor commonly presents the list of patients under care along with some pre-selected information such as severity of illness scores, workload indices and preconfigured alerts or alarms, the latter used to help decision making and prioritizing issues for attention. Other monitors are dedicated to the presentation of real time textual or graphical data or diagnostic images and waveforms. One monitor usually supports the ability to selectively view patients via high resolution live video feeds from the patient room with remote zooming and panning capabilities. In its ideal implementation, Tele-ICU should facilitate a remotely-located multi-disciplinary team of highly qualified critical care experts to be virtually brought to the patient bedside.

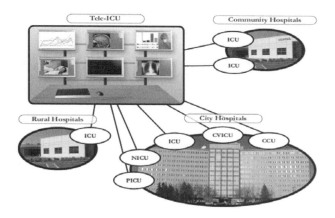

Figure 1. Simplified Tele-ICU structure

1. Methods

A literature search was conducted in PubMed using search phrase "Telecommunication OR Telemedicine OR Telehealth OR Telemetry" OR "Tele consultation" OR "Remote Consultation" OR "Remote Monitoring". The result was restricted to "Critical Care" OR "Intensive Care" OR "ICU", human subjects and English language. Prior to 1999 articles were mostly related to basic remote access techniques to monitor select aspects of ICU care via telephone consultation and telemetry. In year 2000 the first trial of Tele-ICU care was published. From 1999 until the end of 2009, 369 publications were identified of which 49 articles were selected for detailed review on the basis of relevant content after reviewing abstracts. These articles, which were mostly from United States and none from Canada, covered topics of patient outcome and quality impacts, staffing and organizational issues, rural access and costing issues [2].

---

[2] For the detailed search method and a complete list of bibliography please contact the corresponding author.

2. Results and discussions

The North American critical care community faces significant challenge to the delivery of quality care. Driving this are two important inter-related issues – an increasing demand for quality clinical service and shortages of experienced human resources to provide such service.

2.1. Increasing Demands for Quality

The Institute of Medicine report "To Err is human…", revealing the extent of life and financial loss as a result of suboptimal quality of care in the United States, followed by the Canadian adverse events study, reporting on the burden of preventable adverse events on the Canadian healthcare system, set the stage for further investigations in patient safety and quality improvement initiatives. Patients are significantly more likely to experience adverse events in the ICU relative to other parts of the hospital. The incidence of adverse drug events in ICU patients is approximately twice that of non-ICU patients. Ventilator Associated Pneumonia (VAP) is estimated to be responsible for 230 deaths per year and an annual cost of $46 million in Canada [1]. Malnutrition, poor pain management and the spread of antibiotic resistant micro-organisms are additional important and preventable adverse events in the ICU which consume precious and scarce resources [2]. To address these quality concerns, a number of quality improvement initiatives were established, including the Canadian Safer Healthcare Now!" and the Canadian ICU Collaborative, with a mandate to engage clinicians in measuring and enhancing the quality of care in ICU systems.

2.2. Effects of ICU Organization and Staffing on Quality

A growing body of scientific evidence suggests that quality of care in ICUs is strongly influenced by the organization of ICU staff. A lower nurse-to-patient ratio was associated with increased prevalence of VAP and higher ICU Length of Stay (LOS) [3]. Increased nurse-patient ratios were associated with reductions in the ICU infections and hospital mortality [4]. ICUs with mandatory intensivist coverage, complaints with Physician Staffing (IPS) standard, were associated with a 30% reduction in hospital mortality, a 40% reduction in ICU mortality, a considerable reduction of LOS and a significant improvement in processes of care and staff and family satisfaction [5]. The IPS standard has been recommended by the US National Quality Forum Safe Practices Recommendations, American College of Critical Care Medicine, the Joint Commission on Accreditation of Healthcare Organizations and the Leapfrog group and is now included in the pay-for-performance proposal by Medicare and Medicaid [6]. The Leapfrog group has suggested that 54,855 annual deaths could be prevented if the IPS safety standard was implemented in all ICUs across the United States [7].

Despite the published evidence about the advantages of the IPS standard, its widespread implementation has been challenging. In 2008 only 31% of hospitals in the US met this recommendation, up from 10% in 2002 (mostly attributed to the modification of the standard to consider virtual staffing of ICUs in small community hospitals using Tele-ICU [8]). In Canada in 2006, only 15% of ICUs had staff physicians in-house overnight, and 40% of ICUs had no dedicated physicians for substantial portions of the day. An imbalance between the supply and demand of certified intensivists, registered nurses and allied health care professionals are causing shortages that will seriously challenge the provision of standard health services to large populations of seriously ill patients [9]. Underlying contributing factors include increase in the demand for critical care resources given a growing and aging population in relation to retiring human health resources and a decreasing supply of new expertise. In addition, growing expectations for critical care clinicians to dedicate increasing amounts of time to important non-clinical activities, such as quality improvement, education and research compound the problem. These shortages are already reported to be associated with staff burnout which adversely affects quality of care [10].

2.3. Potential Advantages of Tele-ICU

More vigilant monitoring leading to an early detection of potential adverse events is a Tele-ICU attribute which may help hospitals achieve quality improvements similar to those achieved by closed-ICUs while using fewer intensivists [11]. Decreased ICU and hospital mortality and LOS has been reported by some of the early adaptors [12]. Another attribute of Tele-ICU, although not directly related to the technology, is quality improvement through facilitation of improved compliance with evidence-based clinical practices guidelines [3]. Significant reduction of ventilation days has been reported as a result of using Tele-ICU to improve compliance with VAP bundle [3]. Tele-ICU is also reported to add educational value via more effective real-time teaching by constructing libraries of educational cases. Its financial benefits are uncertain and hard to measure. Reductions in LOS and increased ICU capacity, prevention of expensive complications such as VAP and savings in medication costs could drive net savings though the cost of setup and operation are substantial. Tele-ICU can also be a helpful tool during public health emergencies, where standard tertiary care facilities are overwhelmed, for disaster planning, and at situations where a full ICU team can not be made available (e.g. Cruise Ships and military operations). Facilitating the provision of initial resuscitation and critical care for patients in remote locations could be of particular advantage in many parts of Canada.

2.4. Potential Disadvantages of Tele-ICU

The perceived disadvantages of Tele-ICU mostly arise from inserting a layer of technology between patients and clinicians. Removing experienced care givers from the bedside to create a pool of resources to staff Tele-ICU centers is an additional common concern [3]. Physicians typically are cited as the greatest barriers to implementation of telemedicine applications mostly due to concerns for compromised autonomy and reduced patient contact and medico-legal risks [3]. Financial benefits are uncertain and setup and operational costs are significant. Successful Tele-ICU programs depend on the presence of clinical information systems and robust networks. Often such systems are limited in smaller hospitals where paradoxically often greater proportional benefit may be delivered. Patent disputes between companies offering commercial solutions likely prevent other solution providers to enter the market and have caused reluctance among health system leaders to invest in a Tele-ICU system.

---

[3] Due to space limitation the reference can be obtained by contacting the author.

3. Conclusions

Tele-ICU has the potentials to enhance the access and quality of critical care services; however its impacts on staffing shortages, patient confidentiality and costs and organizational issues have not yet been well evaluated yet. Almost all Tele-ICU implementations and studies are from the United States and usually supported by industry vendors. This may have limited generalizability to a Canadian environment due to the differences in funding and models of care. Further studies are required to assess the possible negative impacts and evaluate the potential benefits of introducing this mode of care delivery into the publicly funded Canadian healthcare system in order to generate valuable information to guide decisions for its proper implementation and application in Canada.

References

[1] J. G. Muscedere, C. M. Martin, D. K. Heyland. The impact of ventilator-associated pneumonia on the Canadian health care system. *J.Crit.Care* 2008 Mar **23**(1):5-10.

[2] D. J. Cullen, B. J. Sweitzer, D. W. Bates, E. Burdick, A. Edmondlson, L. L. Leape. Preventable adverse drug events in hospitalized patients: a comparative study of intensive care and general care units. *Crit.Care Med.* 1997 Aug **25**(8):1289-1297.

[3] S. Hugonnet, J. C. Chevrolet, D. Pittet. The effect of workload on infection risk in critically ill patients. *Crit.Care Med.* 2007 Jan **35**(1):76-81.

[4] R. L. Kane, T. A. Shamliyan, C. Mueller, S. Duval, T. J. Wilt. The association of registered nurse staffing levels and patient outcomes: systematic review and meta-analysis. *Med.Care* 2007 Dec **45**(12):1195-1204.

[5] O. Gajic, B. Afessa, A. C. Hanson, T. Krpata, M. Yilmaz, S. F. Mohamed, et al. Effect of 24-hour mandatory versus on-demand critical care specialist presence on quality of care and family and provider satisfaction in the intensive care unit of a teaching hospital. *Crit.Care Med.* 2008 Jan **36**(1):36-44.

[6] P. J. Pronovost, M. W. Jenckes, T. Dorman, E. Garrett, M. J. Breslow, B. A. Rosenfeld, et al. Organizational characteristics of intensive care units related to outcomes of abdominal aortic surgery. *JAMA* 1999 Apr 14 **281**(14):1310-1317.

[7] Leapfrog fact. Fact sheet: ICU physician staffing. 2009; Available at: http://www.leapfroggroup.org/media/file/FactSheet_IPS.pdf. Accessed June/17, 2009.

[8] LeapFrog Group. Leadership group hospital survey. 2008; Available at: http://www.leapfroggroup.org/media/file/2008_Survey_results_final_042909.pdf, 2009.

[9] D. C. Angus, M. A. Kelley, R. J. Schmitz, A. White, J. Jr. Popovich, Committee on Manpower for Pulmonary and Critical Care Societies (COMPACCS). Caring for the critically ill patient. Current and projected workforce requirements for care of the critically ill and patients with pulmonary disease: can we meet the requirements of an aging population? *JAMA* 2000 Dec 6 **284**(21):2762-2770.

[10] G. W. Ewart, L. Marcus, M. M. Gaba, R. H. Bradner, J. L. Medina, E. B. Chandler. The critical care medicine crisis: a call for federal action: a white paper from the critical care professional societies. *Chest* 2004 Apr **125**(4):1518-1521.

[11] J. Shaffer, M. J. Breslow, J. W. Johnson, et al. Remote ICU Management Improves Outcomes in Patients with Cardiopulmonary Arrest. *Crit.Care Med.* 2005 **33**(A5).

[12] E. T. Jr. Zawada, D. Kapaska, P. Herr, M. Aaronson, J. Bennett, B. Hurley, et al. Prognostic outcomes after the initiation of an electronic telemedicine intensive care unit (eICU) in a rural health system. *S.D.Med.* 2006 Sep **59**(9):391-393.

Subject Index

International Perspectives in Health Informatics
E.M. Borycki et al. (Eds.)
IOS Press, 2011

Author Index